ADVANCES IN

Pharmacology and Chemotherapy

VOLUME 16

ADVISORY BOARD

ADVANCES IN

Pharmacology and Chemotherapy

EDITED BY

Silvio Garattini

Istituto di Ricerche Farmacologiche "Mario Negri" Milano, Italy

A. Goldin

National Cancer Institute Bethesda, Maryland

F. Hawking

Commonwealth Institute of Helminthology St. Albans, Herts., England

I. J. Kopin

National Institute of Mental Health Bethesda, Maryland

Consulting Editor

R. J. Schnitzer

Mount Sinai School of Medicine New York, New York

VOLUME 16—1979

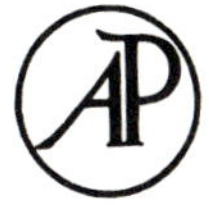

ACADEMIC PRESS New York San Francisco London

A Subsidiary of Harcourt Brace Jovanovich, Publishers

ACADEMIC PRESS, INC.
111 Fifth Avenue, New York, New York 10003

United Kingdom Edition published by
ACADEMIC PRESS, INC. (LONDON) LTD.
24/28 Oval Road, London NW1 7DX

LIBRARY OF CONGRESS CATALOG CARD NUMBER: 61-18298

ISBN 0-12-032916-6

PRINTED IN THE UNITED STATES OF AMERICA

79 80 81 82 83 84 9 8 7 6 5 4 3 2 1

CONTENTS

Contributors to This Volume ix

New Experimental Antimalarial Drugs

Robert S. Rozman and Craig J. Canfield

I. Introduction 1
II. Biology of the Parasite 3
III. Quinolinemethanols 5
IV. Phenanthrenemethanols 17
V. Quinazolines 27
VI. Drugs Entering Efficacy Trials 32
VII. Concluding Remarks 37
References 38

Mechanisms of Action of Benzodiazepines

William Schallek, W. Dale Horst, and Walter Schlosser

I. Introduction 45
II. Historical Background 46
III. Biochemistry 50
IV. Neuropharmacology 61
V. Psychopharmacology 69
VI. Discussion 79
Addendum 82
References 84

Resistance of Animal Helminths to Anthelmintics

J. D. Kelly and C. A. Hall

I. Introduction 90
II. Definitions 91
III. Occurrence of Anthelmintic Resistance 95
IV. Physiological Characteristics of Resistant Helminths 103
V. Selection for Resistance 114
VI. Diagnosis of Resistance 119
VII. Control of Resistant Helminths 122
VIII. Conclusions 125
References 126

Diethylcarbamazine and New Compounds for the Treatment of Filariasis

Frank Hawking

I. Chemistry . . . 130
II. Absorption, Excretion, Distribution, and Metabolism . . . 135
III. Pharmacology . . . 138
IV. Antifilarial Activity . . . 145
V. Toxicity . . . 164
VI. Clinical Use . . . 171
VII. Review of Other Antifilarial Compounds . . . 180
VIII. Conclusion . . . 187
References . . . 188
Addendum . . . 194

Pharmacology and Toxicology of Halogenated Anesthetics

Thomas H. Corbett

I. Introduction . . . 195
II. Halogenated Hydrocarbons . . . 196
III. Halogenated Ethers . . . 203
IV. Summary . . . 211
References . . . 211

Magnetically Responsive Microspheres and Other Carriers for the Biophysical Targeting of Antitumor Agents

Kenneth J. Widder, Andrew E. Senyei, and David F. Ranney

I. Introduction . . . 213
II. Goals and Problems of Targeted Cancer Chemotherapy . . . 215
III. Biodegradable Encapsulation Carriers . . . 218
IV. Exposed Carriers and Targeted Natural Products . . . 261
V. Summary . . . 264
References . . . 265

cis-Diamminedichloroplatinum(II): A Metal Complex with Significant Anticancer Activity

Daniel D. Von Hoff and Marcel Rozencweig

I. Introduction . . . 273
II. Discovery . . . 274
III. Chemical and Physiochemical Properties . . . 274
IV. Biological Properties . . . 275

V. Mechanism of Action 277
VI. Experimental Antitumor Activity 277
VII. Animal Toxicity 279
VIII. Drug Metabolism and Distribution 281
IX. Clinical Studies 282
X. Summary and Conclusions 293
References 294

SUBJECT INDEX 299

CONTRIBUTORS TO THIS VOLUME

Numbers in parentheses indicate the pages on which the authors' contributions begin.

CRAIG J. CANFIELD (1), *Division of Experimental Therapeutics, Walter Reed Army Institute of Research, Walter Reed Army Medical Center, Washington, D. C. 20012*

THOMAS H. CORBETT* (195), *Department of Anesthesiology, The University of Michigan Medical Center, Ann Arbor, and Department of Anesthesiology, Wayne County General Hospital, Eloise, Michigan*

C. A. HALL (89), *New South Wales Department of Agriculture, Veterinary Research Station, Glenfield, New South Wales, Australia 2167*

FRANK HAWKING (129), *Commonwealth Institute of Helminthology, St. Albans, England AL1 3EW*

W. DALE HORST (45), *Pharmacology Department, Research Division, Hoffmann-La Roche, Inc., Nutley, New Jersey 07110*

J. D. KELLY (89), *Department of Veterinary Pathology, University of Sydney, Sydney, Australia 2006*

DAVID F. RANNEY† (213), *Departments of Microbiology-Immunology and Surgery, and the Northwestern University Cancer Center, Northwestern University Medical and Dental Schools, Chicago, Illinois 60611*

MARCEL ROZENCWEIG (273), *Cancer Therapy Evaluation Program, National Cancer Institute, Bethesda, Maryland 20014*

ROBERT S. ROZMAN (1), *Division of Experimental Therapeutics, Walter Reed Army Institute of Research, Walter Reed Army Medical Center, Washington, D.C. 20012*

WILLIAM SCHALLEK (45), *Pharmacology Department, Research Division, Hoffmann-La Roche, Inc., Nutley, New Jersey 07110*

* Present address: 4271 Pratt Road, Ann Arbor, Michigan 48103; current affiliation: Flower Hospital, Toledo, Ohio.

† Present address: Department of Pathology, University of Texas Health Science Center, 5323 Harry Hines Blvd., Dallas, Texas 75235.

WALTER SCHLOSSER (45), *Pharmacology Department, Research Division, Hoffmann-La Roche, Inc., Nutley, New Jersey 07110*

ANDREW E. SENYEI (213), *Department of Pathology and the Northwestern University Cancer Center, Northwestern University Medical School, Chicago, Illinois 60611*

DANIEL D. VON HOFF (273), *National Cancer Institute, Medicine Branch, Clinical Building 12N226, National Institute of Health, Bethesda, Maryland 20014*

KENNETH J. WIDDER (213), *Department of Pathology and the Northwestern University Cancer Center, Northwestern University Medical School, Chicago, Illinois 60611*

ADVANCES IN

Pharmacology and Chemotherapy

VOLUME 16

ADVANCES IN PHARMACOLOGY AND CHEMOTHERAPY, VOL. 16

New Experimental Antimalarial Drugs*

ROBERT S. ROZMAN AND CRAIG J. CANFIELD

Division of Experimental Therapeutics
Walter Reed Army Institute of Research
Walter Reed Army Medical Center
Washington, D.C.

I. Introduction 1
II. Biology of the Parasite 3
III. Quinolinemethanols 5
A. WR 30,090 5
B. WR 142,490 11
IV. Phenanthrenemethanols 17
A. WR 33,063 17
B. WR 122,455 21
C. WR 171,669 25
V. Quinazolines 27
A. WR 158,122 27
VI. Drugs Entering Efficacy Trials 32
A. WR 184,806 32
B. WR 180,409 35
VII. Concluding Remarks 37
References 38

I. Introduction

Malaria is a parasitic disease that has brought misery and death to many millions of people in tropical and subtropical regions. The social, economic, and political impact of malaria through the centuries has been severe. There was no effective treatment for the disease until quinine, the active principal of cinchona bark, was introduced into Europe over three centuries ago. This remarkable drug became accepted as the treatment of choice for malaria and its use was limited only by its availability.

Supplies of quinine were severely curtailed by World War I, and this shortage provided the impetus for an organized effort to develop synthetic antimalarial drugs in Germany. This effort led to the discovery of pamaquine, mepacrine, and chloroquine. However, the value of these synthetic agents was not fully realized and quinine remained the mainstay of antimalarial chemotherapy.

* This report represents contribution No. 1479 to the U.S. Army Research Program on Malaria.

ISBN 0-12-032916-6

It was not until World War II, when quinine supplies were again threatened, that a program to exploit synthetic antimalarial drugs was started in the United States. This led to the widespread use of mepacrine, the rediscovery of chloroquine, and the discovery of primaquine. The abrupt termination of this program following the war interrupted the development of many promising leads. However, some antimalarial drug synthesis by the drug industry continued during ensuing years, leading to the commercial development of drugs such as proguanil and pyrimethamine.

The malaria problem appeared to be solved. Chloroquine and these latter two drugs were rapidly effective against the erythrocytic stages of all species of *Plasmodium,* and primaquine was effective against exoerythrocytic stages. Complacency resulting from the widespread success of these drugs was abruptly shattered, however, when *Plasmodium falciparum* resistance to chloroquine was reported from widely separate geographic areas in the early 1960s. In addition, many strains of these parasites were also resistant to the other available drugs.

Because U.S. military personnel were involved in one of these areas of parasite resistance (Southeast Asia), the U.S. Army organized a new program in 1963 to develop drugs effective against these drug-resistant strains (Tigertt, 1969). It has proven to be the most massive antimalarial development program in history, with over 235,000 chemical compounds being examined to date.

From the inception of the program many thousands of compounds were shown to have good antimalarial activity in the animal test screens. A complex series of secondary tests successfully reduced the number of compounds for introduction into humans. These steps included evaluation of comparative efficacy and comparative toxicity in several animal models (Kinnamon and Rothe, 1975; Canfield and Rozman, 1974). Following introduction into humans, development of some drugs was discontinued because they were found to be poorly tolerated at doses necessary for antimalarial efficacy or they demonstrated less antimalarial activity when compared to the most active drugs. However, a number of highly active new antimalarial drugs emerged.

The scope of the present review is limited to the most promising of these newer antimalarial drugs. Many of the toxicological data and some of the clinical information on these drugs have had only limited distribution. All of the drugs to be discussed have undergone some clinical testing and have proven highly efficacious in man or are of sufficient interest in a primate model of human malaria to warrant clinical testing.

Older and well-established drugs will not be discussed at length. In addition, combinations of established drugs will not be covered in this review. For these and other antimalarial drugs of interest, attention is called to a number of recent reviews and summaries (Peters, 1970, 1974; Thompson and Werbel, 1972; Steck, 1972; Rozman, 1973; Canfield and Rozman, 1974; Clyde, 1974; Strube, 1975; Hall, 1976).

II. Biology of the Parasite

A brief review of the protozoan parasite, with definitions of drug response, may help in understanding some of the results to be discussed in detail for each drug.

Four plasmodial species are responsible for naturally acquired human malaria. As shown in Fig. 1, *Plasmodium falciparum* does not have a persistent tissue form. *Plasmodium vivax* and *Plasmodium ovale* do have this secondary tissue schizont stage that can cause a long interval between clinical attacks. *Plasmodium malariae* persists as a latent erythrocytic infection. This lack of the secondary tissue phase by *P. falciparum* is of therapeutic importance; once the blood forms are destroyed, a radical cure is obtained.

Several terms directly relating to drug action and the developmental forms of the parasite may be defined as follows.

Causal prophylactic—a drug producing complete prevention of erythrocytic infection by destroying either the sporozoites or the primary tissue forms of the parasite.

Suppressive prophylactic—a drug that prevents or eliminates clinical symptoms and/or parasitemia by early destruction of the erythrocytic forms without affecting the establishment of the exoerythrocytic forms.

Clinical cure—relief by drugs of symptoms of a malaria attack without necessarily complete elimination of the infection.

Radical cure—complete elimination of the malaria parasite from the body by drugs so that relapses cannot occur.

Relapse—renewed manifestation of malarial infection separated from previous manifestations of the same infection by an interval greater than those due to the normal periodicity of the paroxysms.

Recrudescence—renewed manifestation of infection believed due to survival of erythrocytic forms.

As already stated, it can be seen that since *P. falciparum* does not have the persistent tissue forms, complete suppression of the asexual erythrocytic parasites will result in a cure. This is not the case with *P. vivax,* where a tissue reservoir exists.

In evaluating the results of drug therapy both in subhuman models and in human trials, the method of infecting the host is important. As Fig. 1 indicates, mosquito (and thus sporozoite)-induced infection occurs in the liver before the peripheral blood cycles begin. On the other hand, blood (and thus trophozoite)-induced infections bypass the liver and will not

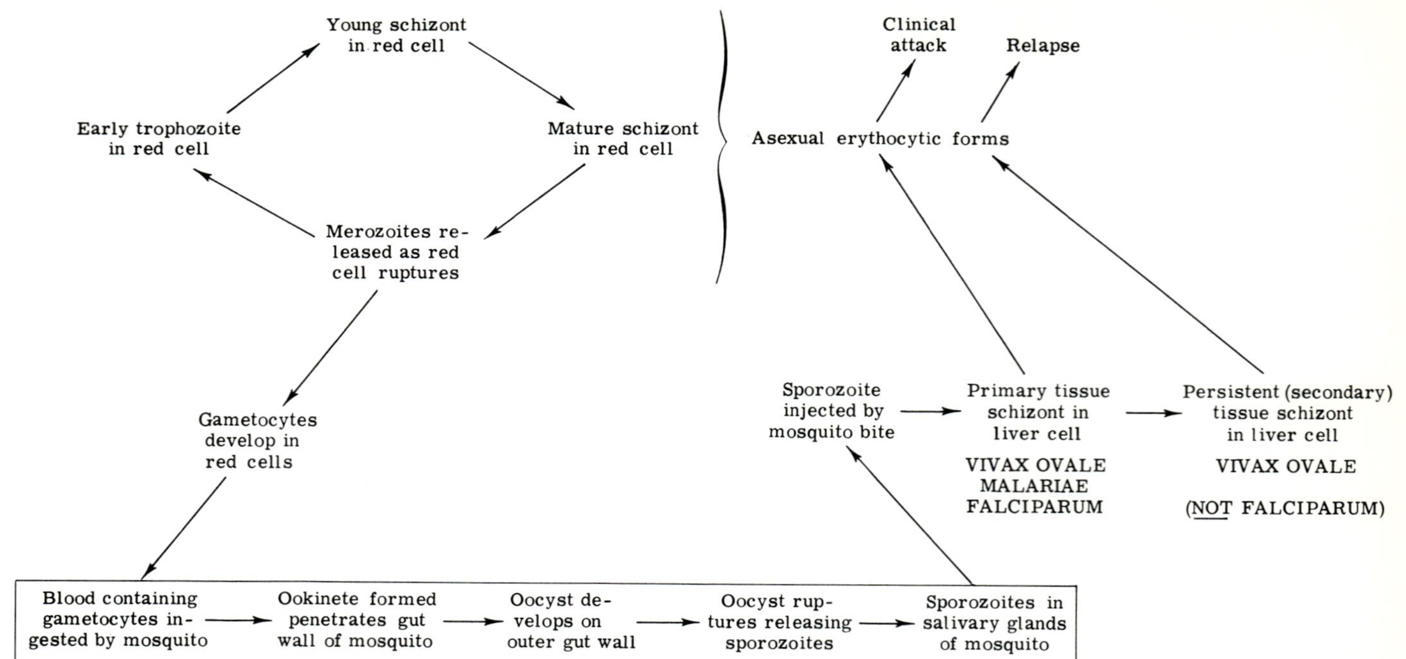

FIG. 1. Life cycle of human plasmodia.

show an effect from a pure causal prophylactic drug. Conversely, the drug may be an effective suppressive agent, but not produce a radical cure in *P. vivax*.

The primary initial animal test for blood schizonticidal activity used in the Army program is a blood-induced *Plasmodium berghei* infection in mice, developed by Dr. Leo Rane (Osdene *et al.*, 1967). The most important subhuman primate screens are blood-induced *P. falciparum* and *P. vivax* infections in the *Aotus* monkey (Schmidt, 1973). Since these systems test drugs against established erythrocytic parasitemias, causal prophylactic effects cannot be determined without modifications. Drugs being evaluated for this effect are initially tested in a sporozoite-induced mouse system (Gregory and Peters, 1970) and confirmed in rhesus monkeys with sporozoite-induced *Plasmodium cynomolgi* infections (Davidson *et al.*, 1976).

The same points must be made about Phase II studies in human volunteers. Some of the infections in volunteers were blood-induced and some were mosquito-induced, depending on the type of drug activity being tested. In both man and animals, different strains of parasites are used. Resistance to drugs in animal parasites is often artifically induced and is well characterized in terms of sensitivity to various drugs. In man, some infections are produced with naturally occurring strains that have developed a resistance to one or more of the antimalarial drugs; these strains originate in different areas of the world. Most of these human strains have had their drug-resistance patterns detailed in relation to degree of resistance to the standard antimalarial drugs. Studies in volunteers with several of these characterized strains are thus effective predictors of response to naturally acquired infections in different areas of the world. These human strains can also be used to infect the *Aotus* monkey, and thus this test system is used to evaluate new drugs against specific drug-resistant strains of the target organism.

Among the classes of compounds that produced effective drugs against resistant strains were the quinolinemethanols. They show considerable promise and will be discussed first.

III. Quinolinemethanols

A. WR 30,090

1. *Chemistry*

Synthesis of WR 30,090 (Fig. 2) was first reported by Lutz *et al.* (1946). This compound was originally synthesized as a part of the World War II antimalarial program, and was assigned Survey Number (SN) 15,068. Be-

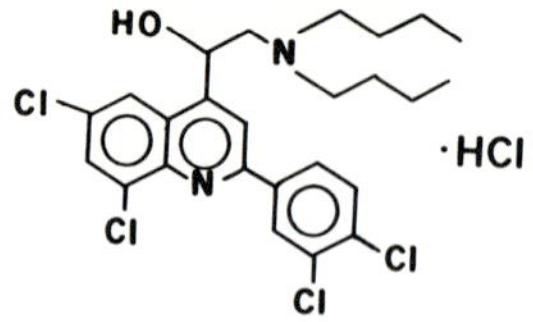

FIG. 2. Drug WR 30,090. α-[(Dibutylamino)methyl]-6,8-dichloro-2-(3,4-dichlorophenyl)-4-quinolinemethanol hydrochloride.

cause the compound was developed late in that war, it was not tested in humans (Wiselogle, 1946) until reactivation of the antimalarial drug development program by the U.S. Army.

Partitioning studies between organic solvents and aqueous buffered solutions showed that WR 30,090 has a very high lipophilicity, with Kp for a number of organic solvents in the general magnitude of 10^3 (Mu *et al.*, 1975).

In vitro studies have shown the hydrochloride salt form to be stable in solution for several days in organic solvents. The free base of WR 30,090 was also relatively stable in these solvents when not exposed to sunlight or to ultraviolet irradiation. When irradiated at ~3000 Å, however, the free base very rapidly decomposed to produce mainly 6,8-dichloro-2-(3′,4′-dichlorophenyl)-4-quinolinecarboxyaldehyde (Okada *et al.*, 1975).

2. *Preclinical Efficacy and Biology*

Efficacy studies published by Wiselogle (1946) showed that orally administered WR 30,090 effectively suppressed *Plasmodium lophurae* in ducks, with a twenty-fold greater potency than quinine. Coatney *et al.* (1953) reported efficacy against *Plasmodium gallinaceum,* with a therapeutic index of 186.5.

Drug WR 30,090 when administered subcutaneously as single doses of 160 mg/kg suspended in peanut oil produced radical cures of all mice infected with *Plasmodium berghei* (Strube, 1975). Temporary suppression of parasitemia was observed at single doses as low as 10 mg/kg. The oral dose of WR 30,090 required to produce 90% suppression of *P. berghei* parasitemia in mice when administered daily to sensitive strains ranged from 0.8 (Thompson, 1972) to 2.7 mg/kg/day (Peters *et al.*, 1975).

The minimum daily oral dose required to cure rhesus monkeys infected with blood-induced *Plasmodium cynomolgi* was 100 mg/kg/day for 7 days (Davidson *et al.*, 1976). Schmidt (1973) found no evidence of cross-resistance with chloroquine in *Plasmodium falciparum*-infected *Aotus* monkeys which were given WR 30,090 orally for 7 days (Strube, 1975).

By contrast, Peters *et al.* (1975) found cross-resistance with the highly chloroquine-resistant RC strain of *P. berghei*. However, they saw little cross-resistance to their moderately chloroquine-resistant NS strain. Essentially the same pattern of cross-resistance was observed by Thompson (1972).

A number of drugs that competitively inhibit chloroquine binding to high-affinity drug receptors (Fitch, 1972) have been shown to have an apparent K_i similar to that of chloroquine.* The apparent K_i for the high-affinity receptor of chloroquine-susceptible *P. berghei* was 5×10^{-7} *M* for chloroquine and 2×10^{-6} *M* for WR 30,090 (Fitch, 1972). This ability to compete for high-affinity binding sites is thought to be a reflection of chloroquine cross-resistance for this parasite.

Another area that was investigated in attempts to predict cross-resistance was the clumping of hemozoin pigment caused by chloroquine in *P. berghei*-infected red blood cells. A number of drugs, including WR 30,090, inhibited chloroquine-induced pigment clumping in *P. berghei* (Warhurst *et al.*, 1972; Warhurst and Thomas, 1975; Einheber *et al.*, 1976). This implied that these drugs compete for the same binding site as chloroquine. Further evidence that WR 30,090 was competing for the chloroquine binding site was found by Einheber *et al.* (1976) who showed disaggregation of fully formed chloroquine-induced hemozoin clumps by WR 30,090.

Warhurst and Thomas (1975) indicated that, in comparison with Fitch's high-affinity binding site, the clumping binding site was more structure specific. The possibility exists that modifications of these several types of sites in chloroquine-resistant *P. berghei* may help explain the inconsistent cross-resistance patterns observed in these studies.

3. *Preclinical Toxicology*

Twenty-day toxicity studies were carried out in rats (Powers, 1968a). Four groups of 5 rats each received 0, 500, 1000, or 2000 mg/kg/day by oral intubation. Appearance and behavior of the rats were normal, but food consumption and body weight gain at the two higher doses were depressed. No other drug-related effects were seen.

An 84-day toxicity study was carried out in rats (Lee *et al.*, 1971a). Four groups of 6 rats each received 0, 250, 500, or 1000 mg/kg/day by oral intubation. No toxicity was associated with the 250-mg/kg/day group. Slight toxic signs were seen in the animals receiving the two higher doses, with a slight depression of food consumption and growth rate.

* The apparent K_i as used here is the association constant for a drug to binding sites in *P. berghei*-infected erythrocytes estimated graphically from Lineweaver–Burk plots.

Fourteen-day oral toxicity studies were carried out in beagles (Lee *et al.*, 1967, 1968a–e) at 12.5, 25, 50, 125, 250, or 500 mg/kg/day. The 12.5-mg/kg/day dose caused no drug-related effects. All other doses produced a drug-related increase in the marrow myeloid/erythroid ratios due to depression of the erythroid series. Dose-related emesis and diarrhea, with decreased food intake, were seen at all but the lowest dose. Possible drug-related atrophy of lymphoid tissue was seen at the higher doses.

A 91-day oral toxicity study was performed in beagles (Lee *et al.*, 1971b). Four groups of 4 dogs each received 0, 10, 20, or 40 mg/kg/day. The weight gain of the treated dogs was somewhat depressed. The major dose-related target organ was the liver, with inflammatory lesions characterized by neutrophil and mononuclear cell infiltration of the portal areas and vacuolar degeneration of the hepatic cord cells. The incidence and severity of naturally occurring inflammatory reactions in the lung, intestinal tract, pancreas, and peripheral lymph nodes may also have been increased by the drug.

Phototoxic potential was investigated in albino mice (Rothe and Jacobus, 1968). The minimum intraperitoneal dose found necessary to produce a phototoxic response was 50 mg/kg. This compared favorably to the 5-mg/kg dose of SN 10,275 [α-(2-piperidinyl)-6,8-dichloro-2-(phenyl)-4-quinolinemethanol], the World War II quinolinemethanol used as a standard (Rothe and Jacobus, 1968). This latter compound had been evaluated in humans, but was abandoned because of its severe prolonged photosensitizing action (Pullman *et al.*, 1948).

4. *Pharmacology*

Aviado and Belej (1970) investigated a number of pharmacological properties of WR 30,090. Protection against chloroform-induced ventricular fibrillation in mice was provided by 100 mg/kg of the drug. Only one-third of the treated mice fibrillated, whereas 82% of the untreated controls fibrillated. No change in cardiac norepinephrine content was associated with WR 30,090 administration.

The same authors measured cardiac output in anesthetized dogs. Drug WR 30,090 infused intravenously decreased cardiac output by approximately one-third at 20 through 40 mg/kg, but the drug was not lethal even at 100 mg/kg.

A limited study of the metabolic fate of WR 30,090-^{14}C in animals and man has been published (Mu *et al.*, 1975). In two anesthetized bile duct-cannulated dogs, 13–15% of the radiolabel appeared in the bile within 4 to 6 hours after intravenous administration, while 3% or less was excreted into urine during that time. Organs from these dogs showed that radiolabel concentrated in liver, spleen, and lung when compared to plasma levels. The heart and kidney also concentrated the radiolabel, but to a lesser extent. Trace amounts were seen in cerebrospinal fluid, saliva, cerebellum, and bone marrow.

Rats excreted the vast majority of radiolabel rapidly in the feces after orally administered WR 30,090-^{14}C, with only trace amounts in the urine (Mu *et al.*, 1975). The extent of absorption from the gastrointestinal tract was not investigated in this species.

A 20-mg dose of WR 30,090 containing a trace amount of WR 30,090-^{14}C was given orally to 1 normal male volunteer (Mu *et al.*, 1975). Plasma levels of radioactivity declined in a biphasic manner, with an apparent terminal half-life of 26 hours. Most of the radiolabel in the 4–8 hour plasma samples was in the form of parent drug. During this 4–8 hour period, the concentration of radiolabel associated with red blood cells was only 10–15% of the level in plasma. Excretion of radiolabel from the body was slow, with less than 2% in the urine and the remainder in the feces. Less than 10% of the radiolabel in the feces and less than 1% of the radiolabel in the urine was associated with the parent drug. An apparent elimination half-life for radiolabel excreted in feces was calculated to be 8–9 days. This, coupled with the data from the cannulated dogs, would indicate an enterohepatic recycling.

5. *Clinical Studies*

Phase I, rising dose, tolerance studies were reported by Martin *et al.* (1973) and J. D. Arnold (personal communication, 1973). Total daily doses increased from 5 mg/day for 3 days to 460 mg 3× per day for 10 days. The drug was very well tolerated, with no subjective complaints or laboratory abnormalities other than four instances of ephemeral phototoxicity that were not dose-related. A total of 47 normal subjects received the drug in these studies.

Phase II studies (Martin *et al.*, 1973) using volunteers infected with various strains of *P. falciparum* showed that 230 mg every 8 hours for 6 days was very efficacious. This regimen cured 6 out of 6 cases of infections of drug-sensitive Uganda I strain, 6 out of 6 cases of chloroquine-resistant Malayan Camp strain, 6 out of 6 cases of chloroquine-resistant Malayan Taylor strain, and the single case of chloroquine-resistant Philippine Per strain. Additionally, cures were obtained in 19 out of 23 cases of chloroquine-resistant Vietnam Smith or Vietnam Crocker strains treated with the foregoing regimen. All 5 cases of chloroquine-resistant Vietnam Marks strain were cured with only 3 days of therapy.

Clyde (1973) treated an additional 23 volunteers infected with a variety of drug-resistant strains of *P. falciparum* and all were cured. His overall experience with WR 30,090 showed a mean lysis time for fever of 66 hours, and a mean parasite clearance time of 67 hours.

Martin *et al.* (1973) also studied efficacy against *Plasmodium vivax*. Blood-induced vivax (Chesson strain) responded rapidly to either 3- or 6-day courses of 460–800 mg daily in divided doses. However, recrudescences occurred in 2 of the 8 cases. Clinical cures were obtained in the 4 mosquito-induced infections similarly treated, although all 4 patients later relapsed, possibly due to persistent exoerythrocytic infections.

Canfield *et al.* (1973) field tested WR 30,090, 230 mg every 8 hours for 6 days, in patients with multidrug-resistant falciparum malaria from Vietnam. Of the 26 men treated, 23, or 88%, were cured, whereas the other 3 men showed an RI response (full clearance of parasitemia with subsequent recrudescence). The mean time for lysis of fever was 80 hours (range 25.5–124 hours). The mean serum drug level during the first 2 treatment days was 0.6 μg/ml, and 1.1 μg/ml on the last day of therapy. No evidence of phototoxicity was seen in any patient. During the follow-up observation periods, 7 patients developed acute *P. vivax* infections. This indicated that the drug was not effective against the persistent exoerythrocytic tissue forms of that parasite.

Field studies of WR 30,090 were extended to Thailand, an area of known multidrug-resistant *P. falciparum* malaria (Hall *et al.*, 1975). The patients were treated with 250 mg every 8 hours for 6 days. Mean fever lysis took 58 hours, whereas mean parasite clearance took 72 hours. A cure rate of 86% (54/63 patients) was achieved. Of the remaining 9 patients, 8 showed an RI response and only 1 had an RII response (marked reduction of parasitemia but no clearance of asexual parasites). Side effects, reportedly associated with WR 30,090, were headache, backache, and dizziness. However, these symptoms are so frequently associated with malaria infection itself that it is impossible to say with any certainty that they were drug-related. Two cases of transient urticaria were possibly associated with WR 30,090 therapy. The drug caused no detectable changes in hematocrit, white blood cell count, or levels of serum glutamic oxalacetic acid transaminase (SGOT), alkaline phosphatase, creatinine, and bilirubin, or in the urinalysis. No phototoxicity was reported.

Potential suppressive prophylactic activity of WR 30,090 was studied by Clyde *et al.* (1973). Eighteen volunteers were given 690 mg once a week for 8 weeks, and 8 volunteers were given 460 mg once a week for up to 8 weeks. On the first day of drug administration, the volunteers were exposed to mosquitoes infected with *P. falciparum,* either the Philippine Per strain, the Malayan Taylor strain, or the Vietnam Smith strain (all chloroquine-resistant strains). Suppressive cures were obtained in 14 of the 18 men in the first group and 6 of the 8 in the second group, for a total of 20 out of 26 or 77%. Serum drug levels ranged from 0.00 to 2.25 μg/ml at 8 hours after dosing, and from 0.05 to 0.35 μg/ml at 24 hours after dosing. No side effects were seen.

An additional 15 men received either 460 or 690 mg once a week for 8 weeks and were exposed to mosquitoes heavily infected with *P. vivax*. Four of the 15 developed parasitemia during treatment, whereas 6 of the remainder developed parasitemia after completion of treatment. This indicated limited suppressive prophylactic activity with this dose regimen and no causal prophylactic activity. Again no drug-related side effects were seen.

In summary, WR 30,090 was well tolerated in oral doses of 460 mg, 3× per day, for 10 days. At 230 mg, 3× per day, for 6 days the drug showed a radical curative rate of approximately 90% against multidrug-resistant *P. falciparum*, which was significantly greater than any single standard drug. At various dosage regimens the drug showed good suppressive activity against *P. vivax* but no tissue schizonticidal activity.

B. WR 142,490

1. *Chemistry*

Synthesis of WR 142,490 (Fig. 3) was first reported by Ohnmacht *et al.* in 1971. The drug, now named mefloquine, is a mixture of the *d*- and *l*-erythro forms. All four configurations, *d*- and *l*-erythro and *d*- and *l*-threo forms, have been isolated (Carroll and Blackwell, 1974) and characterized. Chien and Cheng (1976) varied the N—O distances of the piperidinyl ring to determine the effects on antimalarial activity. Lengthening the potential range of 2.5 to 3.5 Å in the α-2-piperidinyl ring to one of 2.6 to 5 Å in the α-3-piperidinyl configuration greatly reduced antimalarial efficacy.

A method has been described for quantitation of the drug in blood. Grindel *et al.* (1977) extracted with ethyl acetate and determined drug concentrations using high-performance liquid chromatography. Sensitivity with good precision was reported down to 0.05 μg/ml.

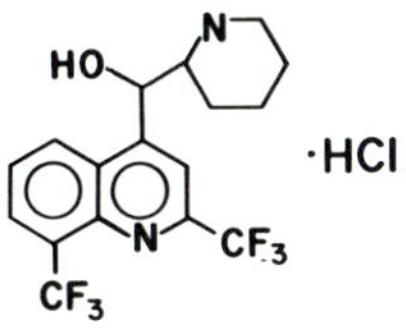

HO, N, ·HCl, N, CF_3, CF_3

FIG. 3. Drug WR 142,490. 2,8-Bis(trifluoromethyl)-α-(2-piperidinyl)-4-quinolinemethanol hydrochloride.

2. *Preclinical Efficacy and Biology*

Drug WR 142,490 effectively cured *P. berghei* infections at 20 mg/kg and above (Ohnmacht *et al.*, 1971) when administered subcutaneously in peanut oil to mice (Osdene *et al.*, 1967). The daily oral dose administered to mice that was effective in producing 90% suppression of *P. berghei* parasitemia was 8.5 mg/kg/day (Peters *et al.*, 1975).

Drug WR 142,490 ranks with the most active 4-quinolinemethanol tested in the *Aotus* monkey–human malaria model (Schmidt, 1973). The daily curative dose (CD_{90}) for *P. falciparum* when given orally for 7 consecutive days was 3.125 mg/kg for both the Malayan Camp CH/Q and the Vietnam Oak Knoll strains and 5.0 mg/kg for the Vietnam Smith strain. For blood-induced *P. vivax,* it was 2.5 mg/kg for both the New Guinea Chesson and Vietnam Palo Alto strains. Of great importance was the observation that curative capacity was a function of the total amount of drug delivered. Identical cure rates were obtained whether the total dose was administered once or was given during 3 or 7 days.

Desjardins *et al.* (1978) quantitatively assessed antimalarial activity utilizing an automated microtiter dilution system in conjunction with continuous *in vitro* culture of *P. falciparum*. No difference in response was seen between the chloroquine-sensitive Uganda I and the chloroquine-resistant Vietnam Smith strains.

Among the correlations attempting to predict cross-resistance of drugs with chloroquine are competitive binding to *P. berghei* high-affinity receptors (Fitch, 1972). Mefloquine and WR 30,090 both have an apparent K_i of 2×10^{-6} *M*, similar to that of chloroquine (5×10^{-7} *M*). Drug WR 142,490 is also apparently capable of competing with chloroquine for *P. berghei* hemozoin clumping sites (Warhurst *et al.*, 1972; Warhurst and Thomas, 1975; Einheber *et al.*, 1976). However, Peters *et al.* (1975) showed little or no cross-resistance to chloroquine in either the highly chloroquine-resistant RC line or the moderately resistant NS line of *P. berghei*.

The development of lines of *P. berghei* resistant to mefloquine has been accomplished by Peters *et al.* (1977a,b). Two procedures were used, the relapse technique and the increasing drug selection pressure method. Resistance developed in the parent N strain slowly to the first and rapidly to the second method. Mixtures of mefloquine with other antimalarials, such as pyrimethamine, sulfaphenazole, or primaquine, caused resistance to development in the parasites more slowly to the component drugs than did the individual drugs.

The mechanism of resistance formation is dependent on the mechanisms through which the antimalarial drug works. These have not been fully elucidated, although many studies have been performed.

One hypothesis is based on the fact that quinoline–acridine type planar molecules such as quinine, chloroquine, and mepacrine all form an intercalated complex with DNA (Hahn *et al.*, 1966). This concept of intercalation (Henry, 1972) has led to the synthesis of a number of good antimalarial drugs (Strube, 1975). However, although it is a very efficient antimalarial, mefloquine has been shown not to bind significantly to DNA (Davidson *et al.*, 1975, 1977).

3. *Preclinical Toxicology*

Oral daily doses for 28 consecutive days were given to both rats and beagle dogs (Lee *et al.*, 1972c,d). No effect in either species was seen at 5 mg/kg/day. In the rat, 30 mg/kg/day caused lymphocytopenia with no other adverse effects. The same dose in dogs caused occasional diarrhea and emesis, and depletion in lymphoid tissues and/or inflammatory changes in the liver characterized by vacuolar degeneration. Doses of 150 mg/kg/day were quite toxic, with accompanying death, in both species. In the rat the major target organs were lymphoid tissue (depression and atrophy) and skeletal and cardiac muscle (inflammation and degeneration progressing to necrosis). Serum transaminase and blood urea nitrogen (BUN) levels were elevated. That dose in the dog caused depression of blood-forming tissues as well as occasional inflammatory and/or vacuolar degenerative changes in the liver, gastrointestinal tract, kidney, and possibly testes. Serum levels of transaminases and alkaline phosphatase were elevated, as was the BUN.

Korte *et al.* (1978) confirmed that daily oral doses of 6 mg/kg or 13.5 mg/kg of WR 142,490 for 28 days were nontoxic to beagles, whereas 30 mg/kg depressed weight gain slightly. At 68 mg/kg, the drug caused mild toxic signs, increased the BUN levels, and caused hepatic degeneration and lymphoid atrophy or depletion.

The effects of oral doses of mefloquine given weekly to rats and beagles for 52 consecutive weeks were determined (Lee *et al.*, 1974a,b). Weekly doses of 5 mg/kg caused no adverse effects in either species. In the rat, 25 and 125 mg/kg/week reduced weight gain with no other effects. In the beagle those doses caused no adverse effects whatsoever.

Minor *et al.* (1976) reported on reproductive studies in rats and mice. Female rats given mefloquine from before mating to weaning produced pups with decreased body weights and survival at 50 mg/kg/day, but these changes were not evident at 5 mg/kg/day. These effects were attributed to malnourishment. Male rats given the drug for 13 weeks had reduced growth and fertility index and epididymal lesions at 50 mg/kg/day but not at 5 mg/kg/day. Drug WR 142,490 produced some anomalies at 100 mg/kg/day, but not at 10 mg/kg/day, when administered from day 6 through day 15 of gestation to both rats and mice. When given drug from gestational day 16 to weaning, some toxicity was produced in rat dams and pups at 70 mg/kg/day, but not at 7 mg/kg/day. Cross-fostering studies indicated that pup toxicity was produced during the postnatal period.

Phototoxicity studies in mice (Rothe and Jacobus, 1968) showed that mefloquine did not produce this reaction (Strube, 1975).

4. *Pharmacology*

Caldwell and Nash (1976, 1977) investigated the cardiovascular and pulmonary effects of intravenously administered mefloquine methanesulfonate salt on anesthetized dogs. At 1 mg/kg/minute for 20 minutes, little or no effect was seen. At 2 or 3 mg/kg/minute for 20 minutes, arterial blood pressure and cardiac contractile force decreased during infusion, returning toward control levels after cessation of infusion. Central venous pressure and pulmonary arterial pressure rose during infusion, returning toward control levels after cessation of infusion. Tidal volume and dynamic airway resistance decreased, and respiratory rate increased during infusion. They returned to normal after infusion, with an overshoot of the airway resistance past control values. Analysis of the time course indicated that the magnitude of the effects was related more to the speed of infusion than to the total dose.

Thus far the fate of radiolabeled WR 142,490 has been published only for the rat. Mu *et al.* (1973, 1975) determined that parenterally administered drug was excreted primarily in the feces. The drug was also concentrated and excreted in the bile and into the gastric juice. For the first 4 days, drug concentrations in rat red cells were 4–6 times higher than plasma levels. This compared to a ratio of approximately 1.7 in human blood. Extensive binding to plasma proteins was seen. Extensive tissue localization of the radiolabel was seen with high tissue-to-plasma ratios noted especially in lung, liver, stomach, kidney, muscle, and fat. On the first day after drug administration, tissue radioactivity was found primarily in the form of parent drug. Interestingly, on day 2, urine and feces samples contained little parent drug, but the radioactivity was present in the form of at least three metabolites.

Liss and Kensler (1976) used whole-body radioautography to follow the fate of the radiolabel after oral administration of mefloquine-^{14}C to rats. They showed long-term binding to melanin in skin and retina as well as deposition in lung and lacrimal gland complex. Deposition in other organs also paralleled those reported by Mu *et al.* (1975).

5. *Clinical Studies*

Phase I, rising dose, tolerance studies were reported by Trenholme *et al.* (1975). Single oral doses increased upward from 5 through 2000 mg. The drug was well tolerated through 1500 mg, but transient dizziness and nausea were reported for 4 out of 8 volunteers receiving either 1750 or 2000 mg. In none of the 42 normal subjects was phototoxicity observed.

Clyde *et al.* (1976) found that weekly doses of 250 mg once per week in 9 volunteers and 500 mg once per week in 4 volunteers for 8 consecutive weeks produced no side effects. In addition, 4 men received oral doses of 500 mg every 2 weeks for 6 to 8 weeks without side effects. Three additional volunteers receiving monthly doses of 1000 mg per dose for either 2 or 3 months reported mild epigastric discomfort but no vomiting or diarrhea after each dose.

A 1-year tolerance study of mefloquine was performed by K. G. Barry and R. C. Reba (personal communication). Weekly doses of 500 mg produced no detectable clinical or laboratory evidence of intolerance.

Phase II studies of radical curative activity have been performed in volunteers infected with *P. falciparum* or *P. vivax*. Trenholme *et al.* (1975) reported on 42 such subjects who received single oral doses of WR 142,490. Two multidrug-resistant strains, Vietnam Marks and Cambodian Buchanan, and the drug-sensitive Ethiopian Taemenie strain, were used. Of 12 subjects with primary infections, all had clearance of parasitemia following a single oral dose of 400 mg, but 10 of these recrudesced. Doses of 1000 mg cured 13 out of 15 subjects, whereas 1500 mg cured 8 out of 8. In partially immune subjects (ones who had previously received partially suppressive doses of other antimalarial drugs), 250 mg cured 1 out of 3, whereas 500 mg cured not only the 2 who recrudesced but also 4 out of 4 additional volunteers.

In addition, 5 partially immune subjects infected with the Chesson strain of *P. vivax* were treated with WR 142,490. Two subjects were cured of blood-induced infections by single doses of 400 or 1000 mg, respectively. In the 3 subjects with mosquito-induced malaria, the drug rapidly cleared the blood of parasites, but parasitemia reappeared in all 3 (Trenholme *et al.*, 1975). This corroborated studies in animals and showed lack of tissue schizonticidal activity, but excellent blood schizonticidal activity.

The radical curative activity of mefloquine was confirmed in a field trial in Thailand with patients who had naturally acquired falciparum malaria

(Hall, 1976). Single oral doses of 1.5 gm cured 29 out of 31 patients. One of the 2 treatment failures was, in retrospect, too ill for any oral medication alone, but was cured by a combination of intravenous quinine and mefloquine. This combination was used in an additional 35 patients, including 5 who were seriously ill, and all were cured (Hall *et al.,* 1977).

Suppressive prophylactic activity of the drug has also been investigated. Rieckmann *et al.* (1974) studied 8 nonimmune volunteers, each of whom received a single 1-gm dose of the drug. At various times after this, from 2 to 21 days, the subjects were bitten by mosquitoes infected with the multidrug-resistant Vietnam Marks strain of *P. falciparum.* Nine control subjects were exposed to the same sporozoite population as the drug-treated volunteers and all became infected. None of the 5 individuals bitten up to 16 days after receiving mefloquine became infected, whereas the 3 bitten after 21 days became infected, although patency was delayed compared to the controls.

A second report (Clyde *et al.,* 1976) confirmed the suppressive prophylactic activity of mefloquine and extended the study using sporozoite-induced challenges of the multidrug-resistant Vietnam Smith strain of *P. falciparum.* Weekly doses of either 250 or 500 mg/week produced suppressive cures in all 14 subjects who were challenged during the first week of drug administration. In addition, fortnightly doses of 500 mg or monthly doses of 1000 mg produced suppressive cures in all 7 men tested.

Suppressive prophylaxis of *P. vivax* was less successful (Clyde *et al.,* 1976). Eight volunteers received weekly doses ranging from 50 to 500 mg/week and were exposed to sporozoites of either the Chesson or El Salvador (Gue.) strains. Parasitemia was completely suppressed at the 250 and 500 mg, but not at the 50 or 100 mg, dose levels during treatment. However, parasitemia developed after cessation of drug administration at the higher doses.

A field trial in Thailand (Pearlman *et al.,* 1977) compared the suppression of *P. falciparum* and *P. vivax* by three different dosage regimens of WR 142,490 and two different dosage regimens of Fansidar® (the combination of sulfadoxine–pyrimethamine, 20:1 by weight). The trial consisted of a 25 week treatment phase with a 12 week follow-up phase. The mefloquine was given orally either 180 mg every week, 360 mg every week, or 360 mg every 2 weeks. Subjects weighing 22–35 kg received half these doses. There were approximately 170 subjects in each drug treatment group who completed the study.

During the chemosuppression period, the control group experienced 53% *P. falciparum* and 81% *P. vivax* infection rates. By contrast, the 180 mg/week mefloquine group showed <1 and <2%, respectively, the 360 mg/week mefloquine group showed <2 and <1%, respectively, and the

360 mg/2 weeks group had no infections. Thus, mefloquine reduced the degree of both falciparum and vivax malaria dramatically. The results with sulfadoxine–pyrimethamine, 1000:50 mg/2 weeks and 500:25 mg/week, showed slightly less efficacy against falciparum malaria and significantly less efficacy against vivax malaria.

In summary, WR 142,490 was well tolerated orally in doses up through 1500 mg for 1 day or in 500 mg weekly doses for 52 weeks. Single daily doses of 1000 mg and above showed a radical curative rate against established *P. falciparum* infections of at least 93%. The suppressive prophylactic activity of the drug against *P. falciparum* and *P. vivax* administered either weekly or biweekly was dramatic.

IV. Phenanthrenemethanols

A. WR 33,063

1. *Chemistry*

Synthesis of WR 33,063 (Fig. 4) was first reported by May and Mosettig (1946). This compound was originally synthesized as a part of the World War II antimalarial program, and was assigned Survey Number (SN) 13,465. Because the compound was developed late in that war, it was not tested in humans (Wiselogle, 1946) until reactivation of the antimalarial drug development program by the U.S. Army.

A series of derivatives of WR 33,063 was prepared consisting of either esters or various salts of WR 33,063 (Harmon *et al.*, 1973). All of these turned out to be less soluble than WR 33,063·HCl, a result opposite to what had been intended. The two optical isomers were resolved using 40% *d*-tartaric acid in aqueous methanol (Pearson and Rosenberg, 1975).

2. *Preclinical Efficacy and Biology*

Efficacy studies published by Wiselogle (1946) indicated that the drug was an effective oral suppressive against *Plasmodium gallinaceum* in the

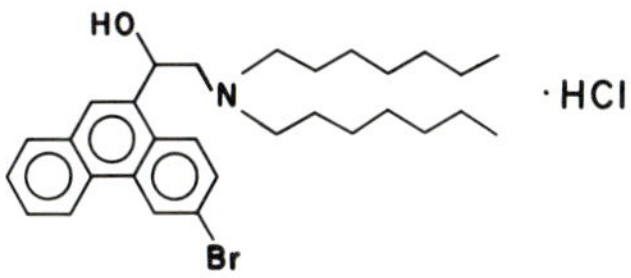

HO N ·HCl Br

FIG. 4. Drug WR 33,063. 6-Bromo-α-[(diheptylamino)methyl]-9-phenanthrenemethanol hydrochloride.

chick. Coatney *et al.* (1953) showed that the drug had efficacy against *P. gallinaceum* with a therapeutic index of 53.4.

Treatment of *Plasmodium berghei*-infected mice given a single subcutaneous injection of peanut oil containing suspended drug (Osdene *et al.*, 1967) produced 4 cures in 5 mice at 320 mg/kg with temporary parasitemia suppression at 40 mg/kg (Harmon *et al.*, 1973). The daily oral dose administered to mice effective in producing 90% suppression of sensitive strains of *P. berghei* parasitemia ranged from 16.7 (Thompson, 1972) to 18.5 mg/kg/day (Peters *et al.*, 1975). The *d*-isomer of WR 33,063 appeared to be somewhat more active than the *l* form against *P. berghei* (Pearson and Rosenberg, 1975).

Drug WR 33,063 was ineffective orally against blood-induced *Plasmodium cynomolgi* infections in rhesus monkeys at 100 mg/kg/day for 7 days (Davidson *et al.*, 1976). In addition, Schmidt showed no curative action at 200 mg/kg/day adminstered orally for 7 days against either the Malayan Camp or Vietnam Smith strains of *Plasmodium falciparum* infection in *Aotus* monkeys (Strube, 1975).

Cross-resistance of WR 33,063 to chloroquine-resistant strains of *P. berghei* in mice has been studied. Thompson (1972) demonstrated that WR 33,063 had a greater than twenty-seven-fold reduction in efficacy against the highly chloroquine-resistant C line. Much the same results were shown by Peters *et al.* (1975) against the highly chloroquine-resistant RC strain, although the degree of cross-resistance was somewhat less.

Drug WR 33,063 has an apparent K_i of 1×10^{-6} M for the *P. berghei* high-affinity drug receptors (Fitch, 1972), similar to that of chloroquine. It also competes with chloroquine for *P. berghei* hemozoin clumping sites (Warhurst and Thomas, 1975; Einheber *et al.*, 1976). A good correlation thus exists between competition with chloroquine-binding sites in *P. berghei* and cross-resistance to chloroquine in this species of *Plasmodium*.

3. *Preclinical Toxicology*

Oral daily doses for 14 consecutive days were given to both rats and rhesus monkeys (Powers, 1968b,c). No drug-related effects in either species were seen at 62.5 mg/kg/day. However, 250 mg/kg/day may have produced mild histological changes in the kidneys of both species. In the rat, histological examination of the group receiving 1000 mg/kg/day confirmed the minimal changes in the kidney and showed mild changes in the spleen and kidney. Otherwise the drug was extremely well tolerated in both species.

Phototoxicity studies in mice (Rothe and Jacobus, 1968) demonstrated that WR 33,063 did not produce sensitivity to ultraviolet light (Strube, 1975).

4. *Pharmacology*

The fate of WR 33,063 was followed by using drug tritiated on the methanolic carbon (Smith and Weigel, 1971a). Total tritium excretion in the urine of owl monkeys ranged up to 4.4%. The fraction present in the urine as tritiated water increased with time in both the *Aotus* monkeys and in humans. Biliary excretion of the radiolabel in the rhesus monkey ranged up to 10% of the dose administered (Smith *et al.*, 1972).

Sadavongvivad and Aviado (1969) studied the effects of WR 33,063 on the biogenic amine content of mouse lung. At doses of 100 or 200 mg/kg, WR 33,063 significantly elevated levels of serotonin and norepinephrine over control values, but did not significantly affect levels of histamine or dopamine.

Ruiz *et al.* (1970) investigated a number of pharmacological properties of WR 33,063. They found no statistically significant effect from WR 33,063 on biogenic amine levels in mouse brain or heart or in rabbit lung. An increase in mouse lung histamine levels over controls was seen at doses from 10 to 200 mg/kg. However, lung histamine levels were much lower in the control mice than this group had previously reported (Sadavongvivad and Aviado, 1969).

Drug WR 33,063 was shown to have no effect on cardiac output, blood pressure, and pulmonary resistance in the anesthetized dog or on pulmonary resistance and blood pressure in the anesthetized rabbit. The drug, when 100 mg/kg was administered, depressed cardiac excitability in mice given chloroform by inhalation (Ruiz *et al.*, 1970).

5. *Clinical Studies*

Phase I, rising dose, tolerance studies were reported by Arnold *et al.* (1973). Total daily oral doses increased upward from 50 mg/day for 3 consecutive days through 4.6 gm/day for 10 consecutive days. A total of 52 normal subjects received the drug during this phase of study. It was very well tolerated in all with only transient mild nausea in 2 volunteers who received 800 mg, 4 × per day, for 10 days. No drug-related abnormalities were seen in the laboratory findings or upon physical examination. No evidence of phototoxicity was seen.

Phase II studies of antimalarial efficacy were carried out by Arnold *et al.* (1973) on 59 volunteers with experimental malaria. It was found that the moderately chloroquine-resistant Camp strain could be cured by as little as 400 mg, 4 × per day, for 3 days, whereas the severely chloroquine-resistant Smith strain required a 6 day regimen of 400 mg, 4× per day. This latter treatment regimen proved quite efficacious for most of the falciparum strains used. Thus, it cured 6 out of 6 Uganda I infections, the single Caribbean Haiti infection, 5 out of 5 Malayan Camp strain infections, 18 out of 22 Vietnam Smith strain infections, 2 out of 4 Vietnam Braithwaite infections, and all 5 Vietnam Marks infections. Except for one volunteer who did not have parasite clearance, clinical responses and parasite suppression were rapid. No clinical or laboratory evidence of adverse drug effects was seen.

Four out of 5 blood-induced Chesson strain *P. vivax* infections were cured with daily doses of 1.6 or 1.8 gm/day for 3 or 6 days (Arnold *et al.*, 1973).

The suppressive prophylactic activity of WR 33,063 was evaluated against the Smith strain of *P. falciparum* (Clyde *et al.*, 1973). Two volunteers received weekly doses of 800 mg of drug and were exposed to heavily infected mosquitoes on the first day of treatment. The drug did not prevent early development of infection.

Canfield *et al.* (1973) field tested WR 33,063, 400 mg every 6 hours for 10 days, in patients with multidrug-resistant falciparum malaria from Vietnam. Of the 25 patients treated, 23, or 92%, were cured, but 1 showed an RI response and the other did not respond at all. The mean time for lysis of fever was 48 hours (range 3.5–106 hours). The mean serum drug level during the first 2 treatment days was 1.8 μg/ml, and 6.0 μg/ml on the last day of therapy. The single patient who did not respond had the lowest serum concentrations observed. No evidence of phototoxicity was seen in any patient. During the follow-up observation periods, 6 patients developed delayed acute *P. vivax* infections; the standard chloroquine–primaquine regimen produced cures in all 6.

Segal *et al.* (1974) compared WR 33,063 with quinine sulfate in treating *P. falciparum* infections in 51 adult Thai males. Drug WR 33,063 was given in doses of 600 mg every 8 hours for 6 days and quinine sulfate was given in doses of 540 mg (base) every 8 hours for 6 days. Mean parasite clearance times were about 65–66 hours and mean fever lysis times were about 58–60 hours for both groups. It cured 23 out of 25 patients (92%) with 1 showing an RI response and the other not responding at all. Quinine cured 95% but 4 subjects moved and were not available for follow-up. Side effects reported were less for the group receiving WR 33,063.

Extending the field studies on WR 33,063 in Thailand, Hall *et al.* (1975) further tested antimalarial efficacy in another area of known multidrug-resistant *P. falciparum*. The dose given to 69 patients was 600 mg every 8 hours for 6 days. Mean fever lysis was 54–55 hours, whereas mean parasite clearance was 77 hours. A cure rate of 92% was achieved. Four patients showed an RI response and only 1 did not respond. Side effects, reportedly associated with WR 33,063, were headache, backache, and dizziness. However, these symptoms are so often associated with malaria infection itself that it is impossible to say with any certainty that they were drug-related. The drug caused no detectable changes in hematology, laboratory tests, or in the urinalysis. No phototoxicity was reported. The authors concluded that WR 33,063 was the most effective and least toxic of the drugs tested, which included WR 30,090 and quinine.

In summary, WR 33,063 was well tolerated orally in doses as large as 1.15 gm, 4 × per day, for 10 days. Doses of 1.6 to 1.8 gm/day for 6 to 10 days gave radical cures in about 90% of the *P. falciparum* infections. The drug also produced clinical cures in *P. vivax* infections but demonstrated no tissue schizonticidal activity.

B. WR 122,455

1. *Chemistry*

Synthesis of WR 122, 455 (Fig. 5) was first reported by Nodiff *et al.* in 1971. The drug is a mixture of the *d* and *l* erythro forms. All four forms, *d*- and *l*-erythro and *d*- and *l*-threo configurations, have been isolated and characterized (Carroll and Blackwell, 1974). Chien and Cheng (1973) varied the N—O distances of the piperidinyl ring to determine the effects on antimalarial activity. Lengthening the potential range of 2.5 to 3.5 Å in the α-2-piperidinyl ring to one of 2.6 to 5 Å in the α-3-piperidinyl configuration did not affect antimalarial efficacy.

Other studies (Agharkar *et al.,* 1976) showed that the *dl*-lactate salt of WR 122,455 had an apparent solubility in water 200 times greater than that of the hydrochloride salt. The dissolution rate in 0.1 *N* HCl, as well as the high apparent solubilities of the 2-hydroxethane-1-sulfonate salt in several commonly used parenteral vehicles, has raised the hope for the development of a more bioavailable form of the drug.

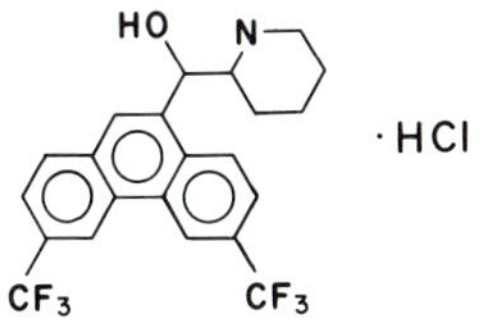

HO N ·HCl

CF_3 CF_3

FIG. 5. Drug WR 122,455. 3,6-Bis(trifluoromethyl)-α-(2-piperidinyl)-9-phenanthrenemethanol hydrochloride.

2. *Preclinical Efficacy and Biology*

Drug WR 122,455 cured all mice of *P. berghei* infection at 80 mg/kg and above (Nodiff *et al.,* 1971) when given subcutaneously in peanut oil (Osdene *et al.,* 1967). The drug compared well with others in Schmidt's *Aotus–P. falciparum* oral test system. Five mg/kg/day for 7 days cured the monkeys of infections of both the Malayan Camp strain and the chloroquine-resistant Vietnam Smith strain (Strube, 1975).

Much investigation has been carried out on the activity of the drug against rodent malaria. Porter and Peters (1976) showed rapid suppression of infection with the chloroquine-sensitive *P. berghei* N strain in mice. The drug affected all of the asexual intraerythrocytic stages, with effective dose levels approximately 3 times those of chloroquine and one-twelfth those of quinine. No causal prophylactic activity was seen.

Peters and Porter (1976) found WR 122,455 to be an effective blood schizonticide against strains of *P. berghei* highly resistant to primaquine, sulfonamides, pyrimethamine, and cycloguanil (Peters *et al.,* 1975). It was active against the moderately chloroquine-resistant NS line but was inactive against the highly chloroquine-resistant RC line. Resistance to WR 122,455 was readily developed in *P. berghei* using a relapse technique. These lines showed cross-resistance to quinine but not to chloroquine, primaquine, sulfonamides, dapsone, pyrimethamine, and cycloguanil. This resistance to WR 122,455 was stable even in the absence of drug selection pressure.

Drug WR 122,455 was one of the series of antimalarials investigated for competition with chloroquine for *P. berghei* hemozoin clumping receptor sites (Warhurst *et al.,* 1972; Warhurst and Thomas, 1975). The affinity of the drug for the site was 40 times that of quinine.

Unlike WR 142,490, drug WR 122,455 interacted strongly with calf thymus DNA (Davies *et al.,* 1975). It thus shared this property of chloroquine, quinine, and mepacrine.

3. *Preclinical Toxicology*

Twenty-eight-day toxicity studies were carried out in rats (Lee *et al.,* 1970b). Five groups of 20 rats each received 0, 12.5, 25, 50, or 100 mg/kg/day by oral intubation. All drug-treated groups showed dose-related anorexia and retardation of weight gain or actual weight loss, with death at the highest dose. The lowest dose caused leukocytosis and neutrophilia. Reticulocytopenia was seen at 25 mg/kg/day, and increased SGOT and serum glutamic pyruvic transaminase (SGPT) levels at 50 mg/kg/day. A possible dose-related increase in incidence and severity was seen in pneumonia, focal hepatitis, interstitial nephritis, myocarditis, encephalitis, myositis and necrosis of skeletal muscle, inflammation of the gastrointestinal tract, and lymphoid depletion in the spleen and lymph node. The target organs were primarily skeletal muscle, lymphoid tissue, and bone marrow.

Twenty-eight-day oral toxicity studies were carried out in beagle dogs (Lee *et al.,* 1970a) at 20, 40, and 80 mg/kg/day. Four dogs were given drug at each dose level. Repeated doses at the lowest level caused some emesis and diarrhea. All dogs of this group had "punched out holes" in the germinal centers of lymph nodes due to lymphocyte necrosis; some had degenerative involvement of the fundic portion of the stomach. The same pattern was seen with higher doses, but was more severe. Leukocytosis was seen. Lymphoid tissue of various organs was damaged. At 80 mg/kg/day, elevation of the marrow myeloid/erythroid ratios was seen, with some depression of erythroid elements and proliferation of maturing neutrophils.

A study on reversability of toxicity in beagle dogs was made (Lee *et al.,* 1970c). Four beagles were given oral doses of 80 mg/kg/day for 28 days. All signs seen in the previous study were present. In addition, there was ophthalmoscopic evidence of hemorrhage and chorioretinitis. However, this was not confirmed on histopathological examination. After drug administration was discontinued, signs gradually disappeared in all dogs. It was concluded that the drug-associated toxicities in beagles were reversible after treatment was discontinued.

Four-week oral toxicity studies were carried out in the rhesus monkey (Powers, 1970). Four groups of 4 monkeys each received 0, 5, 20, or 80 mg/kg/day by gavage. At 5 mg/kg/day there appeared to be no effect. Dose-related toxicity included emesis, diarrhea, and anorexia with associated weight loss. At 80 mg/kg/day, 2 out of the 4 monkeys died during the fourth week. Drug-related toxicity included increased levels of BUN, SGPT, SGOT, and bilirubin with decreased levels of fasting blood sugar, total serum protein, and lymphocyte counts. Histopathological examination, combined with other evidence, indicated that target organs were primarily lymphoid tissue, bone marrow, and liver. No evidence of eye involvement was seen.

4. *Pharmacology*

Tritiated WR 122,455 was given to mice (Rozman *et al.,* 1971). Two-week urinary excretion of radiolabel was less than 5% of the dose, whether given orally, subcutaneously, or intraperitoneally. Fecal excretion of radiolabel continued during the entire 2-week study period. Tissue levels indicated good oral absorption.

Smith and Weigel (1971b) showed that, after oral administration, radioactivity levels peaked in rat blood at 2 days and in monkey blood at 4 to 5 days. Less than 10% of the radiolabel dose was excreted in the urine. In rat the radiolabel concentrated in lung, liver, adrenals, spleen, pancreas, and gonads. In the *Aotus* monkey (Weigel and Smith, 1973) given the radioactive drug orally, blood levels of drug equivalents peaked at 0.5 to 2.7 μg/ml for a number of days. Radiolabel concentrated in the erythrocytes. The greatest amounts of drug equivalents were found in liver and lung, with the highest concentrations found in lung, liver, spleen, bone marrow, and adrenals.

In the rhesus monkey, biliary excretion of radiolabel accounted for a large percentage of the administered dose (Smith *et al.,* 1972). Tritiated water was excreted in urine in small amounts after the tritiated drug was given to *Aotus* monkeys (Smith and Weigel, 1971a), indicating either tritium exchange or metabolism at the methanolic carbon.

5. *Clinical Studies*

Phase I, rising dose, oral tolerance studies were carried out on 33 normal volunteers (Rinehart *et al.,* 1976). Total daily doses increased from a single 320-mg dose through 240 mg, 4 × per day, for 6 days. No significant laboratory or clinical abnormality was seen in any patient, nor was any phototoxicity present. The drug was clinically well tolerated in single doses up through 800 mg. However, 5 out of 10 volunteers receiving 880 through 1520 mg as single doses had mild abdominal cramps and diarrhea. Four subjects tolerated 240 mg, 2 × per day, for 3 to 5 days, but 2 others had mild gastrointestinal symptoms when treated for 6 days. Gastrointestinal symptoms were more severe in 3 additional volunteers who received higher, divided-dose regimens. Symptoms ceased in all cases upon cessation of the drug.

Phase II, antimalarial efficacy studies were carried out in 13 volunteers infected with the Vietnam Smith strain of *P. falciparum* and in 5 volunteers infected with the African Uganda strain. All 5 subjects (4 Smith strain, 1 Uganda strain) who received a 1-day regimen, 440 through 880 mg, had prompt clearance of parasitemia but recrudesced after 3 weeks. The other 8 volunteers received 240 mg, 2 × per day, for 6 days. All were cured.

Clinical response to WR 122,455 was prompt and similar for both the chloroquine-resistant Smith and the chloroquine-sensitive Uganda I strains. Parasite clearance and fever lysis times were 3.1 days and 66 hours, respectively. No adverse effects of the drug were seen.

In summary, WR 122,455 was well tolerated orally at single 800-mg doses but produced some mild gastrointestinal symptoms at 240 mg, 2 × per day, for 6 days. However, a 100% cure rate of *P. falciparum* infection was obtained with the latter dosage regimen in the relatively few patients thus far treated.

C. WR 171,669

1. *Chemistry*

Synthesis of WR 171,669 (Fig. 6) was first reported by Colwell *et al.* (1972). Of the phenanthrene derivatives reported, WR 171,669 was the most potent upon initial antimalarial screening.

2. *Preclinical Efficacy and Biology*

Drug WR 171,669 cured all mice of blood-induced *P. berghei* infection at 20 mg/kg and above (Colwell *et al.*, 1972) when given subcutaneously in peanut oil (Osdene *et al.*, 1967). Suppressive activity was seen at 5 mg/kg.

The drug was less potent than WR 122,455 in Schmidt's *Aotus–P. falciparum* oral test system. Treatment with 20 mg/kg/day for 7 days was the minimum curative dosage regimen against the Malayan Camp strain (Strube, 1975).

In vitro, no difference in response was seen between the chloroquine-sensitive Uganda I and the chloroquine-resistant Vietnam Smith strains of *P. falciparum* (Desjardins *et al.*, 1978). The potency *in vitro* was in the same range as that of mefloquine.

The effect of the drug on chloroquine-induced pigment clumping in *P. berghei* was investigated (Einheber *et al.*, 1976). This drug not only inhibited the hemozoin pigment clumping in *P. berghei,* it also reversed the clumping caused by chloroquine. Thus, both phenanthrenemethanols investigated by the authors had essentially the same effect.

3. *Preclinical Toxicology*

Twenty-eight-day toxicity studies were carried out in rats (Lee *et al.*, 1972e). Four groups of 6 rats each received 0, 25, 100, or 400 mg/kg/day

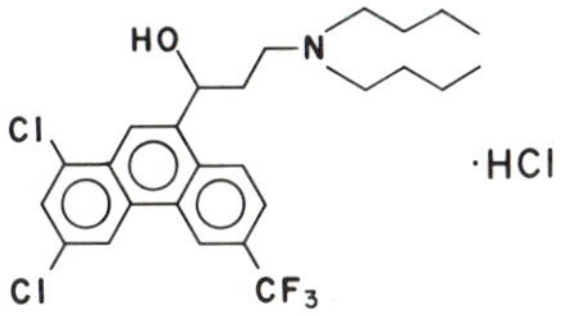

HO N Cl Cl CF_3 ·HCl

FIG. 6. Drug WR 171,669. γ-(Dibutylamino)-1,3-dichloro-6-(trifluoromethyl)-9-phenanthrenepropanol hydrochloride.

by oral intubation. Repeated oral doses of 25 mg/kg/day caused no adverse effects. The incidence and severity of toxic effects in the two higher dose groups appeared to be dose-related, with death occurring in the highest-dose group. Appetite reduction and retardation of weight gain or actual weight loss were seen. Also observed were thrombocytosis and elevation of SGOT, BUN, and/or SGPT levels. Leukocytosis was also seen in the highest-dose group. Morphological lesions included lymphoid depletion and central necrosis in lymph nodes, vacuolar degeneration in the spleen, reticuloendothelial cell hyperplasia in spleen and thymus, some thymic atrophy, and an elevation in the marrow myeloid/erythroid ratios due to myeloid hyperplasia. Myositis and necrosis of skeletal muscle were also observed.

Twenty-eight-day oral toxicity studies were carried out in beagle dogs (Lee *et al.*, 1972f) at 5, 15, 60, and 240 mg/kg/day. Four dogs were treated at each level. Repeated doses at the lowest level did not produce any adverse effects. In the other groups, a dose-related increase in incidence and severity of toxic effects was seen. The drug was lethal to 2 dogs in the 60-mg/kg/day group during the fourth week and to 3 dogs at the 240 mg/kg/day level after the eighth day. There was reduction of appetite associated with reduced weight gain or loss of weight. Diarrhea, emesis, and some ataxia were seen. The peripheral neutrophil/lymphocyte ratio increased. Also observed were reticulocytopenia and depression of bone marrow with an elevation in the myeloid/erythroid ratio. Elevations of the SGPT and BUN levels were observed. Tissue lesions included atrophy and necrosis of lymphoid tissues, thymic involution, vacuolar degeneration of the kidney, catarrhal gastroenteritis, and atrophy or necrosis of skeletal muscle.

4. *Pharmacology*

When radiolabeled WR 171,669 was given orally to rats (Hiremath, 1974), plasma levels of radioactivity peaked at 4 to 8 hours. Radiolabel was found to concentrate in lung, adrenal, spleen, liver, kidney, and heart. Similar studies in the rhesus monkey showed high radiolabel concentrations in liver, lung, cerebrum, cerebellum, lymph nodes, and testes. Excretion of the radiolabel in both species was primarily in the feces.

5. *Clinical Studies*

Phase I, rising dose, oral tolerance studies were carried out on 40 normal volunteers (Rinehart *et al.*, 1976). Total daily doses increased from a single 5-mg dose through 480 mg, 4× per day for 1 day to a maximum of 250 mg, 4× per day, for 6 days. No significant laboratory or clinical abnormality was seen in any patient, nor was any phototoxicity present. The drug was well tolerated when given for only 1 day in doses up through 1260 mg. Three out of 4 subjects given either 1440 or 1920 mg for 1 day in divided doses had abdominal cramps, with mild nausea also reported at the higher dose. Two out of 4 subjects receiving 420 mg, 3× per day, for 2 or 3 days had mild abdominal cramps or nausea. One out of 2 subjects receiving 250 mg, 4× per day, for 5 days experienced epigastric pain. When this regimen was continued for 6 days, both volunteers had gastrointestinal symptoms. Symptoms stopped in all cases upon cessation of the drug.

Phase II, antimalarial efficacy studies were carried out in 6 volunteers infected with the Vietnam Smith strain of *P. falciparum* and in 3 volunteers infected with the African Uganda strain. All 9 patients received 250 mg, 4× per day, for 3 days and all 9 were cured.

Clinical response to WR 171,669 was prompt and similar for both the chloroquine-resistant Smith strain and the chloroquine-sensitive Uganda I strain. Parasite clearance and fever lysis times were 3.5 days and 42 hours, respectively. No adverse effects of the drug were seen.

In summary, WR 171,669 was well tolerated orally at 1260 mg for 1 day and 250 mg, 4 × per day, for 3 days. The latter dosage regimen gave radical cures in 100% of the few *P. falciparum* infections thus far tested.

V. Quinazolines

A. WR 158,122

1. *Chemistry*

The synthesis of WR 158,122 (Fig. 7) was detailed by Elslager and Werbel in 1974. The thiol intermediate, formed by the condensation of the appropriate benzonitrile with chloroformamidine, was oxidized with hydrogen peroxide to produce WR 158,122.

A copolymer of *dl*-lactic acid and glycolic acid was produced as a sustained release vehicle for parenteral administration of WR 158,122 (Wise *et al.*, 1976). Because of the desire to employ a combination of WR 158,122 with sulfadiazine as a repository antimalarial drug, concomitant

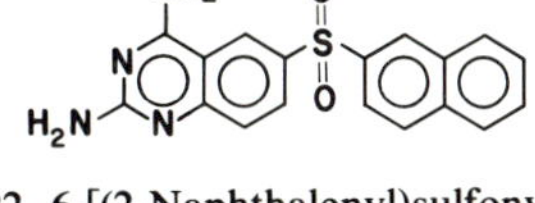

FIG. 7. Drug WR 158,122. 6-[(2-Naphthalenyl)sulfonyl]-2,4-quinazolinediamine.

research has been carried out on copolymers incorporating sulfadiazine (Wise, personal communication).

2. *Preclinical Efficacy and Biology*

Drug WR 158,122 was uniformly curative against *Plasmodium berghei* infections in mice in doses of 10 mg/kg and above (Elslager and Werbel, 1974) when administered subcutaneously suspended in peanut oil (Osdene *et al.,* 1967). Some cures were also produced at 5 mg/kg. Elslager (1975) reported little or no cross-resistance of WR 158,122 against chloroquine-resistant, cycloguanil-resistant, or dapsone-resistant strains of *P. berghei.*

The drug was effective in subcutaneous doses as low as 5 mg/kg in prolonging the lives of chicks infected with *P. gallinaceum* (Elslager and Werbel, 1974).

The antimalarial activity of WR 158,122 alone and in combination with sulfadiazine was extensively studied (Schmidt, 1973) in the *Aotus* monkey system. Daily oral dosing for 7 days produced a diverse response among the various human malaria strains. The CD_{90} for infections with several of these strains were as follows: *P. falciparum* Malayan Camp CH/Q strain (0.39 mg/kg/day), Vietnam Oak Knoll strain (0.098 mg/kg/day), Vietnam Smith strain (>6.25 mg/kg/day); *P. vivax* Chesson strain (0.39 mg/kg/day), Vietnam Palo Alto strain (6.25 mg/kg/day). Of great concern was the very rapid development of resistance to WR 158,122 when subcurative doses were used. This serious drawback, coupled with the demonstrated cross-resistance to pyrimethamine-resistant strains in this test system, led to the investigation of combination therapy.

Sulfadiazine alone in the *Aotus* system effected only transient reduction of parasitemia even at doses of 80 mg/kg. However, the combination of WR 158,122 with 5 mg/kg/day of sulfadiazine produced marked potentiation of WR 158,122 efficacy. The CD_{90} for WR 158,122 against *P. falciparum* strains became 0.025 mg/kg/day for the Camp strain, 0.00156 mg/kg/day for the Oak Knoll strain, and 0.39 mg/kg/day for the Smith strain. For *P. vivax* Palo Alto strain, the CD_{90} was 0.098 mg/kg/day. Thus the efficacy of WR 158,122 was enhanced from sixteen- to sixty-four-fold. Even more important, no resistance to the quinazoline developed in the presence of sulfadiazine.

The minimum curative dose of sulfadiazine for infections of *P. cynomolgi* in rhesus monkeys was 100 mg/kg/day given orally for 7 days (Davidson *et al.,* 1976). The minimum curative dose of WR 158,122 alone in that system was 1 mg/kg/day, whereas the minimum curative dose of the combination was 1 mg:0.1 mg/kg/day (sulfadiazine:WR 158,122), indicating potentiation in this system also (D. E. Davidson, Jr., personal communication).

As with many quinazolines, WR 158,122 has folate antagonistic properties (Elslager, 1975). This characteristic was utilized to develop a sensitive antibacterial assay for determining levels of the drug (Genther and Smith, 1975a). Because of the growth-inhibiting effect of human plasma and the strong binding of the drug to plasma proteins, however, it was necessary to employ matrix controls having quantities of pretreatment human plasma similar to those in the test samples.

Drug WR 158,122 was tested against four bacterial species, three of which required folate and the fourth being *Escherichia coli* (Genther and Smith, 1977). A chloroguanide triazine-resistant strain of each of the folate-requiring species had been developed. Thus the degree of cross-resistance could be measured. A forty-fold cross-resistance was seen with WR 158,122 against the triazine-resistant *S. faecium* and a twenty-five-fold cross resistance against *P. cerevisiae*. Intriguingly, the triazine-resistant strain of *L. casei* was four-fold more sensitive to the drug than was the parent strain. *Escherichia coli* growth was inhibited by WR 158,122 at less than 2% of the dose of sulfadiazine required to produce the same degree of inhibition.

Several studies were carried out on potential mutagenicity of folic acid antagonists (Genther and Smith, 1975b; Genther *et al.*, 1977). Seven folic acid antagonists, including WR 158,122, were negative as mutagens using *Salmonella typhimurium* tester strains. These compounds were then tested for three mutagenic traits in folic acid-requiring *S. faecium* var. *durans*. All the compounds, which also included amethopterin, pyrimethamine, chloroguanide triazine, and trimethoprim, were shown to cause mutations to folic acid independence, rifampin resistance, and resistance to folic acid antagonists.

3. *Preclinical Toxicology*

Repeated daily oral doses of WR 158,122 were given to groups of rats for 28 days (Lee *et al.*, 1972a). Groups of 6 rats each received 0, 125, 250, or 500 mg/kg/day. No drug-related toxic signs, changes in hematology or clinical chemistries, or gross or microscopic abnormalities were seen in the drug groups receiving either 125 or 250 mg/kg/day. The group receiving 500 mg/kg/day had an increase in severity of naturally occurring lesions, but this may not have been drug-related.

Repeated daily oral doses for 28 consecutive days of WR 158,122 were given to groups of 4 beagles each at the following levels: 0.5, 5, 50, 125, 250, or 500 mg/kg/day (Lee *et al.*, 1972b). No drug-related effects were seen at the 2 lowest dose levels. The group receiving 50 mg/kg/day had diarrhea and some emesis by the second week and lost weight. They had progressive reticulocytopenia and leukopenia with hemoconcentration at termination. Minimal lesions in the gastrointestinal tract were evident microscopically, as were atrophy of the thymus and lymphoid tissue decrease. Both erythropoiesis and myelopoiesis in the marrow were severely depressed. Dogs in the group receiving 125 mg/kg had the same types of toxicity but more pronounced. The two highest doses were lethal to the beagles. Toxicities included severe attack on the blood-forming organs as well as degenerative lesions of the gastrointestinal tract, kidney, liver, and myocardium.

Since WR 158,122 is a folic acid antagonist, Lee *et al.* (1972g) studied the effect of folinic acid on toxicity of the drug in beagles. Four beagles were treated orally with 50 mg/kg/day of WR 158,122 and developed the severe toxicity characteristic of the drug. Another group of 4 beagles given 50 mg/kg/day of WR 158,122 was completely protected by concurrent administration of 0.3 mg/kg/day of folinic acid intramuscularly.

The subacute toxicity of sulfadiazine and of the WR 158,122: sulfadiazine combination was also studied in the rat (Lee *et al.*, 1973a). Repeated oral doses for 28 days of 120 mg/kg/day of sulfadiazine alone or 12 mg/kg/day of WR 158,122 alone caused no adverse effects. Repeated doses for 28 days of the drug combination in a 10:1 ratio of sulfadiazine to WR 158,122 caused no adverse effects at either the top dose of 120 mg sulfadiazine: 12 mg WR 158,122 per kilogram per day or at lower doses.

Because of the apparent lack of adverse effect in rats, 5-day high-dose studies were performed in both rats and mice (Lee *et al.*, 1974e). Oral doses of 3000 mg/kg/day of either compound alone, or of 1500 mg sulfadiazine plus 1500 mg WR 158,122 per kilogram per day did not cause any adverse effects in either rodent species.

Since the rat was relatively refractory to WR 158,122 toxicity, a 28-day oral dosing study was carried out in beagle dogs (Lee *et al.*, 1973b). The sulfadiazine: WR 158,122 combination in a 10:1 ratio caused no adverse effects at 1.2 mg: 0.12 mg/kg/day and slightly decreased reticulocyte counts with mild crystalluria at 12 mg: 1.2 mg/kg/day. Doses of 120 mg: 12 mg/kg/day caused toxic signs, including moderate reticulocytopenia and leukopenia, excessive sulfadiazine crystals in the urine, degenerative changes in the intestinal tract, mineralized casts in the renal tubules, and/or mild interstitial nephritis. When given alone, sulfadiazine caused mild transient reticulocytopenia and the appearance of some sulfadiazine crystals in the urine. The other toxicities seen were typical of WR 158,122 alone.

4. *Pharmacology*

The effect of ingested lipids on the bioavailability of WR 158,122 was investigated in dogs (Yesair *et al.*, 1976). Fat emulsions of WR 158,122 increased bioavailability of the drug, but the time course of systemic appearance of drug was delayed. It was also found that drug concentrations in bile were much greater than in portal blood, which in turn exceeded systemic blood levels. The results indicated that the drug was readily absorbed but that the liver efficiently extracted the drug from portal blood and secreted it into the bile. Thus the drug probably has an enterohepatic cycle.

5. *Clinical Studies*

Phase I, rising dose, human, oral tolerance studies were carried out with WR 158,122 by itself (Arnold, 1973a,b,d). A total of 32 volunteers received the drug for 3 days in doses ranging from 5 through 1300 mg/day. No drug-related toxicities were seen in any of the subjects. No clinical or laboratory findings attributable to the drug were seen. No phototoxicity was found at any dose.

Tolerance studies were also carried out in 6 volunteers using the combination of WR 158,122: sulfadiazine in a 1:10 ratio (Arnold, 1974a). Two volunteers received 5 mg/50 mg, 4 × per day, for 3 days, 2 received 25 mg:250 mg, 4 × per day, for 3 days, and 2 received 50 mg:500 mg, 4 × per day, for 3 days. No significant adverse effects or laboratory findings associated with the combinations were seen. One volunteer complained of headache and another of transient anorexia, but these were not considered to be drug related.

Phase II, antimalarial efficacy studies with the chloroquine-sensitive Uganda I strain of *P. falciparum* were carried out in 5 men receiving the 50 mg:500 mg, 4 × per day, drug combination regimen (Arnold, 1975). Three were on a 3-day schedule and the others on a 1-day schedule. Of the first 3, 2 were cured and the third was a probable cure but left the study before the full follow-up period was completed. Average times for fever lysis and full parasitemia suppression were 62 hours and 4.7 days, respectively. The 2 men on the 1-day regimen both exhibited an RI response with recrudescences on days 12 and 14. Fever lysis took 84 hours and clearance of parasites, 2.5 days. One additional volunteer received sulfadiazine, 500 mg, 4 × per day, for 3 days, and had an RII response, indicating that the cures were probably not due to the sulfa drug alone.

Phase II studies with WR 158,122 alone were also carried out using the same strain of *P. falciparum* (Arnold, 1973c, 1974b). A 3-day regimen at either 20 or 75 mg/day evoked an RII response in 3 volunteers. Two volunteers received 250 mg/day for 3 days and exhibited an RI response, with recrudescence on days 10 and 16. Three-day regimens in 3 additional volunteers produced an RI response at 125 mg, 2 × per day, and 250 mg, 4 × per day. The third man was cured at 250 mg, 4 × per day. Thus the cures seen with the drug combination were not likely due to the WR 158,122 portion alone.

In summary, the 1:10 ratio of WR 158,122:sulfadiazine was well tolerated orally at 50 mg:500 mg, 4 × per day, for 3 days. This regimen cured at least 2, and probably also the third, of 3 *P. falciparum* infections. It required 250 mg, 4 × per day, for 3 days of WR 158,122 alone to cure 1 out of 2 falciparum infections, whereas 500 mg, 4 × per day, for 3 days of sulfadiazine alone had little effect in a single subject. It thus appears that the drug combination potentiates the antimalarial effects of the component drugs alone.

VI. Drugs Entering Efficacy Trials

A. WR 184,806

1. *Chemistry*

Synthesis of WR 184,806 (Fig. 8) was first published by Blumbergs *et al.* (1975). The compound represents a modification of the side chain of WR 142,490 at position 4 and has been used as an internal standard in the quantitation of WR 142,490 blood levels (Grindel *et al.,* 1977).

2. *Preclinical Efficacy and Biology*

Treatment of *Plasmodium berghei*-infected mice with drug suspended in peanut oil administered subcutaneously (Osdene *et al.,* 1967) showed that WR 184,806 was curative at 160 mg/kg (Blumbergs *et al.,* 1975). Suppressive activity was reported at doses as low as 10 mg/kg.

Drug WR 184,806 was tested against human plasmodia in the *Aotus* monkey (Schmidt, 1974). Infections of the Vietnam Oak Knoll strain of *Plasmodium falciparum* were cured by a total of 17.5 mg/kg administered orally either as a single dose or divided into three daily doses. However, 17.5 mg/kg divided into seven daily oral doses was insufficient to cure infected monkeys. Infections of that strain were cured by a total of 20 mg/kg

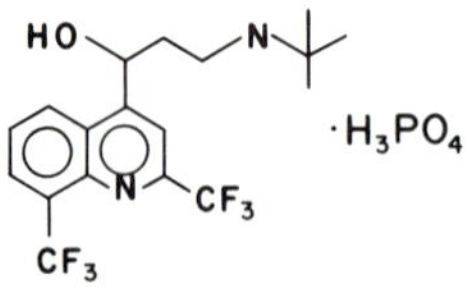

FIG. 8. Drug WR 184,806. γ-(*t*-Butylamino)-2,8-bis(trifluoromethyl)-9-quinolinepropanol phosphate.

administered intravenously either as a single dose or divided into three daily doses. In order to cure infections of the Vietnam Smith strain of *P. falciparum,* oral doses of 5 mg/kg/day for 7 days (35 mg/kg total) or a single 70 mg/kg dose were required. When administered intravenously, 10 mg/kg/day for 3 days (30 mg/kg total) cured infections of that strain.

Blood-induced infections of the Vietnam Palo Alto strain of *Plasmodium vivax* in the *Aotus* monkey were cured by a total oral dose of 17.5 mg/kg whether given as a single dose or divided into three or seven daily doses (Schmidt, 1974). A single intravenous 10-mg/kg dose or 20 mg/kg over 3 days also cured monkeys infected with this strain.

3. *Preclinical Toxicology*

Groups of rats were treated with either 25, 100, 250, 500, or 1000 mg/kg/day orally for up to 28 days (Lee *et al.,* 1974d). The two low doses caused no observable adverse effects. Doses of 250 mg/kg/day were lethal in 8 to 13 days, 500-mg/kg/day doses were lethal in 4 to 9 days, and the highest dose was lethal in 3 to 4 days. Toxic signs prior to death in those animals treated with the higher doses included hypoactivity, anorexia, weight loss, diarrhea, bloody nasal discharge, and convulsions. Also observed in these latter animals were increased neutrophil/lymphocyte ratios and increased levels of SGOT, SGPT, and BUN. Histopathological lesions included pneumonia, severe gastroenteritis, atrophy and/or necrosis of the reproductive organs, depletion or necrosis of lymphoid tissues, thymic involution, and vacuolar degeneration of the hepatic cord cells. The target organs in the rat were thus the lungs, gastrointestinal tract, reproductive organs, lymphoid tissue, and liver.

Groups of beagle dogs were treated orally with either 1, 5, 20, or 80 mg/kg/day for 28 days (Lee *et al.,* 1974c). Repeated doses of 1 or 5 mg/kg/day did not cause any observable adverse effects. Emesis was seen during the first week in the group receiving 20 mg/kg/day. No significant toxicity was seen in these dogs, either in hematology, clinical chemistries, or gross or microscopic examination. Repeated doses of 80 mg/kg/day resulted in death during the sixth through nineteenth day. Toxic signs prior to death included emesis, anorexia, weight loss, ataxia, and tremors. One dog had clonic convulsions. Also observed were lymphocytopenia, reticulocytopenia, and elevated levels of SGOT, SGPT, and alkaline phosphatase. Histopathological lesions included inflammatory and/or degenerative changes in the gastrointestinal tract, liver, and kidney; thymic involution and lymphoid depletion; and bone marrow depression, especially of the erythroid series. The target organs in the beagle were thus the gastrointestinal tract, liver, kidney, lymphoid tissues, and bone marrow.

4. *Pharmacology*

Studies were carried out on the fate of radiolabeled WR 184,806 in the mouse (Grindel *et al.*, 1975, 1976). The drug was well absorbed orally at doses of 10 mg/kg. Plasma levels of drug peaked at 0.4 to 0.5 μg/ml and erythrocyte levels, at 1.5 to 1.8 μg/ml. *In vitro,* parent drug was strongly bound to mouse plasma proteins; *in vivo,* the radioactivity in plasma was associated primarily with metabolites. The radiolabel concentrated in the lungs, liver, skeletal muscle, kidneys, small intestine, and residual carcass. Within these tissues the radioactivity was present predominantly as parent drug rather than as metabolites. The radiolabel was excreted primarily in the feces (ca. 70%) with lesser amounts in the urine (ca. 26%) within 96 hours. By 8 hours after drug administration, unchanged drug represented the minority of radiolabeled material being excreted in the feces and at least four metabolites were present.

5. *Clinical Studies*

Phase I, oral tolerance studies were carried out in two parts. The first was a double-blind, rising, single-dose study with 45 healthy volunteers (Reba and Barry, 1976a). Of these, 23 received placebos, whereas the remainder received single oral doses ranging from 5 through 1400 mg. No symptoms or findings of adverse drug effects were observed in any of the 12 volunteers receiving less than 100 mg. Two out of the 4 subjects receiving 1000 mg complained of lightheadedness. This symptom, with some combination of difficulty in concentrating, headache, nausea, insomnia, and unusual dreams appeared dose-related in the 4 volunteers receiving 1200 mg and the 2 receiving 1400 mg. All symptoms were mild and lasted less than 24 hours. None of the volunteers had significant drug-related abnormalities in hematology, clinical chemistries, urinalyses, or electrocardiogram. No phototoxicity was observed in any subject.

Special tests were performed on subjects at higher-dose levels. No drug-related orthostatic intolerance was seen. There was no evidence that the drug affected the vestibular mechanism as determined by electronystagmography analysis. One subject may have had a drug-related temporary decrease in the amplitude of accommodation upon ophthalmological evaluation.

The second portion of the Phase I, oral toxicity testing consisted of multiple oral dosing in 29 subjects (Reba and Barry, 1976b). Thirteen volunteers received placebo and 16 received the drug for 3 consecutive days. Doses increased from 100 mg every 8 hours through 400 mg every 8 hours for a total of 900 through 3600 mg. An additional 4 subjects received 250 mg every 6 hours for a total of 3000 mg. No symptoms attributable to the drug appeared in the 6 volunteers receiving a total dose of 900 through 1800 mg. Possible drug-related sleep disturbance was reported in 1 volunteer at 2250 mg, and some brief blurring of vision in one at 2700 mg. At 3000 mg, 2 volunteers reported headaches and 1 of these reported an increase in vivid dreams. At 3600 mg, both subjects had subjective balance disturbances on the third day of dosing. In all subjects the symptoms were mild, temporary, and without associated physical or laboratory abnormalities. No drug-related abnormalities in hematology, clinical chemistries, urinalyses, or electrocardiogram were seen. No phototoxicity attributable to the drug was observed.

B. WR 180,409

1. *Chemistry*

Synthesis of WR 180,409 (Fig. 9) was first reported by LaMontagne *et al.* in 1974. They resolved both the erythro and threo forms, the threo configuration being WR 180,409.

2. *Preclinical Efficacy and Biology*

Drug WR 180,409 was uniformly curative against *P. berghei* infections in mice at doses of 20 mg/kg and above (LaMontagne *et al.*, 1974) when injected subcutaneously suspended in peanut oil (Osdene *et al.*, 1967). The threo epimer (WR 180,409) was more active in this system than was the erythro epimer.

Schmidt (1976) reported antimalarial efficacy results in the *Aotus* monkey test system. The drug given either orally or intravenously for 3 or 7 days at a total dose of 17.5 mg (base)/kg routinely cured the monkeys of blood-induced infections of the Vietnam Smith strain of *P. falciparum* or the Vietnam Palo Alto strain of *P. vivax*. Single-dose treatments required at least 35 mg/kg to produce cures consistently.

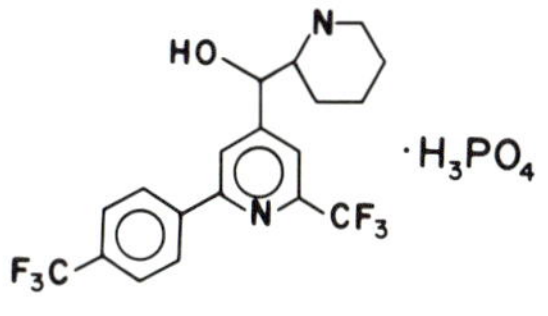

HO, N, $\cdot H_3PO_4$, N, CF_3, F_3C

FIG. 9. Drug WR 180,409. 2-(Trifluoromethyl)-6-(4-trifluoromethylphenyl)-α-(2-piperidinyl)-4-pyridinemethanol phosphate.

3. *Preclinical Toxicology*

Twenty-eight-day oral toxicity studies were carried out in rats (Lee *et al.*, 1976a,b). Groups of rats received either 10, 20, 30, or 90 mg/kg/day of drug. Doses of 10 or 20 mg/kg/day produced no adverse effects. Two of the rats in the 30-mg/kg/day group died after 10 days; 3 of the 10 rats in the highest-dose group died after 9 days. Drug-related and dose-related toxic signs were weight loss with reduced food intake, and hemorrhage around the eyes and nose. There were increases in erythrocyte counts, hematocrits, hemoglobin concentration, and platelet counts with decreases in reticulocyte counts and peripheral neutrophil/lymphocyte ratios. Also seen were elevations in levels of SGOT, SGPT, alkaline phosphatase, and/or BUN. The highest dose also caused necrosis of skeletal muscle, lymphoid depletion of the thymus and spleen, and an increase in incidence and severity of naturally occurring lesions in the lung. Thus the target organs in the rat were skeletal muscle and lymphoid tissues.

Twenty-eight-day oral toxicity studies were also carried out in beagle dogs (Lee *et al.*, 1976c,d). Groups of dogs received either 5, 15, 30, or 45 mg/kg/day of the drug. Repeated administration at the three lower-dose levels did not cause any adverse effects. Doses of 45 mg/kg/day reduced food intake and weight gain and caused occasional emesis. Mild necrosis of lymphoid tissue was seen in the tonsils of all the dogs receiving the highest-dose level, whereas 1 had severe involution of the thymus with atrophy of the germinal centers, lymphoid depletion, and cellular infiltration of the lymph nodes. The target organs in dogs were the lymphoid tissues.

4. *Pharmacology*

Radiolabeled WR 180,409 disposition studies were carried out in the mouse (Chung *et al.*, 1976, 1978) and in the rat (Galbraith *et al.*, 1976). In the mouse the radiolabel from a 20-mg/kg oral dose was excreted primarily in the feces (>80%) during a 10 day period while only small amounts (<6%) were excreted in urine. The rat also excreted little radiolabel into the urine. Three major metabolites were separated from mouse excreta and several from rat excreta. In mouse blood, the parent drug concentrated in erythrocytes in amounts 3–4 times those found in plasma, with plasma radioactivity primarily in the form of metabolites. Even so, the drug was found to be very strongly bound to mouse plasma proteins. Regression analysis of parent drug gave elimination half-lives in the mouse of 26.4 hours for plasma and 27.4 hours for erythrocytes.

In the mouse, radiolabel concentrated in the liver, lungs, kidneys, and gastrointestinal tract, with the radiolabel primarily associated with parent drug in most organs and the residual carcasses. In the rat, wide distribution of radioactivity was also seen. The highest concentrations were found in lungs, liver, adrenal glands, and bone marrow.

5. *Clinical Studies*

Phase I, rising, single oral dose, double-blind tolerance studies were carried out in 43 volunteers (Reba and Barry, 1977). Twenty-one subjects received placebo, whereas the remainder received doses increasing from 5 through 1500 mg. No significant symptoms or findings of adverse effects were attributed to the drug in any of the 12 volunteers receiving less than 1000 mg, although brief mild central nervous system symptoms were seen in 3 subjects. Three out of the 4 subjects treated at 1000 mg and 3 out of the 4 volunteers treated at 1250 mg showed various combinations of nausea, vomiting, dizziness, and mild mental "fuzziness." Both subjects given 1500 mg of drug showed the same general symptoms. Symptoms tended to be mild and none lasted 48 hours. None of the volunteers had significant drug-related abnormalities in hematology, clinical chemistries, urinalyses, or electrocardiogram. No phototoxicity was observed in any subject.

VII. Concluding Remarks

Malaria remains a serious worldwide health problem, and chemotherapy is one of the few effective measures for control of the disease. Quinine, a natural product obtained from the cinchona bark, was the first chemotherapeutic agent proven effective against malaria, and it retains an important role in the clinical management of this parasite infection. However, the periodic scarcity of quinine, especially during wartime, coupled with the emergence of plasmodial strains that are relatively resistant to this drug have stimulated the search for effective substitutes—especially among the synthetic chemicals.

Although all three major synthetic drug development programs have been highly successful, several factors have complicated the search for newer and more effective antimalarials: (*1*) the malaria parasite has shown a remarkable ability to develop resistance to antimalarial drugs and many new drugs show cross-resistance to those previously developed; (*2*) novel leads are increasingly difficult to uncover, and efforts to do so often result in more complex organic molecules, with attendant synthetic problems; and (*3*) the development of new drugs must be accompanied by more sophisticated animal toxicity testing prior to clinical trials to minimize potential toxicity to humans.

To meet these problems, continual work is required at various levels to develop new synthetic drugs and to develop new techniques for treating the disease. For example, the mechanisms of antiplasmodial action of many antimalarial chemicals still remain to be fully elucidated at a molecular level. Complete understanding of molecular mechanisms could lead to the design of the "ideal chemical." Other clinical strategies, such as vaccines, may also offer new avenues for control of malaria, but such techniques require much more study and development before they could be operational.

While these frontiers are being explored, a continual program to develop and test new drugs is required. Several years are required between the synthesis of potential antimalarial drugs and their widespread use. The new experimental drugs developed by the U.S. Army, which have been emphasized in this review, represent an important source of new drugs for the immediate future.

Acknowledgments

We would like to thank Drs. Melvin H. Heiffer and Robert E. Desjardins for their suggestions on specific portions of this review.

References

Agharkar, S., Lindenbaum, S., and Higuchi, T. (1976). *J. Pharm. Sci.* **65,** 747.

Arnold, J. D. (1973a). 8 February 1973. U.S. Army Medical Research and Development Command Contract No. DA-49-193-MD-2545.

Arnold, J. D. (1973b). 28 June 1973. U.S. Army Medical Research and Development Command Contract No. DA-49-193-MD-2545.

Arnold, J. D. (1973c). 6 September 1973. U.S. Army Medical Research and Development Command Contract No. DA-49-193-MD-2545.

Arnold, J. D. (1973d). 5 October 1973. U.S. Army Medical Research and Development Command Contract No. DA-49-193-MD-2545.

Arnold, J. D. (1974a). 31 July 1974. U.S. Army Medical Research and Development Command Contract No. DADA-17-74-C-4004.

Arnold, J. D. (1974b). 23 November 1974. U.S. Army Medical Research and Development Command Contract No. DADA-17-74-C-4004.

Arnold, J. D. (1975). July 1975. U.S. Army Medical Research and Development Command Contract No. DADA-17-75-C-5064.

Arnold, J. D., Martin, D. C., Carson, P. E., Rieckmann, K. H., Willerson, D., Jr., Clyde, D. F., and Miller, R. M. (1973). *Antimicrob. Agents & Chemother.* **3,** 207.

Aviado, D. M., and Belej, M. (1970). *Pharmacology* **3,** 257.

Blumbergs, P., Ao, M.-S., LaMontagne, M. P., Markovac, A., Novotny, J., Collins, C. H., and Starks, F. W. (1975). *J. Med. Chem.* **18,** 1122.

Caldwell, R. W., and Nash, C. B. (1976). *Pharmacologist* **18,** 204.

Caldwell, R. W., and Nash, C. B. (1977). *Toxicol. Appl. Pharmacol.* **40,** 437.

Canfield, C. J., and Rozman, R. S. (1974). *Bull. W. H. O.* **50,** 203.

Canfield, C. J., Hall, A. P., MacDonald, B. S., Neuman, D. A., and Shaw, J. A. (1973). *Antimicrob. Agents & Chemother.* **3,** 224.

Carroll, F. I., and Blackwell, J. T. (1974). *J. Med. Chem.* **17,** 210.

Chien, P.-L., and Cheng, C. C. (1973). *J. Med. Chem.* **16,** 1093.

Chien, P.-L., and Cheng, C. C. (1976). *J. Med. Chem.* **19,** 170.

Chung, H., Gillum, H. H., and Rozman, R. S. (1976). *Fed. Proc., Fed. Am. Soc. Exp. Biol.* **35,** 328.

Chung, H., Gillum, H. H., and Rozman, R. S. (1978). *Drug Metab. Dispos.* **6,** 82.

Clyde, D. F. (1973). Annual report. U.S. Army Medical Research and Development Command Contract No. DA-49-193-MD-2740.

Clyde, D. F. (1974). *Bull. W. H. O.* **50,** 243.

Clyde, D. F., McCarthy, V. C., Rebert, C. C., and Miller, R. M. (1973). *Antimicrob. Agents & Chemother.* **3,** 220.

Clyde, D. F., McCarthy, V. C., Miller, R. M., and Hornick, R. B. (1976). *Antimicrob. Agents & Chemother.* **9,** 384.

Coatney, G. R., Cooper, W. C., Eddy, N. B., and Greenberg, J. (1953). *Public Health Monogr. v.s., Public Health Serv.,* **9.**

Colwell, W. T., Brown, V., Christie, P., Lange, J., Reece, C., Yamamoto, K., and Henry, D. W. (1972). *J. Med. Chem.* **15,** 771.

Davidson, D. E., Jr., Johnsen, D. O., Tanticharoenyos, P., Hickman, R. L., and Kinnamon, K. E. (1976). *Am. J. Trop. Med. Hyg.* **25,** 26.

Davidson, M. W., Griggs, B. G., Jr., Boykin, D. W., and Wilson, W. D. (1975). *Nature (London)* **254,** 632.

Davidson, M. W., Griggs, B. G., Boykin, D. W., and Wilson, W. D. (1977). *J. Med. Chem.* **20,** 1117.

Davies, E. E., Warhurst, D. C., and Peters, W. (1975). *Ann. Trop. Med. Parasitol.* **69,** 147.

Desjardins, R. E., Haynes, J. D., Chulay, J. D., and Canfield, C. J. (1978). *Fed. Proc., Fed. Am. Soc. Exp. Biol.* **37,** 379.

Einheber, A., Palmer, D. M., and Aikawa, M. (1976). *Exp. Parasitol.* **40,** 52.

Elslager, E. F. (1975). *Proc. Int. Symp. Med. Chem., 4th, 1974* 227.

Elslager, E. F., and Werbel, L. M. (1974). U.S. Patent 3,853,873.

Fitch, C. D. (1972). *Proc. Helminthol. Soc. Wash., Spec. Issue* **39,** 265.

Galbraith, W. M., Campbell, S., Tillery, K., and Mellett, L. B. (1976). *Fed. Proc., Fed. Am. Soc. Exp. Biol.* **35,** 488.

Genther, C. S., and Smith, C. C. (1975a). *Am. J. Trop. Med. Hyg.* **24,** 559.

Genther, C. S., and Smith, C. C. (1975b). *Am. Soc. Microb., Abstr. Annu. Meet.* p. 10.

Genther, C. S., and Smith, C. C. (1977). *J. Med. Chem.* **20,** 237.

Genther, C. S., Schoeny, R. S., Loper, J. C., and Smith, C. C. (1977). *Antimicrob. Agents & Chemother.* **12,** 84.

Gregory, K. G., and Peters, W. (1970). *Ann. Trop. Med. Parasitol.* **64,** 15.

Grindel, J. M., Leahy, D. M., Molek, N. A., and Rozman, R. S. (1975). *Fed. Proc., Fed. Am. Soc. Exp. Biol.* **34,** 734.

Grindel, J. M., Rozman, R. S., Leahy, D. M., Molek, N. A., and Gillum, H. H. (1976). *Drug Metab. Dispos.* **4,** 133.

Grindel, J. M., Tilton, P. F., and Shaffer, R. D. (1977). *J. Pharm. Sci.* **66,** 834.

Hahn, F. E., O'Brien, R. L., Ciak, J., Allison, J. L., and Olenick, J. G. (1966). *Mil. Med.* **131,** 1071.

Hall, A. P. (1976). *Br. Med. J.* **1,** 323.

Hall, A. P., Segal, H. E., Pearlman, E. J., and Phintuyothin, P. (1975). *Trans. R. Soc. Trop. Med. Hyg.* **69,** 342.

Hall, A. P., Doberstyn, E. B., Karnchanacheta, C., Samransamruajkit, S., Laixuthai, B., Pearlman, E. J., Lampe, R. M., Miller, C. F., and Phintuyothin, P. (1977). *Br. Med. J.* **1,** 1626.

Harmon, R. E., Lin, T. S., and Gupta, S. K. (1973). *J. Med. Chem.* **16,** 940.

Henry, D. W. (1972). *Natl. Med. Chem. Symp. Am. Chem. Soc.* [*Proc.*], *13th, 1972* p. 41.

Hiremath, C. B. (1974). *Fed. Proc., Fed. Am. Soc. Exp. Biol.* **33,** 472.

Kinnamon, K. E., and Rothe, W. E. (1975). *Am. J. Trop. Med. Hyg.* **24,** 174.

Korte, D. W., Jr., Heiffer, M. H., Kintner, L. D., and Lee, C.-C. (1978). *Fed. Proc., Fed. Am. Soc. Exp. Biol.* **37,** 248.

LaMontagne, M. P., Markovac, A., and Blumbergs, P. (1974). *J. Med. Chem.* **17,** 519.

Lee, C.-C., Castles, T. R., Crawford, C. R., and Landes, A. M. (1967). Interim Report No. 13. U.S. Army Medical Research and Development Command Contract No. DA-49-193-MD-2759.

Lee, C.-C., Castles, T. R., Crawford, C. R., and Landes, A. M. (1968a). Interim Report No. 17. U.S. Army Medical Research and Development Command Contract No. DA-49-193-MD-2759.

Lee, C.-C., Castles, T. R., Crawford, C. R., and Landes, A. M. (1968b). Interim Report No. 19. U.S. Army Medical Research and Development Command Contract No. DA-49-193-MD-2759.

Lee, C.-C., Castles, T. R., Crawford, C. R., and Landes, A. M. (1968c). Interim Report No. 23. U.S. Army Medical Research and Development Command Contract No. DA-49-193-MD-2759.

Lee, C.-C., Castles, T. R., Crawford, C. R., and Landes, A. M. (1968d). Interim Report No. 24. U.S. Army Medical Research and Development Command Contract No. DA-49-193-MD-2759.

Lee, C.-C., Castles, T. R., Crawford, C. R., and Landes, A. M. (1968e). Supplement to Interim Report No. 24. U.S. Army Medical Research and Development Command Contract No. DA-49-193-MD-2759.

Lee, C.-C., Castles, T. R., Landes, A. M., Cronin, M. C., and Bristow, R. L. (1970a). Interim Report No. 32. U.S. Army Medical Research and Development Command Contract No. DA-49-193-MD-2759.

Lee, C.-C., Castles, T. R., Landes, A. M., Cronin, M. C., and Bristow, R. L. (1970b). Interim Report No. 35. U.S. Army Medical Research and Development Command Contract No. DA-49-193-MD-2759.

Lee, C.-C., Castles, T. R., Landes, A. M., Cronin, M. C., and Bristow, R. L. (1970c). Interim Report No. 36. U.S. Army Medical Research and Development Command Contract No. DA-49-193-MD-2759.

Lee, C.-C., Castles, T. R., Landes, A. M., Cronin, M. C., Coffelt, J., and Hutchcraft, R. (1971a). Interim Report No. 44. U.S. Army Medical Research and Development Command Contract No. DA-49-193-MD-2759.

Lee, C.-C., Castles, T. R., Landes, A. M., Cronin, M. C., Coffelt, J., and Hutchcraft, R. (1971b). Interim Report No. 45. U.S. Army Medical Research and Development Command Contract No. DA-49-193-MD-2759.

Lee, C.-C., Kintner, L. D., Castles, T. R., Landes, A. M., Cronin, M. C., Hutchcraft, R., and Merle, F. (1972a). Interim Report No. 54. U.S. Army Medical Research and Development Command Contract No. DA-49-193-MD-2759.

Lee, C.-C., Kintner, L. D., Castles, T. R., Landes, A. M., Cronin, M. C., Hutchcraft, R., and Merle, F. (1972b). Interim Report No. 55. U.S. Army Medical Research and Development Command Contract No. DA-49-193-MD-2759.

Lee, C.-C., Kintner, L. D., Castles, T. R., Landes, A. M., Cronin, M. C., Hutchcraft, R., and Merle, F. (1972c). Interim Report No. 56. U.S. Army Medical Research and Development Command Contract No. DA-49-193-MD-2759.

Lee, C.-C., Kintner, L. D., Castles, T. R., Landes, A. M., Cronin, M. C., Hutchcraft, R., and Merle, F. (1972d). Interim Report No. 57. U.S. Army Medical Research and Development Command Contract No. DA-49-193-MD-2759.

Lee, C.-C., Kintner, L. D., Sanyer, J. L., Castles, T. R., Landes, A. M., Cronin, M. C., and Merle, F. (1972e). Interim Report No. 65. U.S. Army Medical Research and Development Command Contract No. DA-49-193-MD-2759.

Lee, C.-C., Kintner, L. D., Sanyer, J. L., Castles, T. R., Landes, A. M., Cronin, M. C., and Merle, F. (1972f). Interim Report No. 66. U.S. Army Medical Research and Development Command Contract No. DA-49-193-MD-2759.

Lee, C.-C., Kintner, L. D., Sanyer, J. L., Castles, T. R., Landes, A. M., Cronin, M. C., and Merle, F. (1972g). Interim Report No. 67. U.S. Army Medical Research and Development Command Contract No. DA-49-193-MD-2759.

Lee, C.-C., Kintner, L. D., Sanyer, J. L., Castles, T. R., Landes, A. M., Cronin, M. C., and Merle, F. (1973a). Interim Report No. 71. U.S. Army Medical Research and Development Command Contract No. DA-49-193-MD-2759.

Lee, C.-C., Kintner, L. D., Sanyer, J. L., Castles, T. R., Landes, A. M., Cronin, M. C., and Merle, F. (1973b). Interim Report No. 72. U.S. Army Medical Research and Development Command Contract No. DA-49-193-MD-2759.

Lee, C.-C., Kintner, L. D., Sanyer, J. L., Castles, T. R., Reddig, T. W., Girvin, J. D., Kowalski, J. J., and Buchberger, G. L. (1974a). Interim Report No. 85. U.S. Army Medical Research and Development Command Contract No. DAMD-17-74-C-4063.

Lee, C.-C., Kintner, L. D., Sanyer, J. L., Castles, T. R., Reddig, T. W., Girvin, J. D., Kowalski, J. J., and Buchberger, G. L. (1974b). Interim Report No. 86. U.S. Army Medical Research and Development Command Contract No. DAMD-17-74-C-4063.

Lee, C.-C., Kintner, L. D., Sanyer, J. L., Reddig, T. W., Girvin, J. D., Buchberger, G. L., and Siefert, W. K. (1974c). Interim Report No. 88. U.S. Army Medical Research and Development Command Contract No. DAMD-17-74-C-4063.

Lee, C.-C., Kintner, L. D., Sanyer, J. L., Reddig, T. W., Girvin, J. D., Buchberger, G. L., and Seifert, W. K. (1974d). Interim Report No. 89. U.S. Army Medical Research and Development Command Contract No. DAMD-17-74-C-4063.

Lee, C.-C., Crawford, C. R., and Seifert, W. K. (1974e). Interim Report No. 92. U.S. Army Medical Research and Development Contract No. DAMD-17-74-C-4063.

Lee, C.-C., Hwang, S. W., Kowalski, J. J., Kintner, L. D., Bhandari, J. C., Reddig, T. W., Girvin, J. D., Kroeger, V. E., and Kemp, R. D. (1976a). Interim Report No. 105. U.S. Army Medical Research and Development Command Contract No. DAMD-17-74-C-4036.

Lee, C.-C., Kowalski, J. J., Kintner, L. D., Bhandari, J. C., Reddig, T. W., Ellis, E. R., and Kemp, R. D. (1976b). Supplement to Interim Report No. 105. U.S. Army Medical Research and Development Command Contract No. DAMD-17-74-C-4036.

Lee, C.-C., Hwang, S. W., Kowalski, J. J., Kintner, L. D., Bhandari, J. C., Reddig, T. W., Girvin, J. D., Kroeger, V. E., and Kemp, R. D. (1976c). Interim Report No. 106. U.S. Army Medical Research and Development Command Contract No. DAMD-17-74-C-4036.

Lee, C.-C., Kowalski, J. J., Kintner, L. D., Bhandari, J. C., Reddig, T. W., and Ellis, E. R. (1976d). Supplement to Interim Report No. 106. U.S. Army Medical Research and Development Command Contract No. DAMD-17-74-C-4036.

Liss, R. H., and Kensler, C. J. (1976). *Adv. Mod. Toxicol.* **1,** 273.

Lutz, R. E., Bailey, P. S., Clark, M. T., Codington, J. F., Deinet, A. J., Freek, J. A., Harnest, G. H., Leake, N. H., Martin, T. A., Rowlet, R. J., Salsbury, J. M., Shearer, N. H., Smith, J. D., and Wilson, J. W. (1946). *J. Am. Chem. Soc.* **68,** 1813.

Martin, D. C., Arnold, J. D., Clyde, D. F., Al Ibrahim, M., Carson, P. E., Rieckmann, K. H., and Willerson, D., Jr. (1973). *Antimicrob. Agents & Chemother.* **3,** 214.

May, E. L., and Mosettig, E. (1946). *J. Org. Chem.* **11,** 627.

Minor, J. L., Short, R. D., Heiffer, M. H., and Lee, C.-C. (1976). *Pharmacologist* **18,** 171.

Mu, J. Y., Israili, Z. H., and Dayton, P. G. (1973). *Fed. Proc., Fed. Am. Soc. Exp. Biol.* **32,** 716.

Mu, J. Y., Israili, Z. H., and Dayton, P. G. (1975). *Drug Metab. Dispos.* **3,** 198.

Nodiff, E. A., Tanabe, K., Seyfried, C., Matsuura, S., Kondo, Y., Chen, E. H., and Tyagi, M. P. (1971). *J. Med. Chem.* **14,** 921.

Ohnmacht, C. J., Patel, A. R., and Lutz, R. E. (1971). *J. Med. Chem.* **14,** 926.

Okada, H., Stella, V., Haslam, J., and Yata, N. (1975). *J. Pharm. Sci.* **64,** 1665.

Osdene, T. S., Russell, P. B., and Rane, L. (1967). *J. Med. Chem.* **10,** 431.

Pearlman, E. J., Doberstyn, E. B., Sudsok, S., Thiemanum, W., Kennedy, R., and Canfield, C. J. (1977). Paper No. 133, 26th Annual Meeting of the American Society of Tropical Medicine and Hygiene, 9–11 November.

Pearson, D. E., and Rosenberg, A. A. (1975). *J. Med. Chem.* **18,** 523.

Peters, W. (1970). "Chemotherapy and Drug Resistance in Malaria." Academic Press, New York.

Peters, W. (1974). *Adv. Parasitol.* **12,** 69.

Peters, W., and Porter, M. (1976). *Ann. Trop. Med. Parasitol.* **70,** 271.

Peters, W., Portus, J. H., and Robinson, B. L. (1975). *Ann. Trop. Med. Parasitol.* **69,** 155.

Peters, W., Howells, R. E., Portus, J., Robinson, B. L., Thomas, S., and Warhurst, D. C. (1977a). *Ann. Trop. Med. Parisitol.* **71,** 407.

Peters, W., Portus, J., and Robinson, B. L. (1977b). *Ann. Trop. Med. Parasitol.* **71,** 419.

Porter, M., and Peters, W. (1976). *Ann. Trop. Med. Parasitol.* **70,** 259.

Powers, M. B. (1968a). 9 February 1968. Final Report. U.S. Army Medical Research and Development Command Contract No. DADA-17-68-C-8069.

Powers, M. B. (1968b). 15 August 1968. Final Report. U.S. Army Medical Research and Development Command Contract No. DADA-17-68-C-8069.

Powers, M. B. (1968c). 21 August 1968. Final Report. U.S. Army Medical Research and Development Command Contract No. DADA-17-68-C-8069.

Powers, M. B. (1970). 22 May 1970. Report No. 35. U.S. Army Medical Research and Development Command Contract No. DADA-17-68-C-8069.

Pullman, T. N., Eichelberger, L., Alving, A. S., Jones, R., Jr., Craige, B., Jr., and Wharton, C. M. (1948). *J. Clin. Invest.* **27,** 12.

Reba, R. C., and Barry, K. G. (1976a). Final Report Experiment 2. U.S. Army Medical Research and Development Command Contract No. DAMD-17-75-C-5036.

Reba, R. C., and Barry, K. G. (1976b). Final Report Experiment 2. U.S. Army Medical Research and Development Command Contract No. DAMD-17-75-C-5036.

Reba, R. C., and Barry, J. G. (1977). Final Report Experiment No. 7. U.S. Army Medical Research and Development Command Contract No. DAMD-17-75-C-5036.

Rieckmann, K. H., Trenholme, G. M., Williams, R. L., Carson, P. E., Frischer, H., and Desjardins, R. E. (1974). *Bull. W. H. O.* **51,** 375.

Rinehart, J., Arnold, J., and Canfield, C. J. (1976). *Am. J. Trop. Med. Hyg.* **25,** 769.

Rothe, W. E., and Jacobus, D. P. (1968). *J. Med. Chem.* **11,** 366.

Rozman, R. S. (1973). *Annu. Rev. Pharmacol.* **13,** 127.

Rozman, R. S., Berman, A., Hutchinson, A., and Cintron-Molero, G. (1971). *Fed. Proc., Fed. Am. Soc. Exp. Biol.* **30,** 335.

Ruiz, R., Belej, M., and Aviado, D. M. (1970). *Toxicol. Appl. Pharmacol.* **17,** 118.

Sadavongvivad, C., and Aviado, D. M. (1969). *Mil. Med.* **134,** 1106.

Schmidt, L. H. (1973). *Trans. R. Soc. Trop. Med. Hyg.* **67,** 446.

Schmidt, L. H. (1974). 9 December 1974. U.S. Army Medical Research and Development Command Contract No. DADA-17-69-C-9104.

Schmidt, L. H. (1976). Final Progress Report. U.S. Army Medical Research and Development Command Contract No. DADA-17-69-C-9104.

Segal, H. E., Chinvanthananond, P., Laixuthai, B., Phintuyothin, P., Pearlman, E. J., Na-Nakorn, A., and Castaneda, B. F. (1974). *Am. J. Trop. Med. Hyg.* **23,** 560.

Smith, C. C., and Weigel, W. W. (1971a). *Pharmacologist* **13,** 269.

Smith, C. C., and Weigel, W. W. (1971b). *Toxicol. Appl. Pharmacol.* **19,** 364.

Smith, C. C., Wolfe, G. F., and Mattingly, S. F. (1972). *Toxicol. Appl. Pharmacol.* **22,** 291.

Smith, C. C., Weigel, W. W., and Wolfe, G. F. (1973). *Fed. Proc., Fed. Am. Soc. Exp. Biol.* **32,** 701.

Steck, E. A. (1972). "The Chemotherapy of Protozoan Diseases," Vol. III, Sect. 4, Chapters XXII and XXIII. US Gov. Printing Office, Washington, D.C.

Strube, R. E. (1975). *J. Trop. Med. Hyg.* **78,** 171.

Thompson, P. E. (1972). *Proc. Helminthol. Soc. Wash., Spec. Issue* **39,** 297.

Thompson, P. E., and Werbel, L. M. (1972). *Med. Chem., Ser. Monogr.* **12.**

Tigertt, W. D. (1969). *Ann. Intern. Med.* **70,** 150.

Trenholme, G. M., Williams, R. L., Desjardins, R. E., Frischer, H., Carson, P. E., Rieckmann, K. H., and Canfield, C. J. (1975). *Science* **190,** 792.

Warhurst, D. C., and Thomas, S. C. (1975). *Biochem. Pharmacol.* **24,** 2047.

Warhurst, D. C., Homewood, C. A., Peters, W., and Baggaley, V. C. (1972). *Proc. Helminthol. Soc. Wash., Spec. Issue* **39,** 271.

Weigel, W. W., and Smith, C. C. (1973). *Proc. Int. Congr. Pharmacol. 5th, 1972* Abstract No. 1488.

Wise, D. L., McCormick, G. J., Willet, G. P., and Anderson, L. C. (1976). *Life Sci.* **19,** 867.

Wiselogle, F. Y. (1946). "A Survey of Antimalarial Drugs, 1941–1945," Vols. 1 and 2. Edwards, Ann Arbor, Michigan.

Yesair, D. W., Chadwick, M., and Granchelli, F. E. (1976). *Fed. Proc., Fed. Am. Soc. Exp. Biol.* **35,** 328.

ADVANCES IN PHARMACOLOGY AND CHEMOTHERAPY, VOL. 16

Mechanisms of Action of Benzodiazepines

WILLIAM SCHALLEK, W. DALE HORST, AND WALTER SCHLOSSER

Pharmacology Department, Research Division
Hoffmann-La Roche, Inc.
Nutley, New Jersey

I. Introduction 45
II. Historical Background 46
A. Benzodiazepines and Neurohumors 46
B. A Note on Ionic Movement 50
III. Biochemistry 50
A. Amino Acid Neurotransmitters 51
B. Corticosteroids and Benzodiazepines 58
IV. Neuropharmacology 61
A. Peripheral Ganglia 61
B. Spinal Cord 62
C. Cuneate Nucleus 64
D. Cerebellum 66
E. Higher Centers of the Brain 67
V. Psychopharmacology 69
A. Biochemistry and Behavior 70
B. Neuropharmacology and Behavior 74
C. Effects on Learning and Memory 75
D. Social Relationships 76
VI. Discussion 79
A. CNS, Behavior, and Anxiety 80
B. Possible Mechanisms of Action 82
Addendum 82
References 84

I. Introduction

Since the introduction of the first benzodiazepine in 1960, these agents have been widely used in the clinical treatment of anxiety. Various members of the series are also used for anticonvulsant, muscle relaxant, and hypnotic effects. Nevertheless, little information as to the mechanisms of action of these compounds was available before 1974.

"Mechanisms" is used in the plural because the actions of a psychotropic agent may be expressed on multiple levels. At the most basic level, the actions of psychotropic agents may be discussed in terms of ionic movement. At the level of biochemistry the same effects may be described in terms of molecular interaction. Effects on the central nervous system are

ISBN 0-12-032916-6

described by neuropharmacology, whereas psychopharmacology describes effects on behavior. Finally, recent research has placed increasing emphasis on the effects of drugs on interactions between animals.

The greatest progress in revealing the mechanisms of action of benzodiazepines has been at the biochemical level. In the first review of the benzodiazepines to appear in these volumes, Zbinden and Randall (1967) suggested that anxiety might be caused by the central release of norepinephrine, and that the antianxiety action of the benzodiazepines might be an antinoradrenergic phenomenon. The next review in these volumes (Schallek *et al.,* 1972) cited evidence that benzodiazepines slowed the central metabolism of norepinephrine, dopamine, and serotonin. The reviewers noted that "the relationship of these findings to the antianxiety activity of the benzodiazepines is still unclear."

At a symposium held in 1974, a series of papers was presented indicating that γ-aminobutyric acid (GABA) might be the key to the actions of benzodiazepines at the biochemical level (Costa and Greengard, 1975). A further development was the finding of endogenous receptors with selective binding for benzodiazepines (Squires and Braestrup, 1977). These and other recent papers will be described in this review. Specifically, the review will include key papers on the mechanisms of action of benzodiazepines that were published during the period between January, 1972 and June, 1977.* For reviews of earlier papers, see Zbinden and Randall (1967), Schallek *et al.* (1972), and Randall *et al.* (1974).

II. Historical Background

A. Benzodiazepines and Neurohumors

The first attempts to find relationships between benzodiazepines and various neurohumors were made on peripheral rather than central responses. In dogs under pentobarbital anesthesia, neither chlordiazepoxide (1–32 mg/kg, i.v.) nor diazepam (1–8 mg/kg) had any significant effect on blood-pressure responses to acetylcholine, epinephrine, or serotonin (Randall *et al.,* 1960, 1961). In cats under chloralose anesthesia, chlordiazepoxide at 2 mg/kg, i.v., had a triphasic effect on the blood-pressure response to norepinephrine. The response showed reduction, potentiation, and reduction over a period of 2 hours (Moe *et al.,* 1962). These workers suggested that the effects might be related to changes in the norepinephrine levels of the heart. Further analysis of these peripheral effects might provide clues to some of the mechanisms involved in the cen-

* Papers published during the second half of 1977 are cited in the Addendum.

tral actions of benzodiazepines (for other studies at the peripheral level, see Section IV,A).

The first inquiry into the biochemical basis of the central effects of benzodiazepines was made by Moe *et al.* (1962). These authors found that the levels of norepinephrine and serotonin in the brain of the rabbit showed no significant changes after injection of chlordiazepoxide, 100 mg/kg i.p.

A major advance in this inquiry appears in experiments reviewed by Zbinden and Randall (1967). Marked behavioral stimulation was noted when rats pretreated with the monoamine oxidase inhibitor iproniazid (40 mg/kg, s.c.) were injected with the amine releaser tetrabenazine (2 mg/kg, s.c.). The number of avoidance responses in 15 minutes increased from 80 before tetrabenazine to 320 after 45 minutes (see Fig. 1). This stimulation was completely blocked if diazepam, 0.05 mg/kg, i.p., was injected 2 hours before the tetrabenazine (an experiment with diazepam at 0.1 mg/kg is shown in Fig. 2). These doses of diazepam are well below the 0.9 mg/kg, i.p., needed to attenuate conflict behavior in the rat.

Further experiments showed that the behavioral stimulation in the iproniazid–tetrabenazine test did not occur if norepinephrine synthesis was blocked with α-methylparatyrosine (AMPT) or disulfiram. Zbinden and Randall, therefore, attributed the stimulation to central release of norepinephrine, the metabolism of which was delayed by inhibition of monoamine oxidase. Since this stimulation was blocked by doses of benzodiazepines that were lower than those active in any other test, Zbinden and Randall called this the "most specific action" of the benzodiazepines. They suggested that anxiety is caused by the central release of norepinephrine, and that the antianxiety action of the benzodiazepines is "a central antiadrenergic phenomenon."

A different mechanism of action for the benzodiazepines was suggested by Stein *et al.* (1973). These authors proposed that these compounds "exert their antianxiety effects by reduction of serotonin activity . . . and their depressant effects by reduction of norepinephrine activity." They measured the antianxiety and depressant effects of benzodiazepines with behavioral tests involving multiple schedules of reinforcement. These techniques are described in more detail at the beginning of Section V. Antianxiety (anticonflict) effects refer to *increased* rates of responding in schedules in which animals receive both reward and punishment; depressant effects refer to *decreased* rates of responding in schedules in which animals receive reward only.

Stein *et al.* found that the depressant and anticonflict effects of benzodiazepines may be separated on chronic administration of these agents. If a rat not previously exposed to drugs was given oxazepam, 20 mg/kg i.p., unpunished responding was suppressed on the first day of drug adminis-

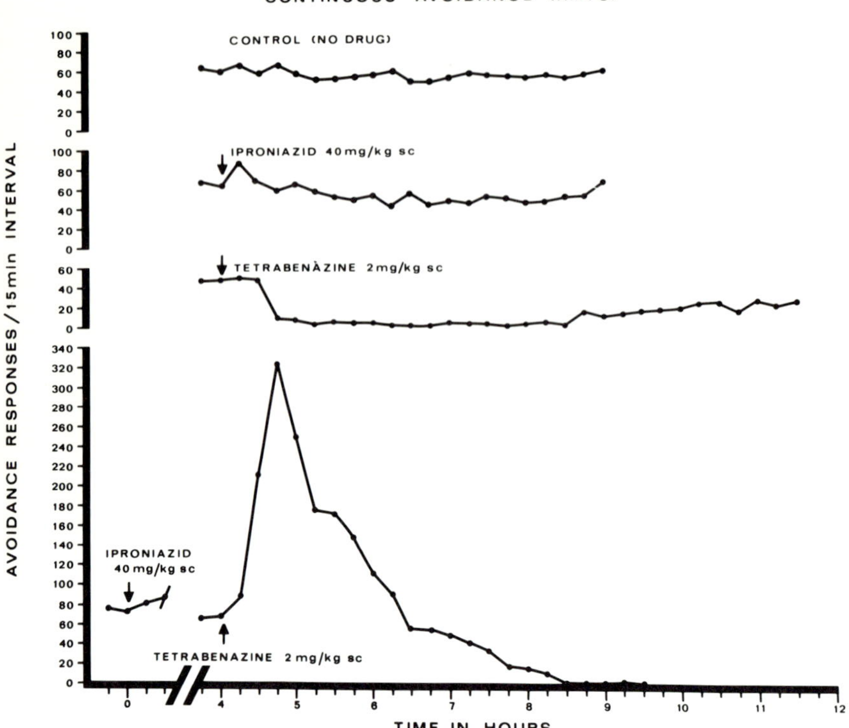

FIG. 1. Effects of iproniazid and tetrabenazine, alone and in combination, on rate of lever pressing of rats in continuous avoidance procedure. Top record: avoidance response rate during a 5-hour control session. Second record: iproniazid alone had no significant effect on behavior. Third record: tetrabenazine alone produced a nearly complete loss of responding. Fourth record: in rats pretreated with iproniazid, tetrabenazine produced marked stimulation, as shown by the increased rate of lever pressing. (Reproduced by permission of Zbinden and Randall, 1967.)

tration, whereas punished responding was greater than in control tests. After six daily doses, unpunished responding returned to control levels, indicating that tolerance had developed to the depressant effect of the compound. No tolerance developed to the anticonflict effect.

Biochemical tests indicate that benzodiazepines decrease the turnover rates of both norepinephrine and serotonin in the brain. Is the antianxiety effect correlated with decreased turnover of either of these neurohumors? Stein *et al.* administered oxazepam to rats under the procedure just described. They then measured the turnover rates of norepinephrine and serotonin in the midbrain and hindbrain. Rats sacrificed after the first daily dose showed significant decreases in the turnover rates of both nore-

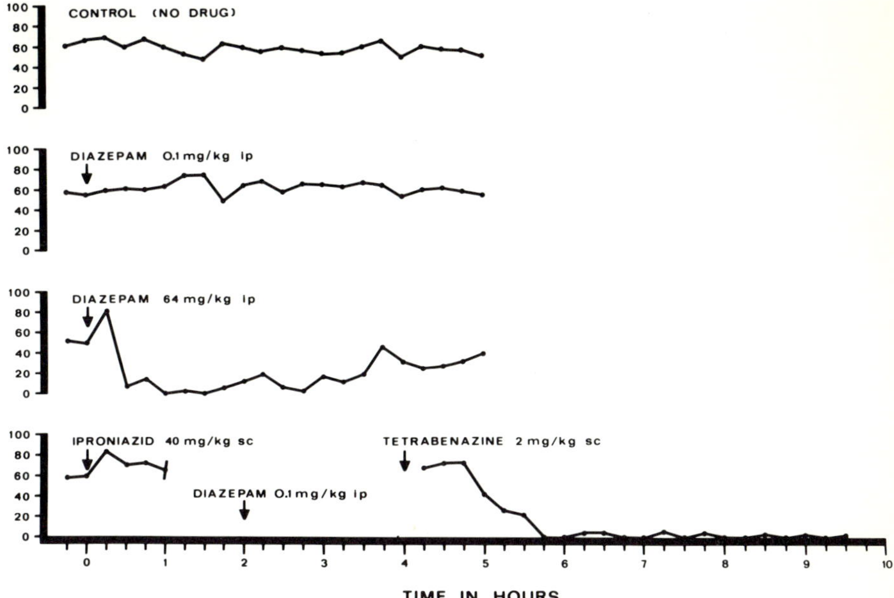

FIG. 2. Effect of diazepam on the stimulation induced by iproniazid and tetrabenazine (see Fig. 1). Top record: control behavior. Second record: a small dose of diazepam had no effect on avoidance behavior. Third record: a large dose of diazepam markedly suppressed avoidance behavior. Fourth record: in rats pretreated with iproniazid, a small dose of diazepam completely blocked the stimulation induced by tetrabenazine. (Reproduced by courtesy of Mr. E. Boff.)

pinephrine and serotonin. Rats sacrificed after the sixth daily dose showed significant decreases in the turnover rate of serotonin but not of norepinephrine. In other words, following chronic administration of oxazepam, tolerance developed to the reduced turnover rate of norepinephrine but not to that of serotonin. As noted previously, under these conditions tolerance developed to the behavioral depression induced by oxazepam but not to the anticonflict effect. Stein *et al.* suggested that the depressant effect of benzodiazepines is associated with reduced norepinephrine turnover, and the anticonflict effect with reduced serotonin turnover.

A new chapter in the story of the benzodiazepines opened in 1974. Studies from Basel, Moscow, and Washington indicated that benzodiazepines might act by enhancing the effects of the inhibitory transmitter GABA (Polc *et al.,* 1974; Zakusov *et al.,* 1975; Costa *et al.,* 1975). These papers are reviewed in Section III.

B. A Note on Ionic Movement

The first experiment to study the effects of benzodiazepines at the ionic level seems to be that of Liebeswar (1972). The isolated papillary muscle of the guinea pig was mounted in a tissue chamber and perfused with Tyrode's solution. The transmembrane potentials were recorded with glass microelectrodes before, during, and after stimulation of the tissue at a frequency of 0.5–1.5 Hz.

Flurazepam hydrochloride, 2.5×10^{-5} to 2×10^{-4} *M*, had no effect on the resting potential, but prolonged the duration of the action potential, decreased its amplitude, and decreased its maximum rate of rise (MRR). Depression of the MRR reached maximum in 30 to 45 minutes; recovery was complete 2 hours after return to normal Tyrode's solution. Partial recovery occurred during a 20 second pause in stimulation, even though the preparation was still exposed to flurazepam.

The MRR can be taken as a measure of the "rapid sodium inward current." Apparently the action of flurazepam on this preparation involves an interference with the rapid inward movement of sodium ions. Partial recovery during a pause in stimulation suggests that action potentials are necessary for this effect.

III. Biochemistry

Early biochemical studies with benzodiazepines showed that these compounds influenced the *in vivo* rates of utilization, or turnover, of several brain amines. Various benzodiazepines slowed the turnover rates of norepinephrine, dopamine, and serotonin in brain tissue. Amines in the cortex and in certain other portions of the brain appeared to be particularly susceptible to the action of these compounds.

Taylor and Laverty (1969) demonstrated that nitrazepam, diazepam, and chlordiazepoxide (all at 10 mg/kg, s.c.) decreased norepinephrine turnover in the cortex, cerebellum, and thalamus of rat brain but not in the brainstem. These benzodiazepines also suppressed the turnover of dopamine within the striatum. Furthermore, these compounds prevented the increased turnover of brain norepinephrine that occurred when rats were exposed to the stress of electroshock to the feet. In contrast to the effects on turnover, there were no changes in the concentrations of the endogenous catecholamines. It is also possible that benzodiazepines have no direct effect on aminergic neurons, since chlordiazepoxide at 10^{-4} *M* had no influence on the *in vitro* uptake, retention, or release of norepinephrine (Lidbrink and Farnebo, 1973).

The rate of disappearance of intracisternally administered serotonin-^{14}C

in rat brain was reduced by diazepam, 20 mg/kg, i.p. (Chase *et al.*, 1970). This effect was attributed to a reduced rate of serotonin turnover. This conclusion has been confirmed by more refined techniques that permit the determination of serotonin turnover rates in specific brain regions. Thus chlordiazepoxide (20 mg/kg, i.p.), diazepam (5 mg/kg), and flurazepam (5 mg/kg) reduced the turnover of serotonin in mouse tel-diencephalon (Dominic, 1973), whereas, in the rat, chlordiazepoxide (50 mg/kg, i.p.) and diazepam (25 mg/kg) reduced the turnover of this amine in the cortex but not in the rest of the brain (Lidbrink *et al.*, 1974). In spite of reducing the rate of serotonin utilization, 20 mg/kg of diazepam increased brain concentrations of 5-hydroxyindole acetic acid (5-HIAA), the major metabolite of serotonin (Chase *et al.*, 1970). These investigators attributed this increase to an influence of diazepam on the transport mechanisms that move 5-HIAA across the blood–brain barrier.

In addition to these effects on brain amines, diazepam also has effects on acetylcholine. Diazepam decreased the turnover rates of acetylcholine in the midbrain and cortex of the rat, but not in the hippocampus or striatum (Zsilla *et al.*, 1976). Since Consolo *et al.* (1975) found that diazepam failed to influence a number of enzymes involved in the storage and release of acetylcholine, this effect on turnover may be indirect.

The actions of benzodiazepines on biogenic amines have been correlated with various pharmacological effects (Corrodi *et al.*, 1971; Wise *et al.*, 1972). Nevertheless, it is probable that these effects on amines are not the primary mechanisms of action. More recent experiments, describing the influence of benzodiazepines on amino acid neurotransmitters, provide evidence for a primary site of action.

A. Amino Acid Neurotransmitters

Glycine and GABA are two amino acids that function as inhibitory neurotransmitters. Both have been implicated in the actions of benzodiazepines (see Section IV,B). Young *et al.* (1974) demonstrated that benzodiazepines interfered with the *in vitro* binding of strychnine-^{3}H (strychnine is a specific inhibitor of glycine receptors). Other workers, using *in vivo* techniques, failed to find an interaction of benzodiazepines and glycine receptors. Thus diazepam did not prevent strychnine convulsions (Curtis *et al.*, 1976a) nor did strychnine reverse the neuronal depression produced by flurazepam (Dray and Straughan, 1976). Furthermore, the diazepam concentration required to inhibit the binding of strychnine-^{3}H (26 μM) was considerably higher than the concentration producing a pharmacological response (0.14 μM) (Costa *et al.*, 1975).

Other studies indicate that benzodiazepines might act by enhancing the effects of the inhibitory transmitter GABA. Polc *et al.* (1974) studied the depressant effect of diazepam on spinal reflexes. Previous workers found that this effect is accompanied by enhancement of presynaptic inhibition and that GABA is the mediator involved in this form of inhibition. Polc *et al.*, therefore, explored the possible role of GABA in the spinal action of diazepam.

Bicuculline blocks GABA receptors. Diazepam, 1 mg/kg, i.v., enhanced presynaptic inhibition in the spinal cat; this effect was reversed by injection of bicuculline, 0.5 mg/kg. Dose–response relations of diazepam were studied in the presence of increasing doses of bicuculline (Fig. 3). As the bicuculline dose was increased, the diazepam curve moved to the right in a series of parallel shifts; this is indicative of a competitive antagonism between the two drugs.

Aminooxyacetic acid (AOAA) is an inhibitor of GABA transaminase,

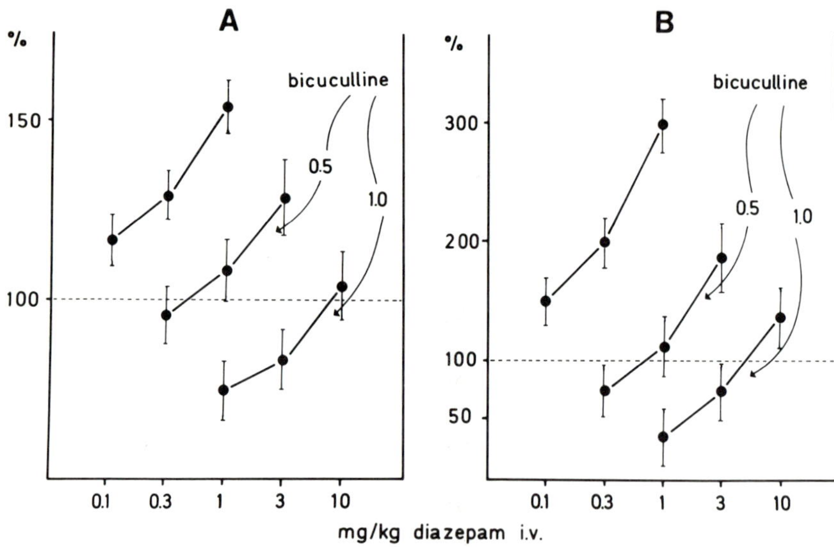

FIG. 3. Influence of two doses of bicuculline on the dose–response curve for the effect of diazepam on (A) dorsal root potential (DRP), and on (B) presynaptic inhibition in spinal cats. Three increasing doses of diazepam were given to a group of untreated controls, and to groups injected with bicuculline 0.5 or 1.0 mg/kg, i.v., immediately before diazepam. Three cats per group; interval between diazepam injections 5 minutes. Means ± S.E.M. are shown. Ordinates show responses expressed as percent of predrug controls. (A) Effect of diazepam on area of DRP evoked by stimulation of nerves to gastrocnemius and biceps muscles and of sural nerve. (B) Effect of diazepam on amplitude of monosynaptic ventral root reflex response to a single shock applied to nerve to gastrocnemius muscle 50 msec after an inhibitory volley in nerve to biceps femoris muscle. [Reproduced from Polc *et al.* (1974) by permission of the authors and publisher.]

an enzyme involved in the degradation of GABA. Treatment with AOAA, 10 mg/kg, i.v., more than doubled the level of endogenous GABA in the spinal cord of spinal cats. Presynaptic inhibition was enhanced. Diazepam, 3 mg/kg, produced a further increase. At 100 mg/kg, thiosemicarbazide (TSC), which is an inhibitor of glutamate decarboxylase (an enzyme involved in the synthesis of GABA) decreased the level of endogenous GABA by more than half. Presynaptic inhibition was reduced. Diazepam, 3 mg/kg, failed to reverse the effects of TSC on the level of GABA or on presynaptic inhibition.

The experiments with bicuculline might suggest a direct action of diazepam on the GABA receptor. However, the enhanced activity of diazepam following an increase in the spinal levels of GABA, and its reduced activity following a decrease in GABA levels, indicate that the action of diazepam is mediated by GABA. Polc *et al.* suggest that diazepam may be able to increase the amount of GABA available for release or to inhibit its inactivation.

Zakusov *et al.* (1975) studied the effects of diazepam on the cortex of the cat. In preliminary experiments, diazepam had a direct depressant effect on the electrical activity of the surgically isolated cortex. Detailed studies were then made on the intracortical response in the intact immobilized cat. The sensory cortex was stimulated with paired pulses of 0.1 msec duration; the interval between pulses varied from 1 to 800 msec. The response in the motor cortex varied with the interval between pulses. At intervals of 1 to 10 msec the second response was depressed, whereas at intervals of 20 to 100 msec the response was enhanced. Diazepam selectively depressed this period of facilitation, the effects ranging from slight depression at 0.1 to complete abolition at 10 mg/kg, i.v.

Zakusov *et al.* investigated the biochemical basis of this action of diazepam. Drugs affecting cholinergic transmission had no specific effects on the intracortical recovery cycle. By contrast, drugs affecting the metabolism of GABA had highly specific effects. Depakine, which increases brain GABA levels through inhibition of GABA transaminase, resembled diazepam by depressing the period of facilitation. Thiosemicarbazide, which decreases brain GABA levels through inhibition of glutamate decarboxylase, differed from diazepam by enhancing the facilitation. Bicuculline had a similar effect. Furthermore, the diazepam depression was abolished by bicuculline, and the bicuculline enhancement was abolished by diazepam (cf. Fig. 3).

Costa *et al.* (1975) reviewed several studies made in their laboratories. To determine whether GABA or glycine is involved in the anticonvulsant activity of benzodiazepines, Costa *et al.* tested the activity of diazepam in rats against the convulsions induced by isoniazid (an inhibitor of GABA synthesis) and against those induced by strychnine (which blocks glycine receptors). The ED_{50} for diazepam against isoniazid convulsions was 0.14 μM/kg, i.p., and against strychnine convulsions 6.0 μM/kg. This forty-fold difference in activity indicates that diazepam has a selective action against seizures induced by changes in the GABA system. The corresponding figures for phenobarbital were 60 and 52 μM/kg, indicating that this compound lacks any such specificity.

These pharmacological experiments indicate that some effects of diazepam are mediated by GABA. Biochemical evidence substantiates these findings. Mao *et al.* (1975) noted that isoniazid increased the level of 3′,5′-cyclic guanosine monophosphate (cGMP) in the cerebellum of the rat; it also decreased the GABA level by inhibiting the conversion of glutamic acid to GABA. Diazepam at 0.52 μM/kg, i.p., prevented the isoniazid-induced rise in cGMP levels; at 1.7 μM/kg, it reduced the cerebellar cGMP levels in animals not treated with isoniazid. Diazepam had no influence on cerebellar GABA levels.

Mao *et al.* (1975) explain these results in the following manner. An inverse correlation between the levels of cGMP and of GABA was found by Mao *et al.* (1974). Hence diazepam seems to enhance or mimic the action of GABA. It could do this either by acting directly on GABA receptors or by increasing the synaptic concentration of GABA. Diazepam does not seem to be a direct GABA agonist, since Snyder and Enna (1975) observed no displacement of GABA from its specific postsynaptic binding sites by diazepam.

Thus far, attempts to find the mechanism by which benzodiazepines potentiate GABA have not been successful. Chlordiazepoxide, at doses as high as 0.5 mM, showed only 18% inhibition of GABA uptake in rat cerebral cortex slices (Iversen and Johnston, 1971; Harris *et al.*, 1973). By contrast, diazepam at a concentration of 0.5 mM inhibited GABA uptake into rat cortical slices by 86% (Harris *et al.*, 1973). Diazepam at a concentration of 50 μM caused 50% inhibition of GABA uptake into synaptosomes prepared from mouse brain (Olsen *et al.*, 1977); the same authors reported that the calcium-independent release of GABA from mouse brain synaptosomes was increased by diazepam (30 μM) but that the calcium-dependent release of GABA was inhibited by this drug at a concentration of 50 μM. W. D. Horst (unpublished) found that diazepam (0.1 mM) increased the K^+ stimulated release of GABA from superfused rat cortical synaptosomes by 23% but that an identical concentration of chlordiazepoxide or flurazepam was without effect.

The benzodiazepines do not appear to have a consistent influence on GABA-transaminase, the major enzyme responsible for GABA catabolism. Sawaya *et al.* (1975) demonstrated that diazepam and clonazepam concentrations of 5 m*M* had no influence on this enzyme, but chlordiazepoxide showed a slight effect.

The lowest dose at which a benzodiazepine influenced GABA uptake, release, or metabolism was 30 μM (Olsen *et al.*, 1977). By contrast, pharmacological activity was observed at 0.14 μM (Costa *et al.*, 1975). Furthermore, few effects on GABA disposition were observed with pharmacologically active benzodiazepines such as chlordiazepoxide. Hence these effects on GABA disposition may have little relevance to the major pharmacological actions of the benzodiazepines. A precise evaluation of these effects must await studies with larger numbers of compounds so that influences on GABA availability may be correlated with clinical efficacy.

Polc and Haefely (1976) observed that benzodiazepines act by enhancing the effect of ongoing activity in GABAergic interneurons. They suggested that this enhancement "could be achieved by sensitizing the subsynaptic membrane to the effect of synaptically released GABA or by augmenting the synaptic concentration of GABA either by delaying its inactivation or by increasing the amount of GABA released per stimulus." Recent experiments allow some choice among these three suggestions. As mentioned in the foregoing, benzodiazepines seem to have inconsistent effects on GABA uptake or catabolism. If benzodiazepines enhanced the activity of GABA by increasing the sensitivity of its receptors, one might expect to find a *decrease* in GABA turnover in brain; if benzodiazepines potentiated the activity of GABA by increasing its release, one might expect to find an *increase* in GABA turnover. Mao *et al.* (1977) showed that diazepam (1 mg/kg, i.p.) reduced the turnover of GABA in the caudate and accumbens nuclei of the rat. The GABA agonist muscimol had the same effect. Although this evidence supports the hypothesis of increased receptor sensitivity, further experiments must be done with other benzodiazepines and with GABA antagonists such as bicuculline and picrotoxin.

The benzodiazepines are known to influence a number of other biochemical processes; for instance, they inhibit phosphodiesterase (Dalton *et al.*, 1974; Schultz, 1974), Na^+-K^+-ATPase and Mg^{2+}-ATPase (Gilbert and Wyllie, 1976), and prostaglandin synthesis (Kunze *et al.*, 1975). The significance of these effects with regard to benzodiazepines' mechanisms of action is not appreciated at this time.

A new approach to benzodiazepine research was taken by Squires and Braestrup (1977) who discovered that labeled diazepam binds with high affinity to specific sites in rat brain tissue. Their study demonstrated that the highest density of binding sites occurs in the frontal and occipital cortex, whereas the lowest levels are in the pons-medulla. The hippocampus

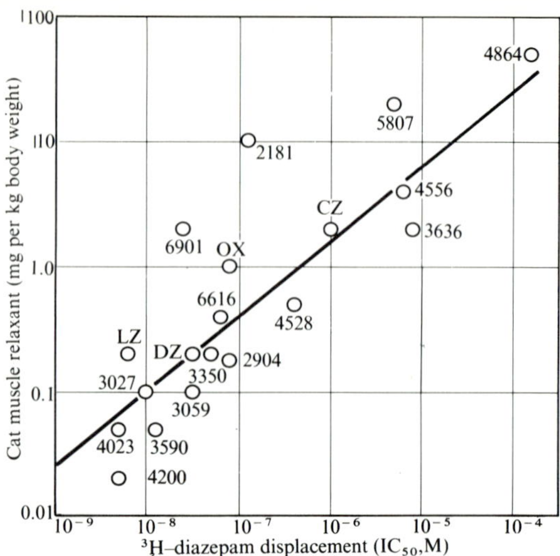

FIG. 4. Correlation between IC_{50} values for diazepam-^{3}H displacement for nineteen benzodiazepines and cat muscle relaxant dosage (mg/kg, p.o.). [The IC_{50} is the concentration of compound causing 50% inhibition of specific diazepam-^{3}H binding (1.6 n*M*) to rat brain membranes.] The cat data are from Randall *et al.* (1974). The best curve fit was assessed by linear regression analysis (r = .891; $P < .001$). Numbers on graph indicate code numbers for Hoffmann-La Roche research compounds. (CZ) Chlordiazepoxide; (DZ) diazepam; (LZ) lorazepam; (OX) oxazepam. [Reproduced from Squires and Braestrup (1977) by courtesy of the authors and publisher.]

has intermediate-binding levels. The diazepam-binding sites described by these investigators have a high specificity for benzodiazepine structures; thus the neurotransmitters acetylcholine, norepinephrine, dopamine, serotonin, GABA, L-glutamate, and glycine do not displace diazepam from its binding sites. Also, psychodepressants such as meprobamate, barbiturates, and ethanol are not effective in this regard. Squires and Braestrup tested many benzodiazepine structures for their effectiveness in displacing labeled diazepam from its binding sites; they found a high correlation between a compound's ability to displace diazepam and its effectiveness as a muscle relaxant in the cat (Fig. 4). These workers "suggest that the brain possesses specific receptors for benzodiazepines which may mediate their pharmacological actions." Furthermore, the natural ligand for these receptors may be "a hitherto undiscovered endogenous transmitter."

Discussion

Biochemical and pharmacological evidence strongly implicates the GABA synapse as a major site of action of the benzodiazepines. An action on the GABA synapse may account for alterations in the effects of other neurotransmitters such as norepinephrine, serotonin, and acetylcholine. One of the most ubiquitous neurotransmitters in brain tissue (Fahn, 1976), GABA is known to impinge upon aminergic and cholinergic neurons throughout the CNS (Iversen and Schon, 1973; Kataoka *et al.*, 1974; Fonnum *et al.*, 1974; Haefely *et al.*, 1975).

There can be no question that the benzodiazepines have a significant impact on GABA function and that this effect may account for many of their pharmacological properties. Nevertheless, the search for the mechanisms of action of these drugs is far from completed. The cellular and molecular events that result in GABA potentiation are completely unknown; several possible sites of action have been proposed by Bloom (1977) and are illustrated in Fig. 5.

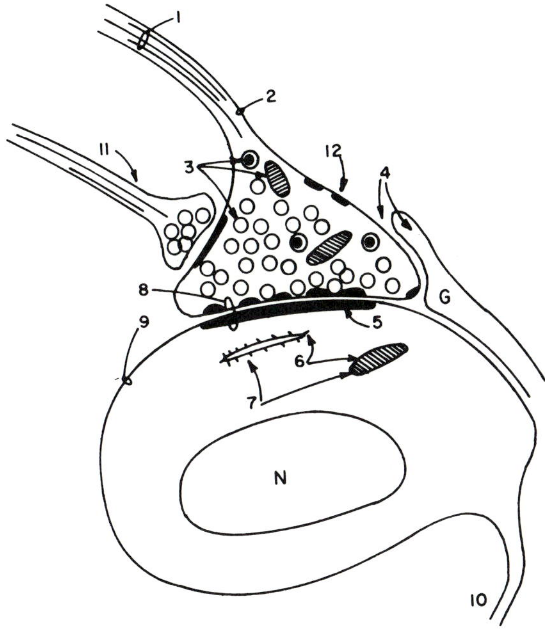

FIG. 5. The enumerated sites indicate possible points in the biological cycle of a central neuron at which benzodiazepines might interact. (1) Axoplasmic transport; (2) excitable components of the membrane; (3) organelles for transmitter synthesis, storage, catabolism, release, and reuptake; (4) Glial–neuronal interaction processes; (5) postsynaptic receptors; (6) organelles that may mediate the postsynaptic response; (7) cytoplasmic–nuclear interactions that regulate transmitter-sensitive gene expression; (8) intrasynaptic events of sensitization and desensitization; (9) integration of simultaneous synaptic potentials; (10) discharge of the target cell and signal propagation; (11) presynaptic element that regulates presynaptic transmitter release; (12) presynaptic autoreceptors. (From Bloom, 1977; copyright 1977 by the American Psychiatric Association. Reproduced by permission of the authors and publisher.)

Benzodiazepines may have direct effects on the activity of neurochemicals other than GABA. Two preliminary reports (Juhasz and Dairman, 1977; Lippa *et al.*, 1977) suggest that alterations in GABA sensitivity do not account for all of the pharmacological activity of diazepam. Most drugs that influence the CNS are known to alter the disposition of more than one neurotransmitter, and there is no evidence to suggest that the benzodiazepines act differently.

The benzodiazepine-binding sites described by Squires and Braestrup (1977) may prove to be a key to the identification and characterization of the cellular components affected by the benzodiazepines. For example, these binding sites might provide a means by which benzodiazepines could alter the sensitivity of GABA receptors. A related problem concerns the ligand that normally acts on these binding sites. Do benzodiazepines act as agonists or antagonists to this ligand? From the biological point of view, the survival value of an endogenous anxiety-producing substance is far greater than that of an anxiety-reducing substance. Hence it is likely that when benzodiazepines bind to these sites, they block the action of an endogenous anxiogenic agent. This possibility opens a new approach to the study of anxiety and to the development of anxiolytic agents.

B. Corticosteroids and Benzodiazepines

A different approach to the biochemical basis of anxiety is taken by Warburton (1974). He begins by defining anxiety in man as "an unpleasant state which is directed toward the future"; it seems to depend on "the amount of uncertainty in the environment."

Experimental evidence suggests that anxiety may result from biochemical changes induced by corticosteroids (CS).Clinical studies show that injection of CS enhances anxiety responses. Animal studies indicate that increased plasma CS levels occur in situations involving "uncertainty and unpredictability."

The hypothalamus, hippocampus, and amygdala may be involved in the control of plasma CS levels. The hypothalamus seems to play a role in a negative feedback system, in which increased plasma CS levels depress the activity of hypothalamic neurons, and this in turn lowers the plasma CS levels. Plasma CS levels may also be lowered by stimulation of the hippocampus, whereas stimulation of the amygdala raises the CS levels. The depressant influences may be mediated by adrenergic systems, whereas the facilitatory influences may be mediated by cholinergic systems. Serotonin may also be involved in these control mechanisms.

Antianxiety agents are known to act on the amygdala and hippocampus, and they also affect turnover rates of norepinephrine and serotonin. Warburton suggests that these actions of antianxiety agents antagonize the anxiety-inducing actions of CS.

Support for Warburton's hypothesis comes from a study by Lahti and Barsuhn (1974). Rats were put under stress by being transferred from the animal room to a laboratory in which a radio was playing loudly. Corticosteroid levels increased from 14.3 in control rats to 77.5 μg/100 ml plasma in test rats.

Pretreatment with diazepam produced a dose-dependent decrease in CS levels. Statistically significant decreases occurred at 5 and 10 mg/kg, i.p.; the CS levels at these doses were 28.3 and 21.7 μg/100 ml plasma. Several other compounds were active. Potencies relative to diazepam (1.0) were as follows: meprobamate, 0.027; phenobarbital, 0.27; chlordiazepoxide, 0.5; nitrazepam, 3.0; a monochlorotriazolobenzodiazepine, 5.67; and a dichlorotriazolobenzodiazepine, 9.95. Inactive compounds included chlorpromazine, phenoxybenzamine, propanolol, atropine, morphine, and imipramine. These results indicate that agents with antianxiety activity reduce stress-induced increases in plasma CS levels in the rat; this action is not shown by a variety of agents with other types of activity.

In a carefully controlled study, Keim and Sigg (1977) measured the effects of psychoactive agents on stress-induced changes in plasma CS levels. "Restraint stress" was induced by placing rats in a plastic cylinder for 30 minutes. The experiments on each drug involved 56 rats. A basal control group of 8 rats received no treatment. The remaining rats were divided into nonstress and stress groups; each group was divided into four subgroups (of 6 rats each) which received placebo and three dose levels of the compound under study.

As shown in Fig. 6, injection of placebo elicited a small rise in plasma CS levels. When placebo-treated rats were subjected to restraint stress, their plasma CS levels increased by approximately 700%. Administration of drugs to unstressed rats was without effect, except for rises in plasma CS levels produced by the highest doses of haloperidol (1 mg/kg, s.c.) and diazepam (10 mg/kg). In the stressed rats, plasma CS levels were significantly decreased by desmethylimipramine (10 and 30 mg/kg), haloperidol (1 mg/kg), diazepam (5 and 10 mg/kg), and phenobarbital (90 mg/kg). In sharp contrast, plasma CS levels were significantly increased by chlorpromazine (10 mg/kg).

To determine whether any part of these drug effects was exerted peripherally, isolated adrenals from drug-treated nonstressed rats were tested for their reactivity to ACTH. *In vitro* release of CS by ACTH was significantly increased in adrenals from rats pretreated with chlorpromazine. Pretreatment with the remaining compounds had no significant ef-

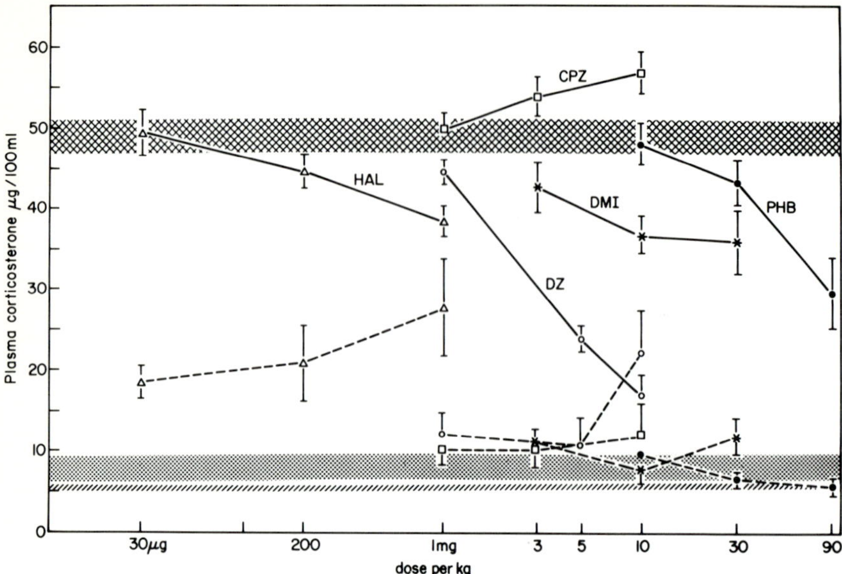

FIG. 6. Effect of psychotherapeutic drugs on basal and stress-induced plasma corticosterone (CS) in rats. Abscissa: log dose of the drugs. Narrow diagonal band (bottom): basal plasma CS ± SEM. Stippled band (middle): plasma CS ± S.E.M. in placebo-injected, non-stressed rats. Cross-hatched band (top): plasma CS ± S.E.M. in placebo-injected rats after 30 minutes restraint. Solid lines connect data points representing mean plasma CS ± S.E.M. after stressing rats pretreated with various drugs; broken lines connect data points obtained when the same drugs were administered to rats without subsequent exposure to restraint stress. Haloperidol (HAL, triangles); Chlorpromazine (CPZ, squares); Diazepam (DZ, open circles); Desmethylimipramine (DMI, asterisks); phenobarbital (PHB, filled circles). [Reproduced from Keim and Sigg (1977) by permission of the authors and publisher.]

fect, indicating that the reduction in stress-enhanced plasma CS levels produced by these compounds was central in origin. The exact mechanism of action has yet to be elucidated. A possible clue lies in the finding that stress-induced reduction of hypothalamic norepinephrine was prevented by diazepam (5 and 10 mg/kg) and by phenobarbital (90 mg/kg).

Discussion

A relatively neglected area in pharmacology and biochemistry involves the effects of chronic administration of drugs. Although in medical practice the psychotropic agents are usually given on a chronic basis, many laboratory experiments are made on an acute basis. As shown in Section II,A, the effects of benzodiazepines on acute administration may differ from their effects on chronic administration. Chronic administration permits endocrine readjustments to take place. Hence corticosteroids may play a role in the clinical efficacy of benzodiazepines.

IV. Neuropharmacology

A. Peripheral Ganglia

The effects of benzodiazepines on the sympathetic ganglia of the bullfrog were analyzed by Suria and Costa (1973, 1975). The excised ganglia were mounted in a plexiglass chamber and perfused with Ringer's solution containing *d*-tubocurarine. A single preganglionic stimulus elicited an excitatory postsynaptic potential (EPSP). This was followed for 1 second by a train of volleys at 40 Hz. A single preganglionic stimulus now produced an EPSP that showed a marked increase in amplitude when compared to the EPSP obtained before the volleys. This increase in size of the response is known as post-tetanic potentiation (PTP).

Drugs were now added to the bath. The PTP was reduced by diphenylhydantoin $10^{-5} M$, by chlordiazepoxide $10^{-6} M$, and by diazepam $10^{-8} M$. There was no change in the response to single shocks. Suria and Costa (1973) suggest that these drug effects are exerted on the presynaptic membrane.

Direct evidence for an action of diazepam on presynaptic terminals was furnished by Suria and Costa (1975). These authors measured the membrane characteristics of the presynaptic terminals with the sucrose gap technique. The terminals were depolarized by diazepam $10^{-6} M$, by dibutyryl–cGMP $10^{-6} M$, and by GABA $10^{-4} M$. These actions were promptly reversed by washing with Ringer's solution, and were antagonized by picrotoxin. The action of diazepam on PTP may involve effects on presynaptic terminals: perhaps diazepam and cGMP "act through a release of GABA."

A different aspect of transmission in the bullfrog ganglion was studied by Suria *et al.* (1975). The EPSP produced by preganglionic stimulation is followed by an inhibitory postsynaptic potential (IPSP). Both potentials exhibit PTP. In contrast to its reduction of the PTP of the EPSP, diazepam $10^{-6} M$ increased the PTP of the IPSP. The latter action was also shown by dibutyryl–cyclic adenosine monophosphate (cAMP) but not by dibutyryl–cGMP.

Suria *et al.* suggest that diazepam may act at two sites: (*1*) a presynaptic site, involving cGMP and EPSP; and (*2*) a postsynaptic site, involving cAMP and IPSP. Diazepam can reduce the efficacy of synaptic transmission both by decreasing the PTP of the EPSP and by increasing the PTP of

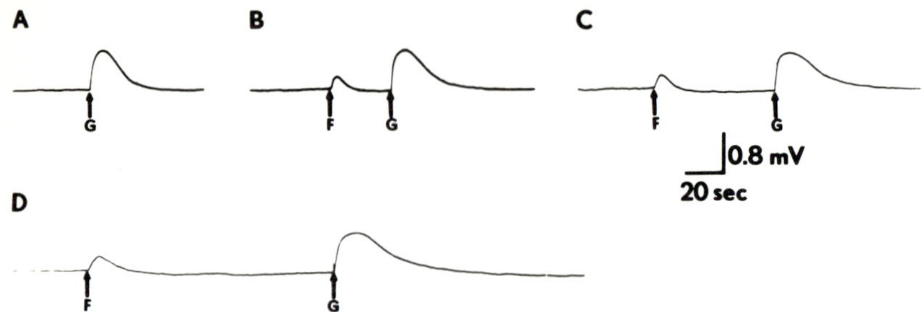

FIG. 7. The effect of flurazepam (1 μM) on the ganglionic response to GABA. Recording electrodes were placed on the surface of the cat superior cervical ganglion and on the crushed end of the postganglionic nerve. Arrows indicate points of injection of flurazepam, F, or GABA, G. (A) Control response to intraarterial injection of 30-nM GABA. (B–D) Depolarizations resulting from intraarterial injection of 1-μM flurazepam (first arrow) followed by 30-nM GABA (second arrow). The intervals between the two injections are 30 seconds in B, 1 minute in C, and 2 minutes in D. The approximate lengths of the GABA-induced depolarizations in A, B, C, and D are 30, 40, 60, and 60 seconds, respectively.

the IPSP. However, these effects of diazepam are exerted on PTP and not on the responses to single shocks. This indicates that diazepam may "interfere with the results of excessive release of the transmitter" but not with normal ganglionic function. Action on such "excessive release" may be involved in the anticonvulsant effect of diazepam; perhaps it is also involved in the antianxiety effect.

Some recent experiments on ganglia suggest that benzodiazepines may act indirectly through a reduction of GABA uptake into ganglionic glia cells. Schlosser *et al.* (1977) observed that intra-arterial injection of flurazepam, 1 μM, not only induced a brief depolarization of the cat superior cervical ganglion, but also prolonged the depolarization induced by GABA (Fig. 7). It is interesting to note that W. D. Horst (unpublished observations) found a reduction of brain glial cell uptake of GABA following flurazepam treatment. A similar mechanism could account for the action of flurazepam on GABA at the ganglionic synapse.

B. SPINAL CORD

1. *Direct Effects*

Because of our advanced knowledge of its sensory and motor physiology and its ease of accessibility, the spinal cord has been used for an intensive study of the actions of benzodiazepines. In the spinal cat, diazepam (0.5 mg/kg, i.v.) had no significant effect on the monosynaptic reflex, whereas polysynaptic reflexes were depressed by 50%. In contrast to the depressant effects of diazepam and chlordiazepoxide on PTP in the frog sympathetic ganglia, neither agent depressed the monosynaptic PTP in mammalian spinal preparations (Swinyard and Castellion, 1966; Schlosser, 1971). This is in contrast to the action of diphenylhydantoin (10–40 mg/kg, i.v.) that reduces the PTP's not only of the ganglionic EPSP but also of the monosynaptic reflex (Esplin, 1957).

At the segmental level, two major inhibitory processes can be distinguished. The first is postsynaptic inhibition; this system is blocked by strychnine and appears to have glycine as its neurotransmitter. The second process is presynaptic inhibition, which is blocked by picrotoxin and appears to have GABA as its neurotransmitter.

Using *in vitro* techniques, Young *et al.* (1974) described an interaction of twenty-one benzodiazepines with glycine receptors from the brainstem and spinal cord of the rat. This interaction was evaluated by measuring the ability of the benzodiazepines to displace the binding of strychnine-^{3}H. Median effective doses (ED_{50}'s) were glycine, 25 μM, diazepam, 26 μM, and chlordiazepoxide, 200 μM. The rank order of potency of the twenty-one compounds correlated ($p < .005$) with their rank order in a variety of pharmacological tests.

These results are in conflict with findings from *in vivo* experiments. In the spinal cat, diazepam (1.5 mg/kg, i.v.) did not interfere with postsynaptic inhibition of the monosynaptic reflex (Schmidt *et al.*, 1967; Schlosser, 1971). Using the anesthetized cat, Curtis *et al.* (1976a) found no reduction in the firing of interneurons following iontophoretic administration of chlordiazepoxide, whereas ejection of glycine produced a clear inhibition. Furthermore, the interaction between strychnine and glycine on dorsal horn interneurons was not significantly affected by diazepam, 3 mg/kg, i.v. Hence *in vivo* experiments provide no evidence for an action of benzodiazepines on glycine receptors. As noted in Section III,A, glycine does not inhibit diazepam binding to endogenous receptors (Squires and Braestrup, 1977).

The second spinal-inhibitory mechanism involves GABA as the putative mediator. Inhibitory interneurons form axoaxonic synapses on the terminals of primary afferent (sensory) fibers (see No. 11 in Fig. 5). The release of GABA by the interneurons produces a depolarization of the primary afferent nerve terminals, a process resulting from an increase in chloride permeability. The resultant depolarization of the afferent fiber reduces or blocks the release of the excitatory transmitter. Thus presynaptic inhibition is a mechanism that can modulate and reduce the amount of incoming sensory information. A number of investigators have reported that benzodiazepines produce a striking enhancement of presynaptic inhibition (Schmidt *et al.*,1967; Schlosser, 1971; Stratten and Barnes, 1971;

Polc *et al.*, 1974). Diazepam in therapeutic doses has been reported to increase the dorsal root reflex and the dorsal root potential; it also increases the presynaptic inhibition. All these actions are manifestations of enhanced primary afferent depolarization.

The marked effects of the benzodiazepines, diazepam in particular, on presynaptic inhibition suggest a possible link between the action of these compounds and the inhibitory neurotransmitter GABA. Stratten and Barnes (1971) noted that the reduction of the dorsal root potential produced by the GABA antagonist picrotoxin could be reversed by intravenous injection of diazepam. Similar studies with bicuculline, another GABA antagonist, have been reported (Schlosser *et al.*, 1973; Polc *et al.*, 1974). A series of experiments by Polc *et al.* demonstrated the role of GABA in the effects of diazepam on spinal reflexes (see Section III,A).

2. *Supraspinal Control of Spinal Reflexes*

A number of spinal activities were studied in decerebrate and spinal cats by Polc *et al.* (1974). The threshold dose of diazepam for depression of monosynaptic and polysynaptic reflexes was 0.1 mg/kg, i.v., in decerebrate cats, and 0.3–0.5 mg/kg in spinal cats. By contrast, the threshold dose for enhancement of dorsal root potentials and of presynaptic inhibition was 0.1 mg/kg in both decerebrate and spinal cats. These findings suggest that supraspinal areas might be involved in the depressant action of diazepam on spinal reflexes, whereas the enhancement of dorsal root potentials and presynaptic inhibition might be largely a spinal action.

The mesencephalic reticular facilitatory and the medullary reticular inhibitory systems have been implicated in some of the spinal effects of diazepam (Przybyla and Wang, 1968). Diazepam given intravenously (0.1 mg/kg) or into the vertebral artery (0.01 mg/kg) was capable of reducing facilitation and inhibition of the kneejerk caused by stimulation of the two brainstem systems in decerebrate cats. In addition, diazepam caused a reduction in the spontaneous rate of firing of neurons located in the mesencephalic reticular facilitatory system and simultaneously reduced the polysynaptic extensor reflex. Hence depression of the brainstem facilitatory system by diazepam may be involved in the depressant effect of this agent on spinal reflexes.

C. Cuneate Nucleus

The cuneate nucleus of the cat has a relatively simple organization (Walberg, 1965; Norton, 1973). Primary afferent fibers from the forelimb ascend in the dorsal columns to impinge on cuneate nucleus relay cells (Fig. 8). Here they form excitatory synapses in which the putative neuro-

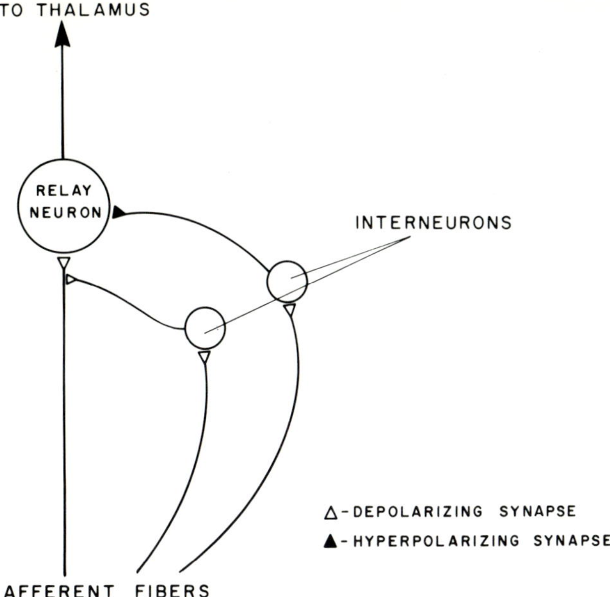

FIG. 8. Schematic diagram illustrating the synaptic organization within the cuneate nucleus. Primary afferent fibers excite the cuneothalamic relay cells (relay neuron), which, in turn, send projections to the contralateral thalamus. Interneurons form either axoaxonal synapses with primary afferent terminals (presynaptic inhibition) or axodendritic and axosomatic synapses with relay neurons (postsynaptic inhibition). In each case, GABA is the suggested transmitter.

transmitter is glutamate (Curtis and Johnston, 1974). The afferent fibers from the forelimb send collaterals to interneurons within the cuneate nucleus. Some interneurons produce postsynaptic inhibition by hyperpolarization of the relay cells, whereas others produce presynaptic inhibition by depolarization of primary afferent endings. At both sites, GABA appears to be the transmitter. This contrasts with the situation in the spinal cord where glycine is the suggested transmitter for postsynaptic inhibition and GABA functions only at the presynaptic site.

Polc and Haefely (1976) investigated the effects of diazepam (0.1–3.0 mg/kg, i.v.) and flunitrazepam (0.01–0.3 mg/kg, i.v.) on the activity of the cuneate nucleus of the cat. The benzodiazepines had no effect on the excitatory mechanism in the cuneate nucleus. However, both compounds produced a dose-dependent enhancement of presynaptic inhibition. These drugs also antagonized the reduction of presynaptic inhibition produced by two GABA receptor blockers, picrotoxin and bicuculline. By contrast, they did not reverse the block of presynaptic inhibition produced by thiosemicarbazide and 3-mercaptopropionic acid, two inhibitors of GABA biosynthesis. This result suggests that the presence of GABA is essential for the action of benzodiazepines on presynaptic inhibition. (Data in Section III,A indicate that benzodiazepines may enhance the sensitivity of GABA receptors.)

Postsynaptic inhibition in the spinal cord is not affected by diazepam (Schmidt *et al.*, 1967; Schlosser, 1971). In the cuneate nucleus, however, where GABA is the suggested inhibitory transmitter, diazepam effectively increased postsynaptic inhibition and also reversed the depression of postsynaptic inhibition induced by picrotoxin (Polc and Haefely, 1976).

D. Cerebellum

Much knowledge of cerebellar function has developed during recent years (Eccles *et al.*, 1967). It appears that the cerebellum is responsible for the preprogramming of movement and that GABA is involved in the regulation of cerebellar function at several levels of organization. The major output of the cerebellum is from Purkinje cells; these are GABAergic neurons that inhibit various nuclei (interpositus, dentate, and fastigial). The Purkinje cells, in turn, are inhibited by stellate and basket cells that have GABA as their transmitter.

The first report on the effects of benzodiazepines on cerebellar function was that of Julien (1972). Julien reported that in cats diazepam (1 mg/kg, i.v.) induced an increase in the rate of discharge of the Purkinje cells from an average control rate of approximately 20 Hz to a maximal rate of 80 Hz. At a higher dose (2 mg/kg, i.v.) the discharge rate increased to 120 Hz. Since the Purkinje cells represent the entire output of the cerebellar cortex and since these cells have a strong inhibitory effect on subcortical nuclei, Julien suggested that the augmentation of Purkinje cell activity may account for the anticonvulsant action of diazepam.

More recent studies do not support these results. Pieri and Haefely (1976) observed in the rat that diazepam and clonazepam in low doses (0.03–0.1 mg/kg, i.v.) consistently and reversibly depressed the firing rate of the Purkinje cells. They suggested that the reduced firing rate of the cerebellar Purkinje cells, producing a decreased output from the cerebellar cortex, may mediate (at least in part) the ataxia and muscular hypotonia observed with these benzodiazepines.

As mentioned earlier, GABA is the mediator of basket cell inhibition of cerebellar Purkinje cells. Curtis *et al.* (1976b) found that in the cat the duration of this inhibition was prolonged by diazepam, 0.5 mg/kg, i.v. (see

Fig. 7 for another situation in which the duration of action of GABA is prolonged by a benzodiazepine). Curtis's group could not confirm the proposed antagonism of benzodiazepines to GABA-mediated inhibition of cerebellar Purkinje cells *in vivo* (Steiner and Felix, 1976) and *in vitro* (Gähwiler, 1976).

E. Higher Centers of the Brain

The effects of benzodiazepines and barbiturates were compared on the electrical activity of the cortex (EEG) in restrained unanesthetized monkeys (Schallek and Johnson, 1976). The gross behavior of the animals was also observed. Diazepam (0.5–2.0 mg/kg, p.o.) and flurazepam (10–40 mg/kg) produced a mixture of fast and slow patterns in the EEG; both compounds caused sedation in some monkeys and restlessness in others. Pentobarbital (5–15 mg/kg) and phenobarbital (20–40 mg/kg) produced a general slowing of the EEG; the only behavioral change that was observed was sedation. The effects of the barbiturates were attributed to depression of the reticular activating system; the effects of the benzodiazepines were attributed to depression of both the reticular activating system and the hippocampus.

Several workers sought to find subcortical brain areas on which benzodiazepines might act. Ruch-Monachon *et al.* (1976) studied the pontogeniculo-occipital (PGO) waves in curarized cats. These waves appear in the pons, lateral geniculate body, and occipital cortex of cats that have been pretreated with depletors of either brain serotonin or brain norepinephrine. Apparently both these transmitters inhibit the generation of PGO waves.

The first experiments were made in cats pretreated with norepinephrine depletors; presumably the serotonin mechanisms were relatively intact. The serotonin precursors, tryptophan and 5-hydroxytryptophan, decreased the number of PGO waves. By contrast, chlordiazepoxide slightly increased the number of waves. However, chlordiazepoxide did not seem to act as a serotonin antagonist, since it did not interfere with the action of the serotinin precursors.

The remaining experiments were made in cats pretreated with serotonin depletors; presumably the norepinephrine mechanisms were relatively intact. Chlordiazepoxide (3 mg/kg, i.v.) increased PGO activity in these animals to a greater extent than in those pretreated with norepinephrine depletors. This suggests that benzodiazepines might interfere with noradrenergic transmission. Since no direct action of benzodiazepines on noradrenergic synaptic transmission is known, the action may be indirect.

To explore this possibility, three groups of cats were prepared. Each group had bilateral lesions in one of the following structures: medial forebrain bundle, ventral part of septum, or anterior basolateral part of amygdala. All three lesions blocked the action of chlordiazepoxide on PGO waves recorded from the lateral geniculate bodies. The action of chlordiazepoxide on PGO waves was also blocked by atropine.

Ruch-Monachon *et al.* concluded from these and other experiments that the action of benzodiazepines on PGO waves involves the following mechanism: activation of a pathway originating in the limbic brain and descending via the medial forebrain bundle to the locus coeruleus in the brainstem. Here the pathway inhibits noradrenergic neurons, thus releasing PGO activity. The action of atropine indicates that a muscarinic synapse is located on this pathway. Additional tests showed that the effects of GABA on PGO waves are similar to those of benzodiazepines. Perhaps GABA is the inhibitory transmitter that acts on the neurons of the locus coeruleus.

Direct evidence for a role of the limbic system in the action of diazepam comes from experiments in which the compound was administered by intracerebral injection (Nagy and Decsi, 1973). Cats were prepared with cannulas and electrodes chronically implanted in various parts of the brain. Rage responses were induced by injection of carbachol into the hypothalamus; the response was quantitated by measuring the duration of vocalization (growling and hissing) in a 20-minute session.

Preliminary experiments with intraperitoneal injection of diazepam showed that 2.3 mg/kg was the ID_{50} (dose reducing duration of vocalization by 50%). This dose also caused slowing of the EEG. Experiments with intracerebral injection showed that the greatest inhibitory effect was obtained from the anterior area of the amygdala. The ID_{50} for this area was 16.4 μg; this dose also slowed the EEG. Higher doses were needed to produce these effects when the drug was injected into other areas of the amygdala or into the hypothalamus; no significant effect was obtained from the hippocampus. These actions were specific for diazepam, since neither levopromazine (20 μg) nor phenobarbital (100 μg) had any effect when injected into the anterior amygdala.

The effects of systemic injection of diazepam on the rage response and on the EEG can be duplicated by injection of the drug into the amygdala. These two effects of diazepam seem to require the presence of the drug in only this area of the brain. It would be worthwhile extending these experiments to determine whether injection of diazepam into the amygdala will affect responses that are not induced by intrahypothalamic carbachol. (Other observations on the amygdala are described in Section V,B.)

V. Psychopharmacology

During the period 1960–1973, psychopharmacologists characterized the behavioral effects of the benzodiazepines (see reviews by Schallek *et al.*, 1972; Randall *et al.*, 1974). Two outstanding effects are the following:

1. Benzodiazepines block various forms of aggressive behavior, such as electrically induced fighting in mice, vicious behavior induced by lesions of the brain in rats, and the spontaneous aggressiveness of vicious cats and monkeys (see Section V,D).

2. Benzodiazepines release a wide variety of previously suppressed responses. Thus lever pressing for a milk reward may be suppressed by administering an electric shock at the same time as the milk. Lever pressing is restored by chlordiazepoxide but not by chlorpromazine. This restoration of suppressed responses, which is usually attributed to release from inhibition, is known as *disinhibition*.

Disinhibition is readily seen in conflict tests. These tests often involve schedules with multiple components. For example, during the unpunished component (signalled by a white light), a rat presses a lever for food reward. During the punished component (signalled by a red light), a lever press may produce both food reward and an electric shock. In control tests (no drug), a trained rat presses the lever at a steady rate during the unpunished phase, whereas responding is suppressed during the punished phase.

The effects of diazepam on this procedure are illustrated in Fig. 9. The ordinate shows the response rate as percentage of the control rate; the

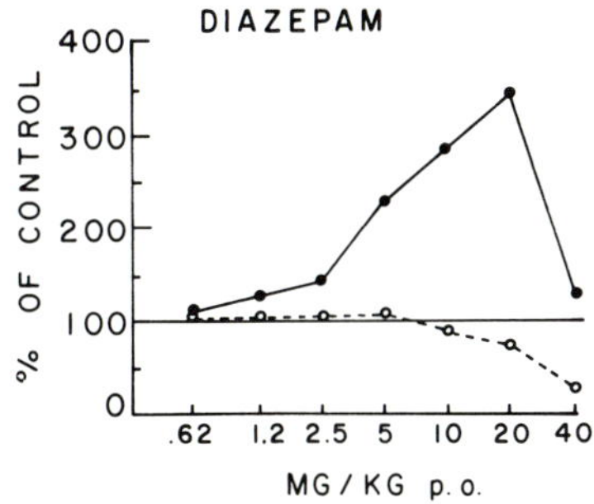

FIG. 9. Dose–response curves for diazepam in multiple schedule test with punished and unpunished responding. The ordinate shows response rate, and the horizontal line at 100% represents the control level. The solid line represents punished responses, and the broken line unpunished responses. Each point shows the mean response of 5 rats. (Reproduced by courtesy of Dr. J. Sepinwall.)

horizontal line at 100% represents the control level. The abscissa shows the drug dose in milligrams per kilogram (by mouth). The experimental points are mean values for groups of 5 rats. The dashed line shows the response of the animals during the unpunished component. Diazepam has almost no effect up to 10 mg/kg. There is a slight reduction in response rate at 20 mg/kg, and a marked reduction at 40 mg/kg. This reduction in rate represents the depressant effect of higher doses of the compound.

A different story is told by the solid line, which shows the response rate during the punished component of the schedule. An increased response rate is evident at 1.25 mg/kg. The rate increases with dose up to 20 mg/kg; the rate with this dose is over 3 times the control rate. This form of disinhibition is referred to as the anticonflict effect of the drug. At 40 mg/kg the rate is close to the control level; at this dose the anticonflict effect is giving way to the depressant effect.

The anticonflict effect seems to be a specific attribute of antianxiety agents, since it is not observed with other psychotropic agents such as *d*-amphetamine, chlorpromazine, or morphine. Furthermore, there is a good correlation between the minimum effective doses in the rat conflict test and the clinical doses used in treating psychoneurotic patients (Cook and Davidson, 1973).

A. Biochemistry and Behavior

In recent years, psychopharmacologists have tried to determine the biochemical basis of the behavioral effects of benzodiazepines. One of the first studies of this type was by Stein *et al.* (1973). As described in Section II, these authors found evidence that the depressant effects of benzodiazepines may be related to changes in norepinephrine turnover, and the anticonflict (antianxiety?) effects to changes in serotonin turnover.

Basing their work on these findings, Quenzer and Feldman (1975) tested the effects of chronic administration of chlordiazepoxide on three models of aggressive behavior in the rat.

1. The mouse-killing response of rats was blocked by a single dose of chlordiazepoxide, 50 mg/kg, i.p. Tolerance developed on successive days of dosing, predrug activity returning by the seventh day.

2. Shock-induced aggression (SIA) refers to fighting between members of a pair of rats placed on a grid through which electric shocks are delivered to their paws. Fighting was reduced by a single dose of chlordiazepoxide, 15 mg/kg, i.p. No tolerance developed during 10 days of daily dosing.

3. Septal rage refers to the increased irritability of rats with lesions in the septal area of the brain. The rage response was reduced by a single

dose of chlordiazepoxide, 25 mg/kg, i.p. No tolerance developed during 3 consecutive days of drug treatment.

These results suggest that the reduction of mouse-killing by chlordiazepoxide might be related to changes in norepinephrine turnover, whereas the effects on SIA and on septal rage might be related to changes in serotonin turnover. To test for a possible role of serotonin in the action of chlordiazepoxide on SIA, Quenzer and Feldman gave the drug to rats treated with either a precursor or an agonist of serotonin. If the action of the drug involved blockade of serotonin synthesis, the blockade might be overcome by pretreatment with the serotonin precursor 5-hydroxytryptophan. If the action of the drug involved blockade of serotonin receptors, the blockade might be overcome by the serotonin agonist α-methyltryptamine. Neither the precursor nor the agonist reversed the reduction in SIA induced by chlordiazepoxide. Hence these experiments provide no support for the hypothesis that the action of chlordiazepoxide on SIA depends on changes in the rate of serotonin turnover.

Graeff (1974) investigated the possible roles of serotonin, acetylcholine, and histamine in the anticonflict action of the benzodiazepines. The effects of chlordiazepoxide were compared with those of two serotonin antagonists (cyproheptadine and methysergide), atropine, pentobarbital, and three antihistaminics. The tests were made on rats performing under a conflict schedule in which lever pressing for water was concurrently suppressed by electric shock. Five of the eight compounds increased the rate of responding. The maximum increase in rate for each drug and the dose at which it occurred are listed in Table I. The antihistaminics depressed the rate of responding.

The large increases in rate produced by the serotonin antagonists suggest that blockade of central serotonin receptors may be involved in the release of behavior suppressed by punishment. The smaller increase pro-

TABLE I

COMPOUNDS INCREASING THE RATE OF RESPONDING IN ANTICONFLICT EXPERIMENTS ON RATS[a]

Compound	Dose (mg/kg, i.p.)	Maximum rate increase as % of control
Chlordiazepoxide	5.6	248
Cyproheptadine	5.6	218
Pentobarbital	10	192
Methysergide	3	163
Atropine	3	136

[a] Graeff (1974).

duced by atropine suggests that blockade of central muscarinic synapses may play a similar but smaller role. These mechanisms may be involved in the release of punishment-suppressed behavior by chlordiazepoxide and pentobarbital (cf. Cook and Sepinwall, 1975, discussed in the following).

The possible role of cholinergic systems in the behavioral effects of benzodiazepines was investigated by Miczek (1973). The strategy was to compare the effects of chlordiazepoxide and scopolamine in a variety of behavioral situations; if blocking of muscarinic synapses is involved in the action of chlordiazepoxide, the effects of the two drugs in each situation should be similar.

Rats were placed on a multiple schedule involving an unpunished component in which lever presses were rewarded with food pellets, and a punished component in which every lever press produced both a food pellet and an electric shock. The rate of unpunished responding was significantly decreased by scopolamine at 0.5–1 mg/kg, i.p., whereas chlordiazepoxide at 10–33 mg/kg, i.m., had no significant effect. The rate of punished responding was significantly decreased by scopolamine at 0.5 and 1 mg/kg, whereas chlordiazepoxide at 25 and 33 mg/kg produced a significant increase in rate.

In a further test, Miczek trained squirrel monkeys to obtain dextrose solution by licking a tube. The response was then suppressed by administering an electric shock each time a monkey licked the tube. The intake was significantly increased by scopolamine at 0.02 mg/kg, but was decreased at 0.1 and 0.5 mg/kg. By contrast, chlordiazepoxide showed a dose-related increase at 1, 5, and 10 mg/kg. The effects of scopolamine differed from those of chlordiazepoxide in three different situations. Miczek concluded that the effects of these compounds do not resemble each other sufficiently to infer a common mechanism of action (cf. Ghoneim and Mewaldt, 1977, discussed in Section V,C).

What role do catecholamines play in the behavioral effects of benzodiazepines? Beer and Lenard (1975) treated rats with intracerebroventricular 6-hydroxydopamine, thereby depleting brain norepinephrine by 91% and brain dopamine by 73%. The rats showed marked decrements in shock-avoidance behavior. These decrements were largely eliminated by injection of diazepam, 3 mg/kg, i.p. Hence, at least in this situation, the restoration of previously suppressed responding by diazepam does not depend on intact catecholaminergic systems.

The influence of a variety of biochemical mechanisms on the behavioral effects of benzodiazepines was described by Cook and Sepinwall (1975). Observations were made on rats trained on a multiple schedule that included punished (conflict) and unpunished components. The biochemical background is discussed in Section III.

1. *Phosphodiesterase Inhibition*

No consistent relationship was found between the activity of nine benzodiazepines as phosphodiesterase inhibitors and their activity in the rat anticonflict test.

2. *Glycine Receptors*

The attachment of compounds to glycine receptors is measured in terms of their displacement of strychnine binding *in vitro*. There was no significant correlation between the strychnine displacement data for ten benzodiazepines and their activity in the rat anticonflict test.

3. *γ-Aminobutyric Acid*

Aminooxyacetic acid raises brain GABA levels through inhibition of GABA transaminase. No anticonflict activity was seen when AOAA was administered to rats, nor was there any evidence of synergism between diazepam and AOAA. These experiments use only one approach to study a possible role of GABA in the anticonflict activity of benzodiazepines. Nevertheless, Cook and Sepinwall suggest that, although GABA may be involved in the relaxant, ataxic, and anticonvulsant effects of benzodiazepines, "no evidence currently exists for a role in the anticonflict (antianxiety) activity" (cf. Stein *et al.*, 1975, discussed next).

4. *Serotonin*

In some (but not all) experiments, pretreatment of rats with the serotonin depletor *p*-chlorophenylalanine (PCPA) blocked the anticonflict activity of chlordiazepoxide. Two serotonin antagonists, cinanserin and methysergide, showed distinct anticonflict activity; additive effects were seen when methysergide was given in combination with chlordiazepoxide. These and other experiments suggest that "serotonin may have a role in the antianxiety properties of benzodiazepines."

Stein *et al.* (1975) suggested that benzodiazepines may affect serotonin-containing neurons indirectly. The primary action may be on GABA-containing neurons; increased release of GABA might cause decreased release of serotonin. This hypothesis was tested in rats by injection of the GABA antagonist picrotoxin. At a dose of 2 mg/kg, picrotoxin significantly reduced the rate of punished responding with oxazepam, whereas there was no significant effect on the rate of unpunished responding. These preliminary results are consistent with the hypothesis that some of the effects of benzodiazepines on serotonin-containing neurons are mediated by GABA.

B. Neuropharmacology and Behavior

Some relationships between the effects of chlordiazepoxide on neuronal activity and on conflict behavior were observed by Umemoto and Olds (1975). Their experiments were made on rats with recording electrodes chronically implanted in four brain areas (amygdala, hippocampus, hypothalamus, geniculate nuclei). An electrode in the central gray region was used for aversive stimulation. The animals were first trained to press a lever for food reinforcement. They were then habituated to a 10-second flash of light; this was later used as a conditioned stimulus (CS). Finally, an 0.2-second electrical stimulation in the central gray region was applied at the end of each CS. After some experience with this aversive stimulation, the rats stopped pressing the lever during the CS.

Chlordiazepoxide (5 and 10 mg/kg, i.p.) restored lever pressing in about half of the animals. The background rate of discharge (neuronal activity during the 10 seconds preceding the CS) showed a dose-related decrease in the amygdala and hypothalamus. The peak effect was 16–35 minutes after drug injection, which was also the time when behavioral disinhibition was most often observed. The rate of discharge during presentation of the CS was significantly reduced in the amygdala by both doses of chlordiazepoxide, and in the hippocampus by the higher dose. Peak effects occurred 6–35 minutes after injection.

Chlorpromazine, which was tested at 1 and 2 mg/kg, produced no behavioral disinhibition. The background rate of discharge showed a dose-related decrease in the hypothalamus and geniculate nuclei. The principal effect on discharge during presentation of the CS was a reduced rate in the hippocampus following injection of the higher dose.

Diazepam was also tested in these experiments. The results were somewhat irregular, possibly because of the low solubility of this compound in aqueous media.

In summary, chlordiazepoxide produced behavioral disinhibition. At the same time it decreased background discharge in the amygdala and hypothalamus, and CS-related discharge in the amygdala and hippocampus. Chlorpromazine, which did not cause behavioral disinhibition, decreased background discharge in the hypothalamus and geniculate nuclei, and CS-related discharge in the hippocampus. These data imply that there may be some correlation between the reduced rate of discharge of neurons in the amygdala and the disinhibitory action of chlordiazepoxide. Furthermore, the reduced discharge rate of these neurons during the period of behavioral disinhibition suggests that there is some correlation between their normal activity and behavioral inhibition (other studies on the amygdala are described in Section IV,E).

Simultaneous measurement of drug effects on behavior and on neuronal activity is an important contribution to pharmacology. Umemoto and Olds (1975) conclude that their findings "point in the direction that future work will have to take" in order to explain the neuropharmacological basis of the antianxiety effects of the benzodiazepines.

C. Effects on Learning and Memory

Several clinical studies have tested benzodiazepines as amnesic agents to impair the memory of painful procedures (e.g., Frumin *et al.*, 1976; George and Dundee, 1977). In a study using healthy volunteers, Ghoneim and Mewaldt (1977) found that neither diazepam (0.3 mg/kg, i.v.) nor scopolamine (8 μg/kg, i.m.) affected the recall of information learned prior to drug administration. By contrast, both compounds impaired the learning of new material. Physostigmine (32 μg/kg, i.m.) antagonized the memory deficits produced by scopolamine but not those produced by diazepam. Evidently, the amnesic action of scopolamine involves a cholinergic system, whereas that of diazepam involves a different mechanism (cf. Miczek, 1973, in Section V,A). However, much further work with other compounds and in other situations will be necessary before the full significance of these findings will be apparent.

Only a few workers have tested the effects of benzodiazepines on learning and memory in animals. Soubrie *et al.* (1976) studied rats that were placed for 1 minute in an enclosure in which they could receive unavoidable electric shock. The rats were then returned to their home cages. The test session occurred 4 days later, when the animals were placed in the enclosure for 3 minutes without shock. Undrugged controls that had received shocks showed a 78% decrease in mobility in comparison with controls that had received no shocks. A dose-related reversal of this inhibition was seen with chlordiazepoxide, diazepam, and lorazepam, but not with chlorpromazine. The reversal occurred if diazepam (10 mg/kg, i.p.) was administered 2 minutes before the shock session, but not if it was administered 2 minutes after the session. Soubrie *et al.* suggest that the benzodiazepines may act on the registration phase of the memory process (note that both Ghoneim and Mewaldt in man and Soubrie *et al.* in the rat found that diazepam impaired the learning of material presented after drug administration).

A different type of study is that of Fox *et al.* (1977). These authors present evidence that benzodiazepines "enhance adult learning when administered at low doses during early development." Six benzodiazepines were tested in mice. Three treatment groups were used for each drug (with appropriate controls):

Group F received the drug *in utero* only, the compound being administered in the diet to the gravid females. At birth the pups were fostered to untreated mothers.

Group C received the drug *in utero* and during lactation, the pups being nursed by their treated mothers. Weaning occurred at 3 weeks of age.

Group D received the same treatment as Group C, but in addition the pups received the drug in their diet during the fourth and fifth weeks of life.

No further drug treatment was given. At 12 weeks of age the adult males were tested in a Y-maze. They were trained to use either the right or the left arm of the maze to receive a food reward. The criterion of learning was five consecutive correct choices.

The results with chlordiazepoxide (0.3 mg/gm food) were representative of the six compounds. Treatment caused an apparent enhancement of learning, which was maximal in Group F and then declined as the length of drug exposure increased. This was shown by both the percent of mice reaching criterion (control, 68.2–70.6; Group F, 89.7; Group C, 81.8; Group D, 73.5) and by the mean number of trials to criterion (control, 21.06–22.84; Group F, 14.00; Group C, 15.73; Group D, 21.79). Motor activity, as measured by the mean latency and duration of response, showed no tendency to decline with increasing exposure to the drug.

Fox *et al.* conclude that drug effects on learning ability and on motor activity follow different time courses. They note that "the facilitation of learning may be due to drug effects on emotional and/or motivational processes, rather than learning per se." At this time it would be futile to speculate further on the results of this pioneer study.

D. Social Relationships

Although psychoactive agents are often used to improve the social adaptation of patients, there has been little study of the effects of these agents on social behavior in animals. Earlier studies showed that benzodiazepines decreased aggression in rodents (Valzelli, 1973) and in primates (Delgado, 1973). However, under certain conditions aggression might be increased (DiMascio, 1973).

In a later paper, Zwirner *et al.* (1975) studied aggression between groups of mice. Three male mice were placed in each half of a cage divided in the middle by an opaque barrier. During a separation period of 21 days, one mouse in each group became dominant. On removal of the partition, the mice first sniffed each other and then engaged in "tail rattling" and in vicious fighting. The fighting was usually between the two dominant mice, or between a dominant mouse of one group and a submissive mouse of the other group.

Intergroup aggression was inhibited by five out of six known compounds. The ED_{50}'s were chlorpromazine, 2.2, *d*-amphetamine, 3.2, atropine, 6.2; pentobarbital, 10, and imipramine 24 (mg/kg, p.o.). In contrast to these agents, chlordiazepoxide (0.3, 1, and 3 mg/kg) caused a marked increase in fighting. Zwirner *et al.* suggest that "chlordiazepoxide may have a biphasic effect on aggressive behavior, an initial stimulating effect at low doses, perhaps due to response disinhibition, and a depressive effect at higher doses which runs parallel with increased muscular relaxation and generalized behavioral depression."

Other workers studied drug effects on social relationships in primates. Delgado *et al.* (1976) observed the effects of diazepam in 4 rhesus monkeys. The monkeys were tested alone, when paired with a submissive partner, and when paired with a dominant partner. Measurements were made on spontaneous mobility and on the number of food pellets consumed. Diazepam in doses of 0.1 and 0.3 mg/kg, p.o., had no significant effect on these parameters when the monkeys were tested alone or in a dominant relationship. By contrast, these doses caused significant reductions in both mobility and pellet consumption when the same monkeys were tested in a submissive relationship. For example, when the monkeys were tested alone, the mean numbers of pellets consumed in a 15-minute session were 23 in control tests, and 27 after diazepam 0.1 mg/kg. When the monkeys were in a dominant relationship the corresponding figures were 15 and 15, and in a submissive relationship 7 and 1 ($p < .01$). These experiments indicate that the effect of a compound may vary with the social relationship of the subjects.

Kamioka *et al.* (1977) studied the effects of drugs on "socially induced suppression and aggression" in pairs of male monkeys (*Macaca fascicularis*). A hungry monkey, seated in a restraining chair, was trained to press a lever for food reward. At certain periods, a second monkey, also seated in a restraining chair, was placed face to face to the first monkey, but just out of reach (Fig. 10). During a 7-minute safe period, there was no interaction between the monkeys. During a 3-minute agonistic period, every lever press of the instigator monkey not only resulted in receipt of food reward but also delivered an electric shock to the tail of the attacker monkey.

In control tests, the attacker monkeys displayed threatening behavior during the agonistic periods; lever pressing by the instigator monkeys was completely suppressed. This suppression was reduced by treatment of the instigators with cloxazolam or diazepam at 0.2 mg/kg, p.o., and by chlordiazepoxide or oxazolam at 2 mg/kg. Thus in the hour before administration of diazepam the number of lever presses for 2 monkeys during the safe and agonistic periods was 1605 and 0; in the hour after administra-

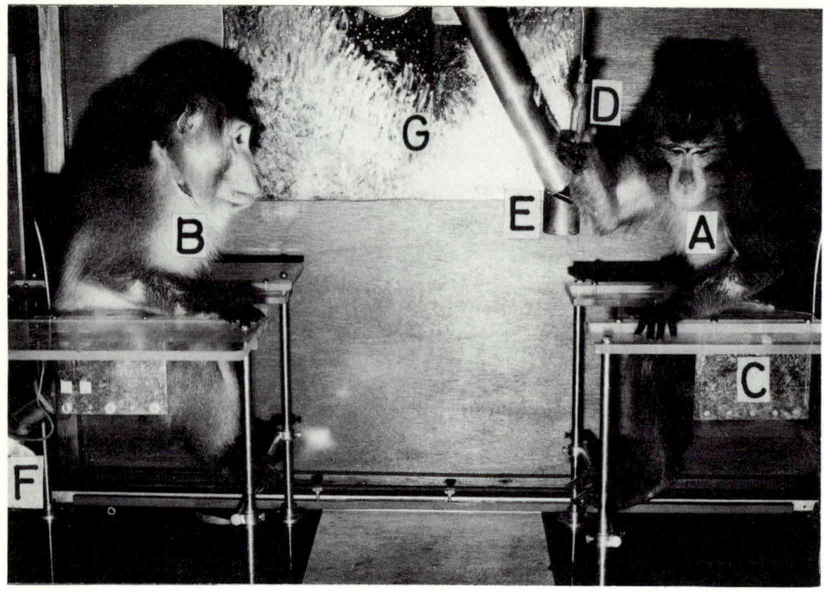

FIG. 10. Inside view of chamber for studying socially induced suppression and aggression in monkeys. (A) instigator; (B) attacker; (C) primate chairs; (D) lever; (E) food dispenser; (F) electrodes; (G) one-way window. (From Kamioka *et al.*, 1977. Reproduced by courtesy of the authors and publisher.)

tion, the corresponding figures were 1830 and 184. When these compounds were administered to the attacker monkeys, there was no change in the lever responses of the instigators. No increase in the number of responses was observed when chlorpromazine (5 mg/kg) and imipramine (10 mg/kg) were given to either the instigators or the attackers.

These experiments involved "socially induced suppression of reinforced responses." This suppression was attenuated by antianxiety agents but not by an antipsychotic or an antidepressant agent. Hence this test may provide "a sensitive measure for evaluating the actions of antianxiety drugs."

The last report in this section describes "diazepam treatment of socially isolated monkeys" (Noble *et al.*, 1976). Monkeys that are reared in total social isolation for 6 or more months show persistent behavioral abnormalities. These include self-directed responses such as self-clasping and rocking, as well as lack of normal exploration and play. Previous studies suggested that rehabilitation of these animals might depend on reduction of anxiety. Noble *et al.*, therefore, tested the effects of diazepam in 3 monkeys. The compound was administered twice daily at a dose of 2 mg/kg by nasogastric intubation; therapy lasted for 3 months. During the first month (eighth month of isolation) the monkeys remained in their isolation chambers; during the second month each animal was placed in a wire cage in which it could see and hear other monkeys but not touch them; during the third month the monkeys were taken twice daily in groups of 3 to a playroom for 30-minute sessions. For 9 months, beginning 1 month predrug and ending 5 months postdrug, the animals were observed twice daily for 10-minute periods; scoring was based on thirty-one behavioral categories.

The results indicated that these social isolates can be partially rehabilitated with diazepam. Two of the 3 monkeys showed significant reductions in self-disturbance behavior, and increases in environmental exploration and in social responses. Relapse followed discontinuation of drug therapy. The results were superior to those obtained in a previous study with chlorpromazine.

Noble *et al.* believe that the efficacy of diazepam in 2 out of 3 subjects indicates that this technique deserves further study as an animal model of anxiety. The failure of the third monkey to respond to drug treatment presents a problem for future research.

VI. Discussion

The previous sections outline what we know about the biochemistry and pharmacology of the benzodiazepines. The next few paragraphs emphasize *what we don't know about the benzodiazepines.*

At the ionic level, our ignorance is almost complete. As already mentioned (Section III,A), the precise mechanism of action of benzodiazepines at the biochemical level is unknown. At the neuropharmacological level, some of the earlier studies described in Section II still require explanation. What is the mechanism of the triphasic action of chlordiazepoxide reported by Moe *et al.* (1962)? What systems are involved in the suppression of the stimulation induced by tetrabenazine in rats that have been pretreated with iproniazid (Zbinden and Randall, 1967)?

More recent studies in neuropharmacology raise further problems. Is presynaptic inhibition involved in the actions of benzodiazepines throughout the CNS or only in certain parts of it? If the benzodiazepines increase presynaptic inhibition, how can we account for signs of facilitation such as the increased EEG frequencies and the behavioral disinhibition produced by these compounds? Are different areas of the brain involved in each of the various actions of the benzodiazepines?

Unsolved problems in psychopharmacology include the following:

How are the effects of benzodiazepines on conflict behavior related to reported effects on aggression, on learning, and on social behavior? What roles do the various neurohumors play in each of these actions? What brain areas are involved? Collaboration between biochemical pharmacologists, neuropharmacologists, and psychopharmacologists may help to solve these problems.

A. CNS, Behavior, and Anxiety

Recent studies indicate that all activity in the CNS is a "dynamic interplay of excitation and inhibition" (Roberts, 1974). Excitatory neurons are often held in check by the tonic activity of inhibitory neurons; when the inhibition ceases, the tonic activity of the excitatory neuron is released. Such disinhibition may be "one of the major organizing principles in nervous system function."

Disinhibition often involves the activity of chains of inhibitory neurons. Thus in the cerebellum the basket cells inhibit the Purkinje cells, which in turn inhibit excitatory cells. The consequences of this arrangement may be shown by the following diagram, in which neurons A_i and B_i are inhibitory, and C_e is excitatory:

$$\rightarrow A_i \rightarrow B_i \rightarrow C_e \rightarrow$$

Assume that under resting conditions A_i is inactive and B_i exerts a tonic inhibitory influence on C_e. On appropriate stimulation, A_i will be activated, thereby inhibiting B_i, which in turn will disinhibit C_e.

Let us assume that GABA is the transmitter released at the terminals of neurons A_i and B_i. Under certain conditions, stimulation of A_i will not release sufficient GABA to inhibit B_i. If benzodiazepines enhance the synaptic activity of GABA, treatment with these compounds will produce inhibition of B_i and disinhibition of C_e. Such disinhibition may account for the increases in EEG frequency and in conflict responding seen in animals following moderate doses of benzodiazepines.

The foregoing assumptions may be illustrated by the experiments of Umemoto and Olds (1975) (Section V,B). These authors studied rats in which responding for food during the presentation of a signal had been suppressed. This suppressed response was restored following administration of chlordiazepoxide; at the same time there was a reduction in the discharge rate of certain neurons in the amygdala.

The initial action of chlordiazepoxide might be on the receptors isolated by Squires and Braestrup (1977). This action, in turn, might enhance the sensitivity of GABA receptors on neuron B_i, so that this neuron could now be inhibited by GABA released from neuron A_i. Inhibition of neuron

B_i (located in the amygdala) could disinhibit neuron C_e, which might be a unit in a brainstem facilitatory system. This could begin a process leading to the restoration of the suppressed behavior.

In addition to the disinhibitory effects of moderate doses of benzodiazepines, there are depressant effects following higher doses (see Fig. 9). These depressant effects might be caused by a direct action of the drugs on neuron C_e. They might also occur if receptors on neuron C_e developed an increased sensitivity to GABA released from B_i or other inhibitory neurons. Of course, the three-neuron chain described here is highly simplified; in reality many more neurons would be involved.

How do these laboratory findings apply to the clinical effects of benzodiazepines? Relaxant, hypnotic, and anticonvulsant effects appear to be depressant in nature. Such effects could be caused either by decreased activity of excitatory neurons or increased activity of inhibitory neurons. Laboratory experiments suggest that an increase in GABA-mediated presynaptic inhibition may be involved. The role of such inhibition in the clinical situation has not yet been determined.

The major unsolved problem with the benzodiazepines is the mechanism of their anxiolytic effect. Experiments described at the beginning of Section V indicate that anticonflict activity seems to be a specific attribute of the benzodiazepines. There is a good correlation between the anticonflict potency of anxiolytics in the laboratory and their potency in the treatment of psychoneurotic patients. As the anticonflict activity of these agents is disinhibitory in nature, this correlation suggests that the antianxiety action is also disinhibitory in nature.

A different view comes from a clinical study by Lehmann and Ban (1970). These authors observed that the initial effect of anxiolytics tended to be "a state of behavioral excitation and facilitation, accompanied by mild euphoria and, sometimes, increased aggressiveness." They attributed these effects to "cortical disinhibition." Following this initial phase, the anxiolytics exerted their "behavioral or emotional inhibition." This study suggests that the disinhibitory phase of the benzodiazepines is a side effect; the anxiolytic action may lie in the inhibitory phase.

These two views of the anxiolytic action of the benzodiazepines may provide some insight into the nature of clinical anxiety. If the antianxiety action is disinhibitory in nature, then at least some forms of clinical anxiety may be correlated with increased central inhibition. If the antianxiety action is inhibitory in nature, then some forms of clinical anxiety may be correlated with decreased central inhibition. These relationships may become clearer when we know more about the roles of inhibition and disinhibition in the CNS. The benzodiazepines may provide a useful tool for this study.

B. Possible Mechanisms of Action

Finally, we here present our current speculations as to the mechanisms of action of the benzodiazepines:

1. The relaxant action seems to involve potentiation of the effects of GABA, which produces increased presynaptic inhibition. Similar mechanisms may be involved in the anticonvulsant effects of benzodiazepines. The mechanism of the hypnotic effect is not yet known.
2. The anxiolytic effect may involve the binding of benzodiazepines to the receptors for an endogenous anxiogenic agent. This binding might block the activity of the endogenous agent.
3. This block may increase GABA activity, which, in turn, would inhibit neuronal systems in which serotonin, norepinephrine, and acetylcholine are transmitters. These systems may be involved in the responses of benzodiazepines observed in neuropharmacological and psychopharmacological tests. Presumably the endogenous agent would have the opposite effect, decreasing the activity of GABA and thereby increasing the activity of the other systems.
4. The antianxiety action of the benzodiazepines may be an inhibitory effect. Disinhibitory actions may be side effects, caused by the blocking of inhibitory neurons before the block extends to excitatory neurons.

Acknowledgments

We wish to thank Dr. Arnold B. Davidson for twice reading preliminary versions of this review and making many helpful suggestions. We also thank Ms. Linda Gregg for patiently typing the original version and its numerous revisions.

Addendum

Some interesting studies on the mechanisms of action of benzodiazepines were published during the second half of 1977.

Ionic Movement

Glass microelectrodes were inserted into single neurons of the sea hare *Aplysia californica*. Flurazepam and other benzodiazepines block the Cl^--dependent fast responses to acetylcholine but not K^+-dependent slow responses (Hoyer, 1977). Experiments with individual muscle fibers of the rat diaphragm indicate that "diazepam increases the resting permeability of the excitable membrane for chloride ions" (Vyskocil, 1977).

Binding Sites

Specific benzodiazepine binding sites are concentrated in the synaptosomal fraction of rat cerebral cortex (Möhler and Okada, 1977a). Some biochemical characteristics of these binding sites are described by Möhler and Okada (1977b) and by Bosmann *et al.* (1977). In human brain the highest densities of the binding sites are in cortical areas (Braestrup *et al.*, 1977).

Neurotransmitters

Several authors find that benzodiazepines potentiate neuronal responses to GABA. Chlordiazepoxide potentiates responses to GABA but not to glycine in neurons from chick spinal cord cultures (Choi *et al.*, 1977). Iontophoretic application of benzodiazepines to the hippocampus of the rat prolongs GABA-mediated recurrent inhibition (Wolf and Haas, 1977). Benzodiazepines have synergistic actions with GABA on single neurons in the sensorimotor cortex of the rabbit (Kozhechkin and Ostravskaya, 1977; Zakusov *et al.*, 1977).

In other experiments, diazepam increases GABA levels in the substantia nigra but not in the caudate nucleus or cingulate cortex of the rat (Pericic *et al.*, 1977). In rats pretreated with amphetamine, ipsilateral circling is induced by unilateral injection of chlordiazepoxide into the GABA-rich zona reticulata of the substantia nigra, but not into the GABA-poor zona compacta (Waddington and Longden, 1977). The action of diazepam in lowering the cGMP content of the rat cerebellum is attributed to activation of GABA receptors (Biggio *et al.*, 1977).

Neuropharmacology

Diazepam facilitates the excitatory input to Purkinje cells in the perfused cerebellum of the frog (Ben-Neria and Lass, 1977). Iontophoretic application of benzodiazepines to cerebellar Purkinje cells of the rat induces firing in a pattern of high-frequency bursts and silent periods (Boakes *et al.*, 1977). Diazepam (1 mg/kg, i.v.) blocks harmine-induced seizure patterns in the spinal cord of the rabbit but not in the cerebellum (de Trujillo *et al.*, 1977). In the hippocampus of the rat, iontophoretic application of medazepam depresses the firing of pyramidal and granule cells (Matthews and Connor, 1977).

Psychopharmacology

Selective lesions to serotoninergic forebrain pathways in the rat reverse the suppressive effects of punishment, suggesting that these pathways may be involved in the anticonflict action of benzodiazepines (Tye *et al.*, 1977). Bicuculline (1 mg/kg, s.c.) antagonizes the anticonflict action of diazepam (1 mg/kg, i.p.), in the rat. This suggests a possible "GABA involvement in the mechanisms of the anxiolytic action of benzodiazepines" (Zakusov *et al.*, 1977).

The behavioral effects of benzodiazepines are reviewed by Dantzer (1977). Experiments indicating a possible role of serotonin in the behavioral effects of benzodiazepines are reviewed by Stein *et al.* (1977), whereas experiments suggesting a role of both noradrenergic and serotoninergic mechanisms are reviewed by Gray (1977).

References

Beer, B., and Lenard, L. G. (1975). *Pharmacol., Biochem. Behav.* **3,** 879.

Ben-Neria, Y., and Lass, Y. (1977). *Experientia* **33,** 1484.

Biggio, G., Brodie, B. B., Costa, E., and Guidotti, A. (1977). *Proc. Natl. Acad. Sci. U.S.A.* **74,** 3592.

Bloom, F. E. (1977). *Am. J. Psychiatry* **134,** 669.

Boakes, R. J., Martin, I. L., and Mitchell, P. R. (1977). *Neuropharmacology* **16,** 711.

Bosmann, H. B., Case, K. R., and DiStefano, P. (1977). *FEBS Lett.* **82,** 368.

Braestrup, C., Albrechtsen, R., and Squires, R. F. (1977). *Nature (London)* **269,** 702.

Chase, T. N., Katz, R. I., and Kopin, I. J. (1970). *Neuropharmacology* **9,** 103.

Choi, D. W., Farb, D. H., and Fischbach, G. D. (1977). *Nature (London)* **269,** 342.

Consolo, S., Garattini, S., and Ladinsky, H. (1975). *In* "Mechanism of Action of Benzodiazepines" (E. Costa and P. Greengard, eds.), p. 63. Raven, New York.

Cook, L., and Davidson, A. B. (1973). *In* "The Benzodiazepines" (S. Garattini, E. Mussini, and L. O. Randall, eds.), p. 327. Raven, New York.

Cook, L., and Sepinwall, J. (1975). *In* "Mechanism of Action of Benzodiazepines" (E. Costa and P. Greengard, eds.), p. 1. Raven, New York.

Corrodi, H., Fuxe, K., Lidbrink, P., and Olson, L. (1971). *Brain Res.* **29,** 1.

Costa, E., and Greengard, P., eds. (1975). "Mechanism of Action of Benzodiazepines." Raven, New York.

Costa, E., Guidotti, A., Mao, C. C., and Suria, A. (1975). *Life Sci.* **17,** 167.

Curtis, D. R., and Johnston, G. A. R. (1974). *Ergeb. Physiol., Biol. Chem. Exp. Pharmakol.* **69,** 97.

Curtis, D. R., Game, C. J. A., and Lodge, D. (1976a). *Br. J. Pharmacol.* **56,** 307.

Curtis, D. R., Lodge, D., Johnston, G. A. R., and Brand, S. J. (1976b). *Brain Res.* **118,** 344.

Dalton, C., Crowley, H. J., Sheppard, H., and Schallek, W. (1974). *Proc. Soc. Exp. Biol. Med.* **145,** 407.

Dantzer, R. (1977). *Biobehav. Rev.* **1,** 71.

Delgado, J. M. R. (1973). *In* "The Benzodiazepines" (S. Garattini, E. Mussini, and L. O. Randall, eds.), p. 419. Raven, New York.

Delgado, J. M. R., Grau, C., Delgado-Garcia, J. M., and Rodero, J. M. (1976). *Neuropharmacology* **15,** 409.

de Trujillo, G. C., de Carolis, A. S., and Longo, V. G. (1977). *Neuropharmacology* **16,** 31.

DiMascio, A. (1973). *In* "The Benzodiazepines" (S. Garattini, E. Mussini, and L. O. Randall, eds.), p. 433. Raven, New York.

Dominic, J. A. (1973). *In* "Serotonin and Behavior" (J. D. Barchas and E. Usdin, eds.), p. 149. Academic Press, New York.

Dray, A., and Straughan, D. W. (1976). *J. Pharm. Pharmacol.* **28,** 314.

Eccles, J. C., Ito, M., and Szentágothai, J. (1967). "The Cerebellum as a Neuronal Machine." Springer-Verlag, Berlin and New York.

Esplin, D. W. (1957). *J. Pharmacol. Exp. Ther.* **120,** 301.

Fahn, S. (1976). *In* "GABA in Nervous System Function" (E. Roberts, T. N. Chase, and D. B. Tower, eds.), p. 169. Raven, New York.

Fonnum, F., Grofova, I., Rinvik, E., Storm-Mathisen, J., and Walberg, F. (1974). *Brain Res.* **71,** 77.

Fox, K. A., Abendschein, D. R., and Lahcen, R. B. (1977). *Pharmacol. Res. Commun.* **9,** 325.

Frumin, M. J., Herekar, V. R., and Jarvik, M. E. (1976). *Anesthesiology* **45,** 406.

Gähwiler, B. H. (1976). *Brain Res.* **107,** 176.

George, K. A., and Dundee, J. W. (1977). *Br. J. Clin. Pharmacol.* **4,** 45.

Ghoneim, M. M., and Mewaldt, S. P. (1977). *Psychopharmacology* **52,** 1.

Gilbert, J. C., and Wyllie, M. G. (1976). *Br. J. Pharmacol.* **56,** 49.

Graeff, F. G. (1974). *J. Pharmacol. Exp. Ther.* **189,** 344.

Gray, J. A. (1977). *Hand. Psychopharmacol.* **8,** 433.

Haefely, W., Kulcsar A., Mohler, H., Pieri, L., Polc, P., and Schaffner, R. (1975). *In* "Mechanism of Action of Benzodiazepines" (E. Costa and P. Greengard, eds.), p. 131. Raven, New York.

Harris, M., Hopkin, J. M., and Neal, M. J. (1973). *Br. J. Pharmacol.* **47,** 229.

Hoyer, J. (1977). *Pharmakopsychiatrie/Neuro-Psychopharmakol.* **10,** 271.

Iversen, L. L., and Johnston, G. A. R. (1971). *J. Neurochem.* **18,** 1939.

Iversen, L. L., and Schon, F. (1973). *In* "New Concepts in Neurotransmitter Regulation" (A. Mandell, ed.), p. 153. Plenum, New York.

Juhasz, L., and Dairman, W. (1977). *Fed. Proc. Fed. Am. Soc. Exp. Biol.* **36,** 377.

Julien, R. M. (1972). *Neuropharmacology* **11,** 683.

Kamioka, T., Nakayama, I., Akiyama, S., and Takagi, H. (1977). *Psychopharmacology* **52,** 17.

Kataoka, K., Bak, I. J., Hassler, R., Kim, J. S., and Wagner, A. (1974). *Exp. Brain Res.* **19,** 217.

Keim, K. L., and Sigg, E. B. (1977). *Pharmacol., Biochem. Behav.* **6,** 79.

Kozhechkin, S. N., and Ostrovskaya, R. U. (1977). *Nature (London)* **269,** 72.

Kunze, H., Bohn, E., and Bahrke, G. (1975). *J. Pharm. Pharmacol.* **27,** 880.

Lahti, R. A., and Barsuhn, C. (1974). *Psychopharmacologia* **35,** 215.

Lehmann, H. E., and Ban, T. A. (1970). "Pharmacotherapy of Tension and Anxiety." Thomas, Springfield, Illinois.

Lidbrink, P., and Farnebo, L.-O. (1973). *Neuropharmacology* **12,** 1087.

Lidbrink, P., Corrodi, H., and Fuxe, K. (1974). *Eur. J. Pharmacol.* **26,** 35.

Liebeswar, G. (1972). *Naunyn-Schmiedeberg's Arch. Pharmacol.* **275,** 445.

Lippa, A. S., Smith, W. V., and Greenblatt, E. N. (1977). *Fed. Proc., Fed. Am. Soc. Exp. Biol.* **36,** 1044.

Mao, C. C., Guidotti, A., and Costa, E. (1974). *Mol. Pharmacol.* **10,** 736.

Mao, C. C., Guidotti, A., and Costa, E. (1975). *Naunyn-Schmiedeberg's Arch. Pharmacol.* **289,** 369.

Mao, C. C., Marco, E., Revuelta, A., Bertilsson, L., and Costa, E. (1977). *Biol. Psychiatry* **12,** 359.

Matthews, W. D., and Connor, J. D. (1977). *J. Pharmacol. Exp. Ther.* **201,** 613.

Miczek, K. A. (1973). *Psychopharmacologia* **28,** 373.
Moe, R., Bagdon, R. E., and Zbinden, G. (1962). *Angiology* **13,** 4.
Möhler, H., and Okada, T. (1977a). *Science* **198,** 849.
Möhler, H., and Okada, T. (1977b). *Life Sci.* **20,** 2101.
Nagy, J., and Decsi, L. (1973). *Neuropharmacology* **12,** 757.
Noble, A. B., McKinney, W. T., Jr., Mohr, C., and Moran, E. (1976). *Am. J. Psychiatry* **133,** 1165.
Norton, A. C. (1973). "The Dorsal Column System of the Spinal Cord—An Updated Review." Brain Inf. Serv., Brain Res. Inst., University of California, Los Angeles.
Olsen, R. W., Lamar, E. E., and Bayless, J. D. (1977). *J. Neurochem.* **28,** 299.
Pericic, D., Walters, J. R., and Chase, T. N. (1977). *J. Neurochem.* **29,** 839.
Pieri, L., and Haefely, W. (1976). *Naunyn-Schmiedeberg's Arch. Pharmacol.* **296,** 1.
Polc, P., and Haefely, W. (1976). *Naunyn-Schmiedeberg's Arch. Pharmacol.* **294,** 121.
Polc, P., Möhler, H., and Haefely, W. (1974). *Naunyn-Schmiedeberg's Arch. Pharmacol.* **284,** 319.
Pryzybyla, A. C., and Wang, S. C. (1968). *J. Pharmacol. Exp. Ther.* **163,** 439.
Quenzer, L. F., and Feldman, R. S. (1975). *Neuropsychopharmacol. Proc. Congr. Coll. Int. Neuropsychopharmacol., 9th, 1974* Excerpta Med. Int. Congr. Ser. No. 359, p. 890.
Randall, L. O., Schallek, W., Heise, G. A., Keith, E. F., and Bagdon, R. E. (1960). *J. Pharmacol. Exp. Ther.* **129,** 163.
Randall, L. O., Heise, G. A., Schallek, W., Bagdon, R. E., Banziger, R., Boris, A., Moe, R. A., and Abrams, W. B. (1961). *Curr. Ther. Res., Clin. Exp.* **3,** 405.
Randall, L. O., Schallek, W., Sternbach, L. H., and Ning, R. Y. (1974). *In* "Psychopharmacological Agents" (M. Gordon, ed.), Vol. 3, p. 175. Academic Press, New York.
Roberts, E. (1974). *Biochem. Pharmacol.* **23,** 2637.
Ruch-Monachon, M. A., Jalfre, M., and Haefely, W. (1976). *Arch. Int. Pharmacodyn. Ther.* **219,** 308.
Sawaya, M. C. B., Horton, R. W., and Meldrum, B. S. (1975). *Epilepsia* **16,** 649.
Schallek, W., and Johnson, T. C. (1976). *Arch. int. Pharmacodyn. Ther.* **223,** 301.
Schallek, W., Schlosser, W., and Randall, L. O. (1972). *Adv. Pharmacol. Chemother.* **10,** 119.
Schlosser, W., Zavatsky, E., Kappell, B., and Sigg, E. B. (1973). *Pharmacologist* **15,** 162.
Schlosser, W., Franco, S., and Kuehn, A. (1977). *7th Annu. Meet., Soc. Neurosci., 1977 Abstracts,* p. 414.
Schmidt, R. F., Vogel, M. E., and Zimmermann, M. (1967). *Naunyn-Schmiedebergs Arch. Pharmakol. Exp. Pathol.* **258,** 69.
Schultz, J. (1974). *J. Neurochem.* **22,** 685.
Snyder, S. H., and Enna, S. J. (1975). *In* "Mechanism of Action of Benzodiazepines" (E. Costa and P. Greengard, eds.), p. 81. Raven, New York.
Soubrie, P., Simon, P., and Boissier, J. R. (1976). *Experientia* **32,** 359.
Squires, R., and Braestrup, C. (1977). *Nature (London)* **266,** 732.
Stein, L., Wise, C. D., and Berger, B. D. (1973). *In* "The Benzodiazepines" (S. Garattini, E. Mussini, and L. O. Randall, eds.), p. 299. Raven, New York.
Stein, L., Wise, C. D., and Belluzzi, J. D. (1975). *In* "Mechanism of Action of Benzodiazepines" (E. Costa and P. Greengard, eds.), p. 29. Raven, New York.
Stein, L., Wise, C. D., and Belluzzi, J. D. (1977). *Handb. Psychopharmacol.* **8,** 25–53.
Steiner, F. A., and Felix, D. (1976). *Nature (London)* **260,** 346.
Stratten, W. P., and Barnes, C. D. (1971). *Neuropharmacology* **10,** 685.
Suria, A., and Costa, E. (1973). *Brain Res.* **50,** 235.
Suria, A., and Costa, E. (1975). *Brain Res.* **87,** 102.

Suria, A., Lehne, R., and Costa, E. (1975). *Neuropsychopharmacol., Proc. Congr. Coll. Int. Neuropsychopharmaco., 9th, 1974* Exerpta Med. Int. Congr. Ser. No. 359, p. 729.
Swinyard, E. A., and Castellion, A. W. (1966). *J. Pharmacol. Exp. Ther.* **151,** 369.
Taylor, K. M., and Laverty, R. (1969). *Eur. J. Pharmacol.* **8,** 296.
Tye, N. C., Everitt, B. J., and Iversen, S. D. (1977). *Nature (London)* **268,** 741.
Umemoto, M., and Olds, M. E. (1975). *Neuropharmacology* **14,** 413.
Valzelli, L. (1973). *In* "The Benzodiazepines" (S. Garattini, E. Mussini, and L. O. Randall, eds.), p. 405. Raven, New York.
Vyskocil, F. (1977). *Brain Res.* **133,** 315.
Waddington, J. L., and Longden, A. (1977). *Naunyn-Schmiedeberg's Arch. Pharmacol.* **300,** 233.
Walberg, F. (1965). *Exp. Neurol.* **13,** 218.
Warburton, D. M. (1974). *Int. Pharmacopsychiatry* **9,** 189.
Wise, C. D., Berger, B. D., and Stein, L. (1972). *Science* **177,** 180.
Wolf, P., and Haas, H. L. (1977). *Naunyn-Schmiedeberg's Arch. Pharmacol.* **299,** 211.
Young, A. B., Zukin, S. R., and Snyder, S. H. (1974). *Proc. Natl. Acad. Sci. U.S.A.* **71,** 2246.
Zakusov, V. V., Ostrovskaya, R. U., Markovitch, V. V., Molodavkin, G. M., and Bulayev, V. M. (1975). *Arch. Int. Pharmacodyn. Ther.* **214,** 188.
Zakusov, V. V., Ostrovskaya, R. U., Kozhechkin, S. N., Markovich, V. V., Molodavkin, G. M., and Voronina, T. A. (1977). *Arch. Int. Pharmacodyn. Ther.* **229,** 313.
Zbinden, G., and Randall, L. O. (1967). *Adv. Pharmacol.* **5,** 213.
Zsilla, G., Cheney, D. L., and Costa, E. (1976). *Naunyn-Schmiedeberg's Arch. Pharmacol.* **294,** 251.
Zwirner, P. P., Porsolt, R. D., and Loew, D. M. (1975). *Psychopharmacologia* **45,** 133.

ADVANCES IN PHARMACOLOGY AND CHEMOTHERAPY, VOL. 16

Resistance of Animal Helminths to Anthelmintics

J. D. KELLY* AND C. A. HALL†

I. Introduction 90
II. Definitions 91
A. Resistance 91
B. Resistance Factors 95
C. Reversion 95
D. Side-Resistance 95
E. Cross-Resistance 95
III. Occurrence of Anthelmintic Resistance 95
A. Sheep 95
B. Cattle 99
C. Horses 100
D. Miscellaneous 102
IV. Physiological Characteristics of Resistant Helminths 103
A. Infectivity and Pathogenicity 104
B. Side- and Cross-Resistance 105
C. Biochemical Aspects 110
V. Selection for Resistance 114
A. Cambendazole Selection of *Haemonchus contortus* 114
B. Glenfield Study 116
C. Armidale Study 117
D. Relationship between Resistance and Inhibited Parasite Development . 117
E. Reversion 118
VI. Diagnosis of Resistance 119
A. Fecal Egg Counts 119
B. Egg Embryonation 120
C. Larval Culture 120
D. Critical Tests 121
VII. Control of Resistant Helminths 122
A. Recommendations for Use of Anthelmintics 122
B. Standards for Anthelmintic Activity 124
VIII. Conclusions 125
References 126

* Department of Veterinary Pathology, University of Sydney, Sydney, Australia 2006.
† New South Wales Department of Agriculture, Veterinary Research Station, Glenfield, New South Wales, Australia 2167.

ISBN 0-12-032916-6

I. Introduction

Healthy livestock represent one of man's most valuable renewable resources. They provide high-quality edible protein, fibers of all types, leather, an enormous variety of useful by-products, and, in the developing countries, motive power and fuel. In order to maintain an adequate supply of such products, given the current rate of increase in human population (4 billion in 1976 to 6.5 billion in the year 2000), it has been estimated that the efficiency of ruminant production will have to be increased by at least 50% over the next two decades (Byerly, 1977). This improvement in production efficiency will have to be achieved without increasing the arable land areas currently used for livestock and without substantially adding to present animal numbers.

The annual world mortality losses from disease are estimated to exceed 50 million cattle and buffalo and 100 million sheep and goats. The effects of nonfatal disease in terms of production loss are extremely difficult to measure. It is reasonable, however, to assume production penalties of the order of 20% (i.e. reduced fertility and growth rates, lowered wool, fiber, and leather production, decreased milk and meat production). In terms of world ruminant protein output (25 million metric tons in 1974), disease-induced production losses conservatively account for at least 5 million metric tons.

World wastage of livestock products due to parasitic disease are estimated at $6 billion annually. In 1974, ruminant livestock products had an estimated value of $150 billion, representing 2% of world gross national product (GNP). Various control measures have been developed, including (*a*) grazing and pasture management, (*b*) nutritional supplementation, (*c*) vaccination of the host, and (*d*) chemotherapy.

The effective control of animal helminthiasis demands an integrated system of planned animal management, chemotherapy and adequate nutritional levels. The crucial role of highly effective anthelmintics is now well established and is likely to become increasingly important as animal industries intensify.

The history of modern ruminant anthelmintics dates from the 1920s and has recently been reviewed by Kelly *et al.* (1976). Arsenite was in common use, followed by copper sulfate, which was later combined with sodium arsenite, mustard, or nicotine. In the early twenties, carbon tetrachloride was introduced and brought about a radical change in the control of *Fasciola hepatica* in sheep and, in addition, was highly effective against *Haemonchus contortus*. The copper sulfate–nicotine mixture was the first useful anthelmintic against *Trichostrongylus* spp. (Gordon, 1935; Gordon and Clunies-Ross, 1936). In the 1930s, several workers demonstrated the strength and weaknesses of the anthelmintics then in use, and the influence of the esophageal groove reflex in cattle and sheep was recognized (Watson, 1944).

Before phenothiazine, treatment against large bowel parasites, especially *Oesophagostomum columbianum* and *Chabertia ovina,* presented problems. The mixture of insoluble copper and arsenical compounds devised by Monnig proved disappointing. Arsenical enemas were highly effective but administration was tedious. These parasites responded to piperazine or 1,8-dihydroxyanthraquinone (then commonly used as a purgative for horses) which was also effective against *Trichuris* spp. (Gordon, 1957).

The advent of phenothiazine in the late 1930s marked the first broad-spectrum anthelmintic and was as revolutionary as the introduction of carbon tetrachloride for the treatment of fasciolosis. The later developments of phenothiazine, related to particle size and purity are noted in Gordon (1962) and Arundel (1963).

Organophosphorus anthelmintics appeared during the late 1950s along with compounds of the bephenium type. Thiabendazole, the first of the benzimidazole anthelmintics (in use from 1961) added further improvement to the control of helminth disease as it has a broad spectrum of activity, high efficiency, and extraordinary safety. It was the first anthelmintic that enabled a true diagnostic application to detect and measure the economic effects of parasitic diseases caused by gastrointestinal nematodes of sheep and cattle. Following the introduction of thiabendazole in 1960, many benzimidazole derivatives have been synthesized (e.g. parbendazole, mebendazole, and albendazole), and such compounds are extensively used to control helminth disease (see Tables I and II).

The introduction of phenothiazine and the benzimidazole broad-spectrum anthelmintics has unfortunately led to the selection of drug-resistant strains of important parasitic helminths. The emergence of an increasing number of resistant helminths is associated with the widespread use and misuse of anthelmintics and poses important problems for the helminth chemotherapist.

II. Definitions

A. Resistance

Resistance is defined as a significant increase in the ability of individuals within a strain to tolerate doses of a compound, which would prove lethal to the majority of individuals in a normal population of the same species.

TABLE I

ANTHELMINTICS FOR SHEEP ENDOPARASITES

Anthelmintic	Dose rate active ingredient (mg/kg)	Spectrum of activity[a]																
		Susceptible[b]															Resistant[b]	
			Abomasum			Small intestine						Large intestine						
		Dictyocaulus	*Haemonchus*	*Ostertagia*	*Trichostrongylus axei*	*Trichostrongylus*	*Nematodirus*	*Cooperia*	*Bunostomum*	*Strongyloides*	*Moniezia*	*Oesophagostomum columbianum*	*Oesophagostomum venulosum*	*Chabertia*	*Fasciola*	*Paramphistome*	*Haemonchus*	*Trichostrongylus colubriformis*
Thiabendazole	44.0		3	3	3	3	3	3	3	3		3	3	3			1	1
Thiabendazole Rafoxanide	44.0 7.5 }		3	3	3	3	3	3	3	3		3	3	3	3		3	1
Parbendazole	20.0		3	3	3	3	3	3	3	3		3	3	3			1	1
Mebendazole	12.5	3	3	3	3	3	3	3	3	3	3	3	3	3	1		1	1

Cambendazole	20.0	1	3	3	3	3	3	3	3	3	3	3	3	3			1	1
Fenbendazole	5.0	3	3	3	3	3	3	3	3	3		3	3	3			1	1
Oxibendazole	10.0		3	3	3	3	3	3	3	3		3	3	3			1	1
Albendazole	3.8 / 4.6	3	3	3	3	3	3	3	3	3	3	3	3	3	2		2	2
Oxfendazole	5.0	3	3	3	3	3	3	3	3	3	3	3	3	3	?		2	2
Thiophanate	44–65	1	3	3	3	3	3	3	3	?		3	3	3			—	—
Levamisole	6.75	3	3	3	3	3	3	3	3	3		3	3	3			3	3
Levamisole / Oxyclozanide	6.75 / 15.0	3	3	3	3	3	3	3	3	3	2	3	3	3	3	3	3	3
Morantel	8.8		3	3	3	3	3	3	3			3	3	3			3	3
Naphthalophos	12.5–50		3	2	3	3											3	—
Rafoxanide	7.5–10.0		3												3		3	—
Phenothiazine	600		3	3	3	3	2	2	3			3	3	3			2	1
Carbon tetrachloride	50		3												3		2	—

[a] Activity: 3 = high; 2 = good; 1 = fair to poor; — = no activity; ? = not tested.

[b] Susceptible or resistant: this classification is used to denote strains of parasites normally susceptible or normally resistant to benzimidazole drugs (e.g., thiabendazole).

TABLE II

ANTHELMINTICS FOR SHEEP INFECTED WITH *Fasciola hepatica*

Anthelmintic	Dose rate active ingredient (mg/kg)	Immature fluke (6 weeks)[a]	Adult fluke (12 weeks)[a]
Carbon tetrachloride	0.05[b]	—	3
Carbon tetrachloride	0.1[b]	2	3
Hexachloroethane	300	1	3
Hexachlorophene	15	2	3
Clioxanide	24–48	3	3
Oxyclozanide	13–18	1	3
Rafoxanide	7–5	3	3
Diamphenethide	100	3	3
Brotianide	5–7.5	3	3
Bromsalans	16–22	2	3
Nitroxynil	10	2	3

[a] Activity: 3 = high; 2 = good; 1 = fair to poor; — no activity.
[b] Values expressed in milliliters per kilogram.

The World Health Organisation standards for describing insecticide resistance indicate that up to a 5 times increase in the normal therapeutic dose is accepted as tolerance and any advance on this is regarded as resistance. It is felt that this ratio is applicable to nematode resistance.

Selection toward resistance can be made by breeding from individuals that survive a discriminating dose of the compound. Consequently, a most important characteristic of resistance is that it is genetically expressed and is inherited. Continuing selection, increases the frequency of resistant individuals within the population, allowing the genetic potential to be expressed at its maximum, although no change in the level of resistance has occurred within the individual.

Resistant individuals are often considered to be present in the normal population, prior to the use of any compound (Hardy Weinberg). The continuous use of any compound eliminates all the susceptible and some of the hybrid individuals from the population. The surviving hybrid and resistant individuals can then mate inter se, increasing the frequency of resistant individuals in the next population.

Resistance may also be induced following survival of individuals that have contacted sublethal doses of the compound. This contact may stimulate the extracellular DNA and RNA to undergo change, which is subsequently transmitted genetically to following generations.

B. Resistance Factors

Dose–response data allow the determination of lethal dose giving a 50% kill (LD_{50}), LD_{90}, etc., which can then be used to calculate resistance factors (RF) as follows:

$$\mathrm{RF} = \frac{\text{concentration of anthelmintic required to kill 50\% of resistant parasites}}{\text{concentration of anthelmintic required to kill 50\% of susceptible parasites}}$$

C. Reversion

Continuous selection pressure does not change the level of resistance within the individual of the species, but it alters the frequency at which these individuals occur within the population. Maximum levels of resistance will be obtained when 100% of the population consists of resistant individuals. This is unlikely to be present in a field population under normal management procedures, and hence if the pressure is withdrawn, the frequency of susceptible individuals will increase, due to their selective advantage in the absence of the the anthelmintic. If withdrawal is for many generations, the population would be expected to become more like the original, and may on an initial test produce results suggesting that resistance does not exist.

D. Side-Resistance

Side-resistance is used to describe the phenomenon when compounds of similar structure and activity show a lowered efficiency against a resistant strain compared to a susceptible strain of the same species.

E. Cross-Resistance

Cross-resistance is used to describe a phenomenon similar to side-resistance but involving compounds of unlike structure and activity.

III. Occurrence of Anthelmintic Resistance

A. Sheep

Several species of ovine nematodes have developed resistance to anthelmintics after repeated exposures (Kelly *et al.*, 1976). Field strains of *Haemonchus contortus* resistant to phenothiazine (coarse particle) were first reported in the United States by Drudge *et al.* (1954, 1957a).

The resistant strain of *H. contortus* (Kentucky strain B) was further characterized by Drudge *et al.* (1957b) as follows:

a. Small daily doses of phenothiazine (approximately 0.5 to 1 gm for 5 to 7 days), normally 100% effective against nonresistant *H. contortus,* had no significant effect on strain B in terms of egg count reductions, larval recovery, and numbers of adult worms remaining at necropsy.

b. The phenothiazine threshold of strain B appeared to be 4–8 times that of nonresistant *H. contortus* using low-level phenothiazine dosage (Drudge *et al.,* 1959).

c. There appeared to be a greater infectivity of resistant strain B *H. contortus* (52.2%) upon exposure of the host when compared with nonresistant strains (33.1%). This observation was subsequently confirmed by Hasche and Todd (1963), and a similar phenomenon has been noted for benzimidazole-resistant *H. contortus* (Kelly *et al.*, 1978).

In later studies on phenothiazine resistance, the following results were obtained:

a. Phenothiazine tends to act selectively against female worms (Drudge *et al.*, 1957a,b).

b. Single therapeutic doses of phenothiazine showed a 2.5-fold difference between the thresholds of resistant and nonresistant *H. contortus* (Drudge *et al.*, 1959). This compares favorably with the 4–8 fold difference recorded for small daily doses. Although this single dose efficacy might be considered satisfactory for practical therapeutics, significantly less effective control of resistant strains has been reported under field conditions using single doses (Leland *et al.*, 1957).

c. Although resistant *H. contortus* is relatively insusceptible to normal therapeutic doses of coarse-particle phenothiazine (16 μm), micronized purified phenothiazine (2–3 μm) has a high level of activity against resistant strains (Hasche and Todd, 1963; Bennett and Todd, 1964; Colglazier *et al.*, 1967). Silangwa and Todd (1964) showed that low-level micronized phenothiazine is more active against third and early fourth stage and adult *H. contortus* (strain B) than against the late fourth or early fifth stages.

d. Phenothiazine-resistant *H. contortus* is fully susceptible to mixtures of copper and nicotine sulfate, several organophosphorus anthelmintics (Levine and Garrigus, 1962), and thiabendazole (Bennett and Todd, 1966).

Since the early 1960s the use of phenothiazine as an anthelmintic for livestock has decreased. In only one known instance (Australia) is it still used in a medicated block for flock or herd therapy. No reports are available to show that phenothiazine resistance exists in any strain of intestinal nematode in this country (Australia), yet it must be conceded that it is not under investigation. Similarly no reports are available from the United

States to indicate the present status of the original phenothiazine-resistant strain of *H. contortus*.

The occurrence of resistance to the newer broad spectrum anthelmintics (e.g. thiabendazole, fenbendazole) was first reported from the United States in 1964. Drudge *et al.* (1964) noted the development of a strain of *H. contortus* tolerant to repeated doses of thiabendazole given at a level of 44 mg/kg of body weight. Later, Partosoedjono *et al.* (1969) isolated the strain and determined in definitive anthelmintic trials that doses of 50 mg/kg were only 34% effective against experimentally established infections in sheep. In field trials with sheep primarily infected with *H. contortus,* Conway (1964) found that fecal egg counts were not reduced nor hematocrit values increased following doses of 50 mg/kg; more favorable results were obtained, however, with doses of 80 mg/kg. Other investigations have reported similar results with *Haemonchus* (e.g., Knight *et al.*, 1967; Colglazier *et al.*, 1969, 1970).

Benzimidazole-resistant strains of *H. contortus* have now been reported from the United States, Chile (dos Santos and Franco, 1967), Australia (Smeal *et al.*, 1968; Kelly *et al.*, 1976), South Africa (Berger, 1975; R. K. Reinecke, personal communication), and West Malaysia (J. D. Kelly, unpublished data) (see Fig. 1). Other species of helminths known to have developed resistance to this group of drugs are *Trichostrongylus colubriformis* and *Ostertagia circumcincta*.

The first report of resistance with *T. colubriformis* was that of Hotson *et al.* (1970) from Australia. Separate strains were isolated from properties on which frequent anthelmintic treatments over a number of years were a routine management practice. These circumstances were similar to those in which drug-resistant strains of *Haemonchus* occurred in the field in Australia (Smeal *et al.*, 1968). At that time, complete elimination of resistant *T. colubriformis* (P strain) required in excess of 200 mg/kg thiabendazole. Benzimidazole-resistant strains of *O. circumcincta* have been recognized in Britain (J. Armour, personal communication) and Australia (Le Jambre, 1974, 1977). In both cases, the parasites are laboratory adapted: the British strain is now completely resistant to thiabendazole after more than fifty passages. The Australian strain, selected with thiabendazole, developed strong resistance that increased its LD_{50} from 9 to 108 mg/kg in eight generations (Le Jambre, 1977).

Field surveys for benzimidazole resistance are not available from any country. In Australia the presence of thiabendazole-resistant *H. contortus* is widespread on the Northern Tablelands of New South Wales, and approximately 75% of the properties surveyed are affected (R. Webb, personal communication). Individual properties are affected with resistant strains on the Central West, Southern Slopes, and South Coast re-

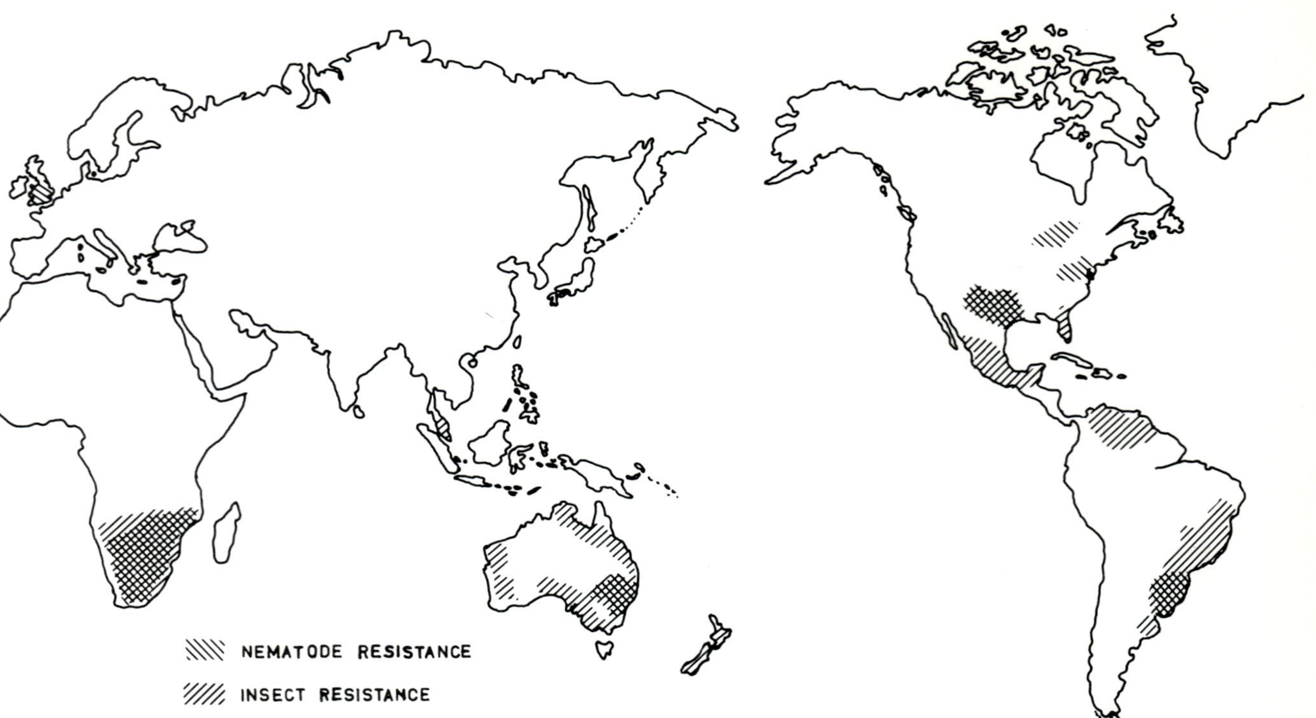

FIG. 1. Regions where anthelmintic and insecticide resistance coexist.

gions of the same state. Resistant *T. colubriformis* has been reported from similar regions in Australia. It would appear that within animals the resistant strains can maintain themselves for many generations without selection pressure. The strains will be transferred from one region to another with the transport of animals and thus spread of infection is assured.

In Southern Africa, four isolates of *H. contortus* are known to be resistant to benzimidazoles (R. K. Reinecke, personal communication, 1977): (*a*) Boshoff strain from the Western Orange Free State; (*b*) Onderstepoort strain; (*c*) Bronkhorstspruit strain from the Eastern Transvaal; (*d*) Marendellas strain from Rhodesia. P. Van Wyk (personal communication, 1977) has also isolated a strain of *H. contortus* resistant to rafoxanide (Tables I and II).

Evidence of resistance to levamisole is scarce, although it is known that a strain of *Trichostrongylus vitrinus* is resistant (R. S. Hogarth-Scott, personal communication). Le Jambre (1977) has selected an Australian strain of *O. circumcincta* that is resistant (after eight generations of multiple selection with thiabendazole, morantel tartrate, and levamisole) to 8 mg/kg levamisole.

A field isolate of *O. circumcincta* has been found in Australia which showed a lower than expected (20%) efficacy following treatment with thiabendazole at 44 mg/kg (Hall, 1979). A lowered efficiency was also shown against levamisole at 7.5 mg/kg, but was fully susceptible to morantel tartrate at 8.8 mg/kg. Another strain of *O. circumcincta* has been recently isolated which is refractory to levamisole (18%) and morantel tartrate (54%) but is susceptible to thiabendazole (95%) (Kelly *et al.* unpublished data). This strain has been designated the PF_4 strain.

A recently isolated field strain of *H. contortus* shows some evidence of resistance in that a dose of 3.25 mg/kg levamisole removed only 65% of an adult worm population established in sheep that were reared worm free (J. D. Kelly, unpublished data). This dose rate is generally considered adequate to kill >95% of normal *H. contortus*. In general, levamisole has high activity against phenothiazine- and benzimidazole-resistant strains of sheep trichostrongyles (Kelly *et al.*, 1976; Campbell *et al.*, 1978).

The only other reports of helminth resistance to anthelmintics are those of *O. circumcincta* to an organophosphate (Douglas and Baker, 1968) and laboratory selected *H. contortus* and *O. circumcincta* to morantel tartrate (Le Jambre *et al.*, 1976; Le Jambre, 1977).

B. Cattle

Herlich (1973) reported on the efficacy of thiabendazole in cattle against a known benzimidazole-resistant ovine isolate of *H. contortus*. Thiabendazole (at 55 mg/kg) was completely ineffective against the ovine isolate in calves. It is interesting to note that thiabendazole at 50 mg/kg removed 39% of the same isolate in infected sheep. A possible explanation for this difference is that helminths may change their susceptibility to anthelmintics when passaged for several generations through animals other than the normal definitive host. Such a change may be one of many physiological alterations required for the parasite to adapt to an alternative host. If this hypothesis is correct, then it has important implications for parasite control in farm management practices where pastures are sequentially stocked with different species of domestic animals (Southcott and Barger, 1973).

Ostertagia ostertagi in cattle may from time to time become inhibited during development from the infective third larval stage to the adult worm. Inhibited development occurs at the fourth larval stage and the phenomenon, which has been termed *hypobiosis,* is not unlike diapause in insects. The exact etiology of inhibition in parasitic nematodes has been variously ascribed to acquired immunity, endocrine changes in the host, environmental preconditioning of infective larvae on pasture, and genetically induced developmental changes in infective larvae (Armour and Bruce, 1974). Inhibited (hypobiotic) larvae are not susceptible to anthelmintics known to be effective against normally developing larvae and adults of *O. ostertagi*.

Recent work with *O. ostertagi* in cattle in Australia has shown a reduced efficiency (28%) for levamisole against adult worms derived from hypobiotic larvae (M. G. Smeal, personal communication), see Table III. This change may be considered as an emerging drug resistance problem, and it is interesting to speculate that hypobiosis in *O. ostertagi* may be partially drug induced (see Section V,D).

C. Horses

The only recognized instances of drug resistance among horse nematodes are the resistance of strongyles to phenothiazine and the benzimidazole anthelmintics. Resistance of large and small strongyle nematodes to phenothiazine has been reported from Britain (Poynter and Hughes, 1958; Gibson, 1960) and the United States (Drudge and Elam, 1961; Drudge, 1965).

In their report, Drudge and Elam (1961) noted the failure of single therapeutic doses of phenothiazine (5 mg/kg) to alter post-treatment strongyle egg counts in feces. The average pretreatment strongyle egg count per gram of feces (EPG) (over 50 mares) was 675 compared with an average EPG of 665 at 2 weeks post-treatment. The majority of eggs passed be-

TABLE III

ANTHELMINTIC EFFICACY OF LEVAMISOLE ON ADULT *Ostertagia ostertagi* DERIVED FROM HYPOBIOTIC LARVAE IN CATTLE[a]

No. inhibited fourth-stage larvae	No. adults	Group mean (adults)	Geometric mean (adults)
	Untreated controls		
1 000	6 250		
1 550	3 150		
1 150	9 750	6 600	6 052
700	4 550		
700	9 300		
	Levamisole-treated		
150	700		
500	2 050		
100	850	2 110	1 706
800	3 950		
800	3 000		

[a] Worm counts assessed 7 days after oral treatment with levamisole at 7.5 mg/kg body weight. Students t test on $\log_{10}$ transformed adult worm counts is $t = 3.008$ on 8 df; $P < 0.05$.

longed to the small strongyle group; significant numbers of *Strongylus vulgaris* and *Strongylus edentatus* were present. Resistance of strongyles to phenothiazine does not appear to cross over to mixtures of piperazine and phenothiazine (Drudge, 1965).

The occurrence of resistance to the benzimidazole group of anthelmintics has been demonstrated only for the small strongyles and this has been reviewed by Round (1976). Resistant strains of equine strongyles were reported from the United States in 1965. In their study, Drudge and Lyons (1965) noted that continuous use of thiabendazole on a stud farm over a 4-year period resulted in a continuing increase in strongyle egg output in both mares and yearlings. By contrast, no significant increase in fecal egg output was observed in horses treated with either trichlorphon or mixtures of phenothiazine, piperazine, and carbon disulfide (these thiabendazole-resistant strains were designated strains B and C). Thiabendazole at 50 mg/kg per os given as a single dose was fully effective against the large strongyles *S. vulgaris* and *S. edentatus*. However, the following species of small strongyles were resistant: *Cyclicocyclus nassatus; Cyathostomum coronatum; Cyathostomum catinatum; Cyclicostephanus longibursatus;* and *Cyclicostephanus goldi*.

Although thiabendazole-resistant strains of equine strongyles are also resistant to other benzimidazoles, for example, mebendazole (Drudge *et al.*, 1974), there is no evidence to date that benzimidazole-resistant strains are cross-resistant to nonbenzimidazole drugs. For example, thiabendazole–piperazine combinations are fully effective against benzimidazole-resistant strongyles. It is important to remember that resistance to thiabendazole "forecasts" resistance to the other benzimidazoles.

Thiabendazole- and mebendazole-resistant strongyles have been reported from Britain by Round *et al.* (1974). In every case, resistant strongyles occurred on farms where regular anthelmintic treatments are a routine management practice. There are no published reports of benzimidazole resistance in countries other than the United States or Great Britain.

In Australia, cases are frequently seen where treatment is not completely effective in removing eggs or is rapidly followed by the reappearance of strongyle eggs in feces. Such a response may be indicative of developing resistance or may be due to (*a*) resumption (by worms) of egg laying, which was temporarily suppressed by the anthelmintic; (*b*) worms that have completed their migration since anthelmintic treatment and matured; (*c*) hypobiotic worms that have resumed development since treatment and begun to produce eggs.

There are no reports of equine nematodes resistant to the pyrantel or morantel group of compounds, nor to piperazine and to the organophosphates dichlorvos, trichlorphon, and haloxon. Levamisole is not very effective against equine intestinal nematodes (Clarkson and Begg, 1970).

D. Miscellaneous

1. *Necator americanus in Man*

Several workers have reported that bephenium hydroxynaphthoate is less effective against *N. americanus* than against *Ancylostoma duodenale* in man (Gilles *et al.*, 1961; Rowland, 1966). Commey and Haddock (1970) studied 5 cases of *N. americanus* which were not responsive to repeat doses of bephenium. In addition, 2 of the cases were also treated with thiabendazole without effect. These results are suggestive of anthelmintic resistance to bephenium and a possible cross-resistance to thiabendazole.

2. *Schistosoma mansoni*

Katz (1973) reported on the isolation of a strain of *S. mansoni* from human infections that was relatively resistant to hycanthone, oxamniquine, and niridazole. Similar reports of hycanthone resistance in murine schistosomiasis have been noted by Lee *et al.* (1971) and Rogers and Bueding (1971). In this latter study, female *S. mansoni* in mice and hamsters, after surviving exposure to relatively high doses of hycanthone produced eggs that gave rise to a generation of schistosomes resistant to hycanthone and two related drugs.

There is no hard evidence for resistance in *Fasciola hepatica* or *Fasciola gigantica,* although Zelentsov (1970) referred to an increasing tolerance of a strain of *F. hepatica* to hexachlorophene. This drug is widely used as a fasciolacide and, apart from the reference cited above, it is still active against this parasite.

3. *Onchocerca volvulus*

The treatment of human onchocerciasis with diethylcarbamazine has been well established (Mazzotti and Hewitt, 1948). Vargas and Tovar (1957) published on a series of 50 cases in which treatment with diethylcarbamazine at 40 mg/kg failed to eliminate microfilariae in 5–10% of patients. They claimed that this represented developing resistance.

IV. Physiological Characteristics of Resistant Helminths

Important physiological and immunological differences have been attributed to subspeciation or strain formation in helminths (Das and Whitlock, 1960; McKenna, 1973). For example, in the eastern United States, *Haemonchus contortus cayugensis* was observed in sheep for 10 years prior to 1960 (Das and Whitlock, 1960), yet by comparison with British strains of the same era, "self-cure" phenomena were not seen, phenothiazine chemotherapy was often inadequate, and "spring-rise" results were different. McKenna (1973) has described differences in "inhibition proneness" between two geographically and morphologically distinct strains of *H. contortus* in New Zealand. It is important to note that a shift in the pathogenicity of *Haemonchus* worms has been shown to accompany adaptive changes. Allen *et al.* (1958), in a comparative study of the pathogenicity of *Haemonchus* worms obtained from wild (Bighorn and Barbary) and domestic sheep, found that in domestic sheep both of the strains from wild ruminants were less pathogenic than the "domestic" strain.

In addition to host and climatic factors, helminths have been able to adapt in response to anthelmintic exposure, that is, the development and/or selection of worm populations resistant to various anthelmintics, e.g., phenothiazine (Drudge *et al.*, 1957a,b), thiabendazole (Drudge *et al.*, 1964; Colglazier *et al.*, 1970), and the related benzimidazoles (Kelly *et al.*, 1976).

A. Infectivity and Pathogenicity

The effect of changes in genetic constitution (associated with the development of drug-resistant helminths) on the pathogenicity and infectivity of *H. contortus* in sheep has been studied by Drudge *et al.* (1957b) and Kelly *et al.* (1978). Drudge *et al.* (1957b) reported that Kentucky strain B *H. contortus,* which is resistant to phenothiazine, had a higher infectivity for sheep (52.2%) than nonresistant strains (33.1%).

A similar phenomenon has been shown to occur with benzimidazole-resistant *H. contortus* (Kelly *et al.*, 1978). In this study, resistant *Haemonchus* had a significantly higher establishment rate in worm-free sheep than nonresistant strains (57.4% vs. 39.6%; Table IV). Resistant *H. contortus* produced significantly more eggs per gram of feces, and sheep infected with this strain developed a significantly greater anemia than those infected with benzimidazole-susceptible *Haemonchus* (see Fig. 2).

The higher infectivity of benzimidazole-resistant *H. contortus* has been correlated with higher exsheathment rates in the host and increased survival of infective larvae on pasture.

The percentage exsheathment of third-stage larvae of *H. contortus* in ruminal fluid is significantly higher (20%) for resistant strains over time (Kelly *et al.*, 1978), allowing increased opportunities for infection of the host. In a related study, experimental pasture plots were seeded with eggs of both susceptible and resistant strains of *H. contortus,* and these pastures were then subsequently assayed at weekly intervals for the presence of infective third-stage larvae. At the end of 12 weeks, a total of 876 larvae per 1200 gm dry matter had been recovered for susceptible *H. contortus* (LD_{50} for thiabendazole = 12.5 mg/kg) compared with 3342 larvae/1200 gm dry matter for the resistant strain (LD_{50} = 175 mg/kg) (see Fig. 3).

These results indicate that while strains of *H. contortus* are selected for

TABLE IV

Group Mean Fecal Egg and Total Worm Counts for Sheep Infected with 10 000 Third-Stage Larvae of Benzimidazole Susceptible (TBZ-S) or Resistant (TBZ-R) Strains of *Haemonchus contortus*

Strain of *H. contortus*	Replicates	Geometric Means: Fecal egg counts (EPG), Week 4	Week 5	Week 6	Total worm counts, Week 6
TBZ-S	A	2 167	6 604	8 416	4 105
	B	9 389	12 694	10 219	3 823
TBZ-R	A	6 443	17 270	25 107	5 941
	B	16 904	22 049	21 627	5 532

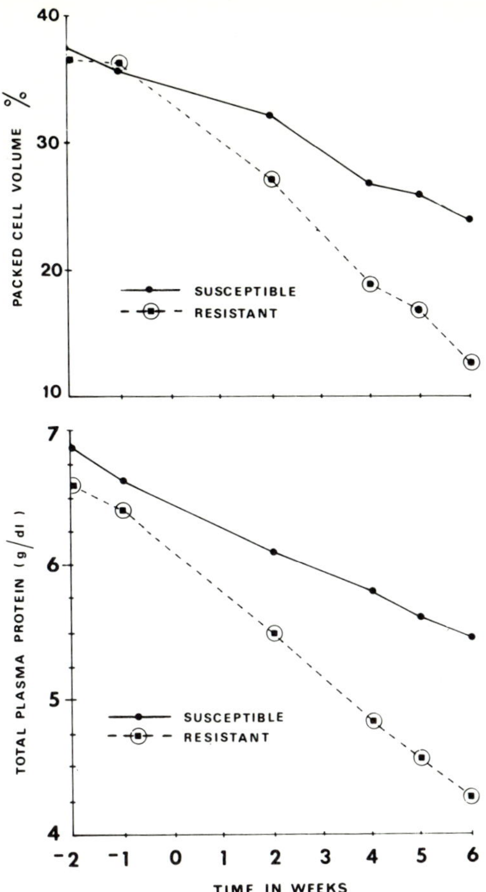

FIG. 2. Comparative pathogenicity of benzimidazole-susceptible and -resistant strains of *Haemonchus contortus* in sheep.

resistance, there can be a simultaneous selection for other physiological characteristics such as increased pathogenicity, infectivity, and larval survival.

B. SIDE- AND CROSS-RESISTANCE

Thiabendazole-resistant strains exhibit marked side-resistance to other benzimidazole anthelmintics, e.g. parbendazole (Hotson *et al.*, 1970; Theodorides *et al.*, 1970; Kates *et al.*, 1971), cambendazole (Colglazier *et al.*, 1972), fenbendazole (Hogarth-Scott *et al.*, 1976; Kelly *et al.*, 1977), and mebendazole and oxibendazole (Kelly *et al.*, 1976) (see Fig. 4).

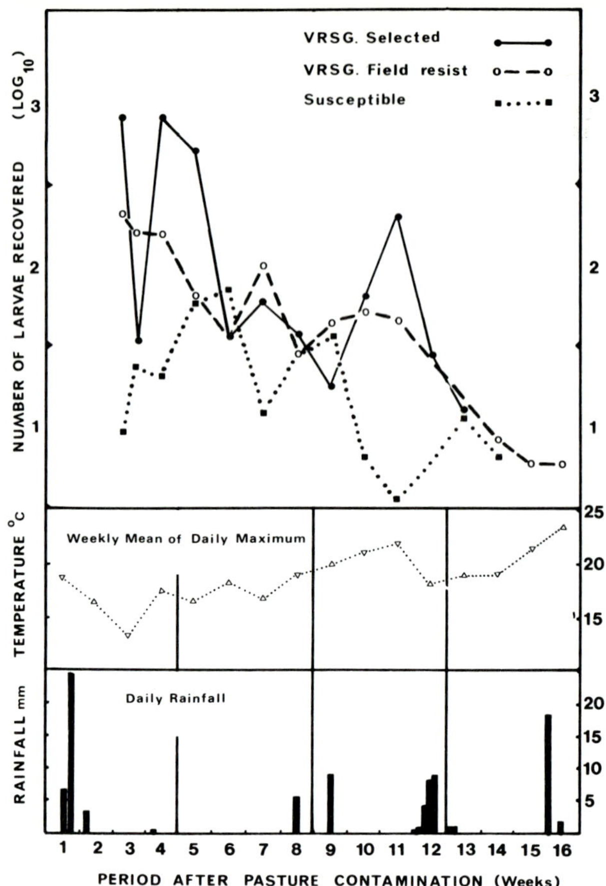

FIG. 3. Patterns of survival for infective larvae of susceptible and resistant strains of *Haemonchus contortus* on pasture. (Taken from Kelly *et al.*, 1978.)

It is of interest to record that Berger (1975) recently reported the occurrence of a parbendazole-resistant field strain of *H. contortus* in South Africa. The strain was isolated from a property on which continuous short-interval nematode control with parbendazole over a period of 6 years had provided the anthelmintic exposure conducive to the development of resistance. Although the parasite had not been exposed to other benzimidazoles, it was, nevertheless, resistant to thiabendazole, fenbendazole, mebendazole, and cambendazole. This resistant strain of *H. contortus* was still fully susceptible to levamisole and haloxon.

In a recent study, Hall *et al.* (1978) compared the anthelmintic activity of benzimidazole drugs and levamisole against benzimidazole-resistant

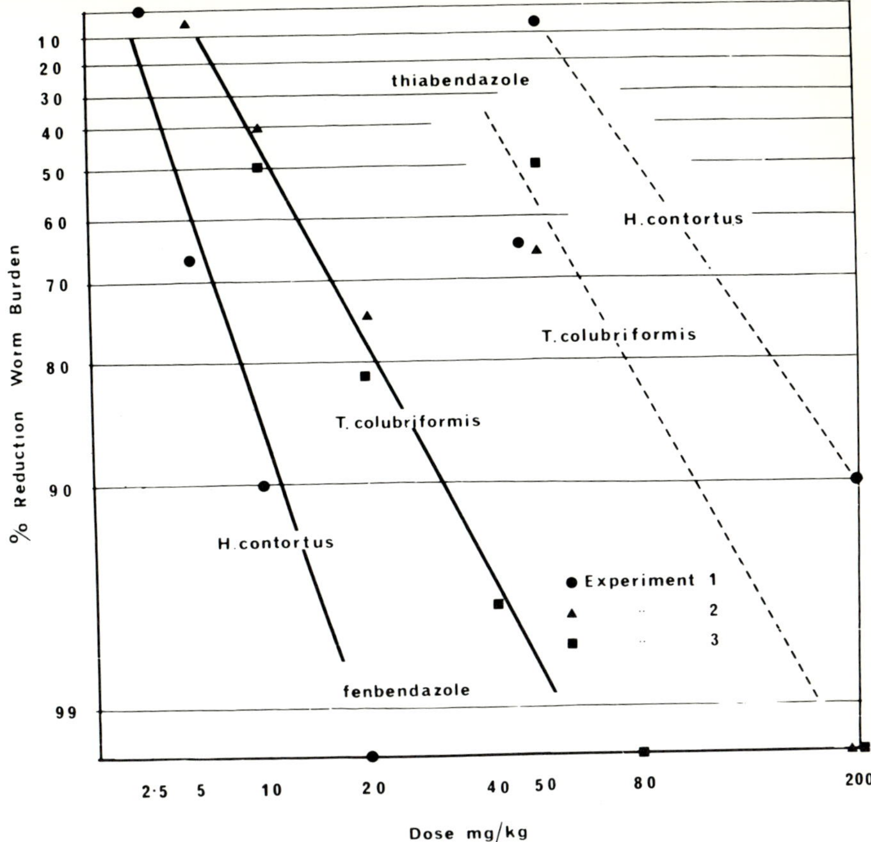

FIG. 4. Dose–response lines for thiabendazole and fenbendazole against benzimidazole-resistant strains (VRSG) of *Haemonchus contortus* and *Trichostrongylus colubriformis* in sheep.

field strains of *H. contortus* and *T. colubriformis* in sheep (see Table V). Although levamisole was 100% active against both parasites, all benzimidazole drugs had reduced efficiencies.

The anthelmintic activity of nonbenzimidazole compounds against benzimidazole-resistant strains of *H. contortus* and *T. colubriformis* has been reported by Campbell *et al*. (1978). Levamisole and morantel were fully active against resistant *H. contortus* and *T. colubriformis*. In addition, naphthalophos, rafoxanide, and phenothiazine were more than 98% active against *H. contortus*. These and the other compounds tested (see Table VI) had low or zero efficiency against benzimidazole-resistant *T. colubriformis*.

TABLE V

EFFICIENCY OF BENZIMIDAZOLE ANTHELMINTICS AGAINST VRSG STRAINS OF BENZIMIDAZOLE-RESISTANT *Haemonchus contortus* AND *Trichostrongylus colubriformis* BY EGG AND TOTAL WORM COUNTS[a]

Compound	Dose rate (mg/kg)	Eggs per gram of feces: Pre-treatment	Eggs per gram of feces: Post-treatment (12 days)	% Reduction	Total worm counts: *H. contortus*	% Reduction	*T. colubriformis*	% Reduction
Thiabendazole	22.00	8 397	6 320	24.7	4 026	—	7 497	—
	44.00	7 826	7 093	7.0	1 915	—	5 579	—
	88.00	4 533	1 280	71.8	1 293	18.9	1 386	74.4
Parbendazole	10.00	6 020	1 880	68.9	831	22.2	7 324	—
	20.00	5 967	1 867	68.8	955	10.5	6 800	—
	40.00	10 210	973	90.5	516	44.2	4 467	17.6
Fenbendazole	2.50	5 780	1 040	82.0	240	77.6	5 129	11.0
	5.00	7 463	587	92.1	142	86.7	2 813	48.1
	10.00	4 740	27	99.4	4	99.6	235	95.7
Mebendazole	6.25	6 360	6 213	2.3	595	44.3	7 378	—
	12.50	7 333	2 280	68.9	582	45.6	2 591	52.2
	25.00	3 193	120	96.2	62	94.2	1 147	78.9
Oxibendazole	5.00	9 080	1 500	15.6	1 067	—	6 543	—
	10.00	8 520	2 240	73.7	1 876	—	5 014	—
	20.00	3 500	347	90.1	373	65.0	1 106	79.6
Cambendazole	5.00	5 534	2 827	48.9	1 040	2.7	6 947	—
	10.00	2 807	347	87.6	89	91.7	2 902	46.5
	20.00	2 908	40	98.6	36	96.7	27	99.5
Oxfendazole	2.25	3 293	320	90.3	129	87.9	5 818	—
	4.50	8 027	147	98.2	18	98.3	3 382	37.6
	9.00	6 293	0	100.0	4	99.6	325	94.0
Albendazole	1.90	6 900	427	93.9	631	40.9	4 298	20.8
	3.80	5 827	80	98.6	93	91.3	1 431	73.6
	7.60	7 673	0	100.0	9	99.2	27	99.5
Thiophanate	22.00	10 013	6 507	35.0	1 941	—	6 884	—
	44.00	5 443	2 547	53.2	1 031	3.5	7 209	—
	88.00	12 480	7 520	73.1	1 147	—	7 205	—
Controls	—	3 315	3 755	—	1 068	—	5 424	—

TABLE VI

EFFICIENCY OF NONBENZIMIDAZOLE ANTHELMINTICS AGAINST VRSG STRAINS OF BENZIMIDAZOLE-RESISTANT *Haemonchus contortus* AND *Trichostrongylus colubriformis* BY EGG AND TOTAL WORM COUNTS[a]

Compound	Dose rate (mg/kg)	Eggs per gram of feces		% Change in egg count (+/−)	Total worm counts			
		Pre-treatment	Post-treatment (12 days)		*H. contortus*	% Change	*T. colubriformis*	% Change (+/−)
Levamisole	6.4	3820	3	−99.9	7	99.2	13	−99.8
Morantel	8.8	2862	28	−99.1	2	99.8	870	−85.6
Naphthalophos	12.5	1979	12	−99.4	4	99.5	4732	−21.5
Rafoxanide	7.5	5555	653	−88.3	0	100.0	6761	(+12.2)
Phenothiazine	530.0	5834	342	−94.2	10	98.8	6845	(+13.6)
Carbon tetrachloride	0.05[b]	2823	406	−85.6	251	71.2	6751	(+12.1)
Controls	—	2830	2998	+ 5.6	871	—	6045	—
Thiabendazole	44.0	5032	1923	−63.2	1076	—	5184	14.0

[a] Taken from Campbell *et al.* (1978).
[b] Expressed as milliliters per kilogram.

C. Biochemical Aspects

Prichard (1970) reported that the enzyme fumarate reductase was inhibited *in vitro* by thiabendazole in a thiabendazole-sensitive strain of *H. contortus*. This effect is known to impair energy production in nematodes and is thought to be one of the major sites of action for benzimidazole compounds.

Inhibition of this enzyme is significantly reduced and this reaction site appears to be less sensitive in resistant strains (Malkin and Camacho, 1972; Prichard, 1973). Romanowski *et al.* (1975) reported that cambendazole inhibited fumarate reductase by up to 40% more in a cambendazole–thiabendazole sensitive strain than in the cambendazole-resistant strain (BPL-2) of Colglazier *et al.* (1974). On the other hand, levamisole is a weak inhibitor, and fumarate reductase was inhibited equally in resistant and sensitive strains. These results parallel the known anthelmintic effect of benzimidazole drugs and levamisole on benzimidazole-resistant and -susceptible helminths and indicate that all benzimidazole anthelmintics have a common site of action.

The concentration of anthelmintics to which parasite tissues are exposed after drenching of the host are unknown. Such information would be of value in explaining differences in efficacy between anthelmintics of the same or different classes. Recent studies by Kelly *et al.* (1977) have shown that fenbendazole is significantly more effective against benzimidazole-resistant *H. contortus* and *T. colubriformis* in sheep following intraruminal administration than after intra-abomasal administration. This effect is not seen against normally susceptible strains when treated with the therapeutic dose rate (see Table VII). Similar responses occur with parbendazole and mebendazole but not with oxibendazole, thiabendazole, or levamisole (see Table VIII).

In a related study, Prichard *et al.* (1978), using thiabendazole-^{3}H and fenbendazole-^{14}C, found the following:

a. Susceptible worms are removed from the infection site commencing 12 hours after anthelmintic administration; resistant worms remain *in situ* (see Fig. 5).

b. Incorporation of radiolabel from fenbendazole was significantly greater in susceptible strains of *H. contortus* and *T. colubriformis* than in resistant worms (see Table IX). No such difference occurred with thiabendazole. (There appears to be no differential incorporation between *H. contortus* or *T. colubriformis*.)

c. Thiabendazole is rapidly absorbed from both the rumen and abomasum, and peak plasma levels are maintained only for very short periods. This is reflected in the lower relative concentrations of thiabendazole found in both resistant and susceptible worms.

TABLE VII

EFFECT OF ROUTE OF ADMINISTRATION ON THE ANTHELMINTIC EFFICACY OF A SINGLE DOSE OF FENBENDAZOLE AGAINST THIABENDAZOLE-RESISTANT STRAINS (VRSG) OF *Haemonchus contortus* AND *Trichostrongylus colubriformis* IN SHEEP[a]

Route of administration (FBZ,[c] 10 mg/kg)	*H. contortus*			*T. colubriformis*		
	Group mean total worm counts			Group mean total worm counts		
	Arithmetic mean	Transformed mean ± SD[b]	Reduction (%)	Arithmetic mean	Transformed mean ± SD[b]	Reduction (%)
Oral	7	40.9 ± 65.84	99.8	362	250.1 ± 24.6	82.0
Intraruminal	0	—	100.0	139	190.6 + 58.5	93.0
Intra-abomasal	800	243.4 ± 121.60	78.0	1451	309.4 ± 25.3	27.0
Controls	3594	354.9 ± 8.60	—	1996	325.4 ± 24.1	—

[a] Taken from Kelly *et al.* (1977).

[b] Transformed = 100 $\log_{10}(x + 1)$, where x = total worm count. Mean derived from groups of 6 animals each.

[c] FBZ = fenbendazole.

TABLE VIII

EFFECT OF ROUTE OF ADMINISTRATION ON THE ANTHELMINTIC EFFICACY OF SEVERAL BENZIMIDAZOLES AGAINST AN INFECTION WITH A THIABENDAZOLE-RESISTANT STRAIN (VRSG) OF *Trichostrongylus colubriformis* IN SHEEP[a]

Anthelmintic treatment	Group mean total worm counts					
	Intraruminal administration			Intra-abomasal administration		
	Arithmetic mean	Transformed mean ± SD[b]	Reduction (%)	Arithmetic mean	Transformed mean ± SD[b]	Reduction (%)
Thiabendazole (66 mg/kg)	1277	182.7 ± 172.0	72	1000	214.4 ± 137.5	79
Oxibendazole (15 mg/kg)	3539	353.8 ± 10.7	21	3832	356.2 ± 15.2	14
Fenbendazole (7.5 mg/kg)	2187	331.8 ± 15.6	51	4152	359.2 ± 16.5	7
Parbendazole (30 mg/kg)	1501	277.7 ± 66.1	66	5077	365.9 ± 23.9	0
Mebendazole (18.75 mg/kg)	1283	289.7 ± 53.0	71	3341	342.6 ± 37.6	26
		IR Mean = 287.2			IA Mean = 327.7	
Levamisole (7.5 mg/kg)	3	—	100	0	—	100
Controls: Arithmetic mean = 4470; transformed mean ± SD = 364.5 ± 7.6						

[a] Taken from Kelly *et al.* (1977).

[b] Transformation = 100 $\log_{10}(x + 1)$, where x = individual total worm count. Means derived from groups of 5 animals ($n = 5$) except controls where $n = 8$.

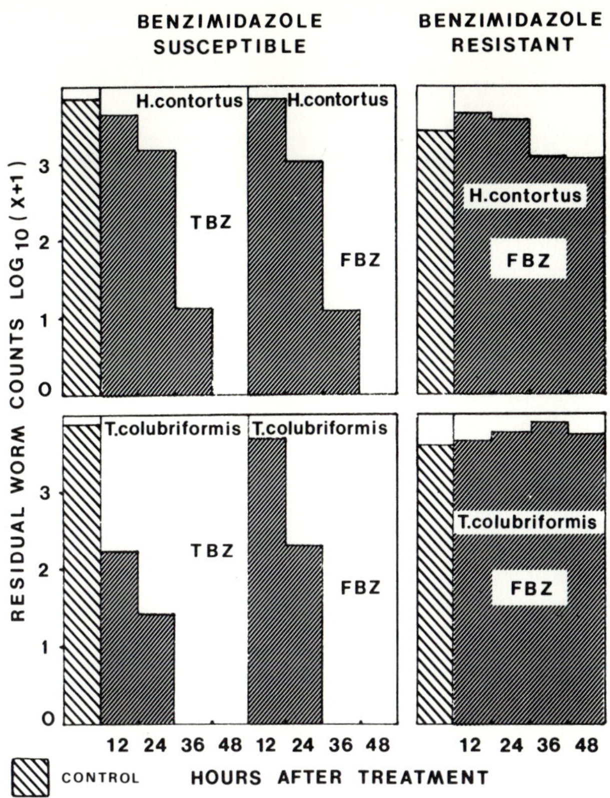

FIG. 5. Effects of thiabendazole (TBZ) and fenbendazole (FBZ) on worm numbers in the gastrointestinal tract at intervals after anthelmintic treatment (TBZ—50 mg/kg; FBZ—5 mg/kg). (Taken from Prichard *et al.*, 1978.)

d. Fenbendazole is slowly absorbed from the rumen and rapidly from the abomasum (see Fig. 6). This suggests that the rumen acts as a reservoir of fenbendazole prolonging the period of high anthelmintic concentration in the host, thus contributing to the relatively high efficacy of this drug against resistant worms. On the other hand, when fenbendazole was administered directly into the abomasum, it was rapidly absorbed, reached peak plasma levels at 8 hours, and then declined rapidly. This rapid absorption and lack of persistence may well explain the poor performance of fenbendazole against resistant strains in sheep, as reported by Kelly *et al*. (1975) and Hogarth-Scott *et al*. (1976), when the compound by-passes the rumen.

TABLE IX

INCORPORATION OF RADIOLABEL INTO *Haemonchus contortus* AND *Trichostrongylus colubriformis* 12 HOURS AFTER ADMINISTRATION OF FENBENDAZOLE-^{14}C OR THIABENDAZOLE-^{3}H[a,b]

	Susceptible worms		Resistant worms	
Anthelmintic[c]	Abomasum[d]	Rumen[d]	Abomasum[d]	Rumen[d]
		H. contortus		
FBZ	396	191	108	36
TBZ	463	144	394	397
		T. colubriformis		
FBZ	281	216	168	141
TBZ	496	95	323	349
		Worms pooled		
FBZ	338	203	138	89
TBZ	479	120	358	373

[a] Taken from Prichard *et al.* (1978).
[b] Values expressed as mean nanogram anthelmintic equivalent per milligram nitrogen.
[c] FBZ = fenbendazole; TBZ = thiabendazole.
[d] Site of anthelmintic administration.

V. Selection for Resistance

Several unsuccessful attempts have been made artificially to select phenothiazine-resistant nematode strains (Sinclair, 1953; Hasche and Todd, 1963; Silangwa and Todd, 1966; Bennett and Todd, 1966).

A. CAMBENDAZOLE SELECTION OF *Haemonchus contortus*

The first successful demonstration of artificially selected drug resistance in trichostrongylid nematodes was by Kates *et al.* (1973). They reported that a cambendazole (CBZ)-sensitive strain of *H. contortus* (BPL-2) became partially resistant to cambendazole after four successive exposures in experimentally infected lambs.

In the first exposure, worm-free lambs were infected p.o. with 5000 third-stage larvae of a cambendazole-sensitive *H. contortus* strain. Twenty-seven days later, lambs were dosed with the anthelmintic at 5 mg/kg. Feces were then collected between 1 and 4 days post-treatment and cultured. Larvae cultured from the feces of treated lambs were used for the second exposure infection. This procedure was repeated for four successive generations (over a period of 7 months) and the doses of cambendazole used were 5, 5, 10, and 20 mg/kg. The response of the second to fourth successive generation of *H. contortus* exposed to the drug indi-

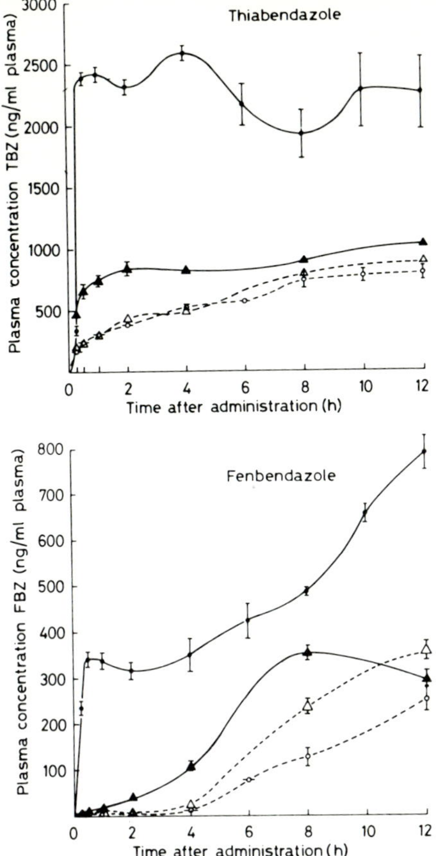

FIG. 6. Mean concentration of radiolabel ± standard deviation (nanograms anthelmintic equivalent) in the plasma of sheep infected with *Haemonchus contortus* and *Trichostrongylus colubriformis*. (●—●) Intra-abomasal and (○---○) intraruminal administration to sheep with benzimidazole-susceptible parasites; (▲—▲) intra-abomasal and (△---△) intraruminal administration to sheep with benzimidazole-resistant parasites. Top—after thiabendazole-^{3}H administration; bottom—after fenbendazole-^{14}C administration. (Taken from Prichard *et al.*, 1978.)

cated that the parasite was developing cambendazole resistance. After the fourth exposure a critical controlled test showed the following efficiencies:

	CBZ-pressured strain (%)	CBZ-sensitive strain (%)
CBZ (20 mg/kg)	71.5	97.7
CBZ (40 mg/kg)	92.7	99.9

Further experimental development of this cambendazole-resistant strain of *H. contortus* (BPL-2) using cambendazole (up to 60 mg/kg) for a further five generations was reported by Colglazier *et al.* (1974). After the tenth drug exposure, twofold (40 mg/kg) and threefold (60 mg/kg) increments of the normal therapeutic dose (20 mg/kg) of cambendazole resulted in efficiencies of 45 and 72%, respectively whereas these dose levels were still 100% effective against the original cambendazole-sensitive strain. It was also shown that there was no evidence of reversion in anthelmintic sensitivity after two passages in nonmedicated lambs (probably due to an insufficient number of generations without anthelmintic selection for reversion to show).

The experimentally produced cambendazole-resistant strain (BPL-2) is side-resistant to chemically related benzimidazoles. Colglazier *et al.* (1975) tested cambendazole (20 mg/kg), thiabendazole (50 mg/kg), mebendazole (20 mg/kg), oxibendazole (10 mg/kg), and levamisole (8 mg/kg) against the CBZ-resistant *H. contortus*. None of the benzimidazole anthelmintics had any activity against resistant *H. contortus*. The only nonbenzimidazole drug, levamisole, was 100% effective.

B. Glenfield Study

The response of resistant field strains of sheep trichostrongyles to continuing selection pressure has been studied in Australia by Hall and coworkers at the Veterinary Research Station, Glenfield, and by Le Jambre at the Pastoral Research Laboratory, Armidale.

The strain of benzimidazole-resistant *H. contortus* isolated in Australia by Smeal *et al.* in 1968 has been continuously maintained in the laboratory by passage in worm-free lambs. Similarly, the thiabendazole-resistant strain of *T. colubriformis* was also maintained in the laboratory (Hotson *et al.*, 1970). These strains have been shown by Hogarth-Scott *et al.* (1976) and Kelly *et al.* (1976) to be not only resistant to thiabendazole but to have side-resistance to all other benzimidazole anthelmintics (parbendazole, cambendazole, mebendazole, oxibendazole, fenbendazole, oxfendazole, and thiophanate).

Strains of these two benzimidazole-resistant nematodes have been passaged in worm-free lambs and selected at a dose rate of 70 mg/kg of thiabendazole at each adult generation since 1974. At 5 days post-treatment, the surviving eggs were cultured to provide the infective larvae for the next generation. After a total of eight passages the two strains were reassayed. It was found that the level of resistance for *T. colubriformis* had not changed, but the level of thiabendazole resistance (RF) in *H. contortus* had increased from 6 to 18. An additional eight passages in the second year has shown a similar trend with the resistance in *H. contortus* increasing still more (RF-19-22), whereas *T. colubriformis* remains static.

From these results it is hypothesized that the resistance in *T. colubriformis* is probably controlled by a small number of loci, whereas in *H. contortus* the presence of resistance probably is controlled by many loci (polygenic).

C. Armidale Study

At the commencement of Le Jambre *et al.*'s study (1976), approximately 20% of resistant *H. contortus* survived a 50 mg/kg dose of thiabendazole. The isolate was subsequently selected over six generations for resistance to thiabendazole at 50 mg/kg. At this stage, the LD_{50} had shifted dramatically from 64 mg/kg to >200 mg/kg. After the sixth generation, selection was extended to include morantel tartrate. Assay of the third generation thiabendazole–morantel selected line showed that the LD_{50} for morantel had risen from 2.5 mg/kg (for non-benzimidazole-resistant *H. contortus*) to 5.3 mg/kg. The lowest dose of levamisole (1.6 mg/kg) killed more than 95% of all strains (selected only against thiabendazole or against both thiabendazole and morantel concurrently). Le Jambre *et al.* (1976) concluded that "(*a*) resistance to thiabendazole (TBZ) was due to a single gene; (*b*) resistance to morantel tartrate appeared to be polygenic in nature and due to increased vigour."

More recently, Le Jambre *et al.* (1978) have indicated that TBZ resistance in *H. contortus* is polygenic based on a series of cross-breeding studies.

Similar studies with *O. circumcincta* were reported by Le Jambre (1977). Four lines of *O. circumcincta* were selected as follows:

- Line 1 50 mg/kg thiabendazole (TBZ)
- Line 2 4 mg/kg morantel tartrate (MT)
- Line 3 3.2 mg/kg levamisole (LEV)
- Line 4 multiselected with TBZ + MT + LEV

Ostertagia circumcincta selected with TBZ increased its LD_{50} for adult worms from 9 to 108 mg/kg in eight generations. Lines 2 and 3 developed low levels of resistance to either MT or LEV.

The multiselected *O. circumcincta* showed the same high- and low-resistance levels as did the singly selected lines.

D. Relationship between Resistance and Inhibited Parasite Development

The degree of "inhibition proneness" of a parasite may be influenced by regular anthelmintic treatment. Levamisole treatment of sheep, infected with *O. circumcincta,* may result in increased levels of arrested development in subsequent infections arising from larvae cultured from the feces of such sheep. In his study, Le Jambre (1977) reported that the parent strain of *O. circumcincta* had less than 0.01% of inhibited larval stages. After eight generations of LEV selection, more than 16% of larvae became inhibited in the host and 8% of these were resistant to LEV at doses up to 8 mg/kg. In the multiselected line, all inhibited larvae were resistant to all dose levels up to 100 mg/kg TBZ, 20 mg/kg MT, and 8 mg/kg LEV. In an analogous fashion to the increased pathogenicity of *H. contortus* associated with developing benzimidazole resistance (Kelly *et al.*, 1978), it appears that *O. circumcincta* increases the percentage and resistance of inhibited larvae.

E. Reversion

When anthelmintic treatment gives rise to resistance in the field, a search begins for alternative compounds. An original report of thiabendazole-resistant *H. contortus* on a research station in Australia was made in 1968. A recommendation was made to change the anthelmintic to levamisole. This compound was used continuously for all drenching in the next 5 years until 1973. In this year a report was received of a possible failure in control for levamisole. Animals carrying a natural infection were transferred to the Veterinary Research Station, Glenfield, for further investigation. Infective larvae were produced from these donor animals and given to worm-free lambs, which were then treated with levamisole or thiaben-

TABLE X

Reversion in an Established Benzimidazole-Resistant Strain of *Haemonchus contortus* after Treatment for 5 Years with Levamisole

	Fecal egg counts (% reduction)	
	Levamisole (7.5 mg/kg)	Thiabendazole (44 mg/kg)
First passage	99.8	99.2
Second passage	99.6	80.1
Third passage	99.6	42.3

	Total worm counts (third passage)	
	No. worms after treatment	% Reduction
Control (untreated)	1000	0
Thiabendazole (44 mg/kg)	625	37.5
Levamisole (7.5 mg/kg)	30	97.0

dazole at normal therapeutic dose rates. After three passages the efficiency of levamisole remained at the 99% level, indicating no presence of resistance. With thiabendazole the efficiency fell from 95% at the first passage to less than 50% on the third (see Table X) (C. A. Hall, unpublished data). It is concluded that once benzimidazole resistance is present, partial reversion may occur over a long period, but on reintroduction of the same drug the original level of resistance is rapidly reexpressed.

VI. Diagnosis of Resistance

A change in response to anthelmintic therapy is often first reported as a complaint to the drug manufacturer by the farmer. Animals fail to respond and continue to show symptoms of helminthiasis.

Many of these preliminary observations remain within the commercial organization. Their investigations are usually aimed to prove that the anthelmintic was not at fault and that other explanations are possible. Often the explanation is offered that the dose rate was in error and below the therapeutic level or that, due to seasonal conditions, the infection rate was extremely high.

Such explanations are frequently accepted, as seasonal and management conditions are not repeatable. The same anthelmintic continues to be used, and this aggravates the problem by continuing the selection of individuals that show a level of resistance. Ultimately, there is a major failure to control helminthiasis, when further investigations are undertaken.

A. Fecal Egg Counts

Drudge *et al.* (1957a), reporting on changes in response of sheep nematodes to the action of phenothiazine, were initially made aware of the problem by a failure of the anthelmintic to depress egg counts to the same level as was previously experienced.

Similarly, Kates *et al.* (1973) showed a failure of cambendazole to reduce egg counts when administered to sheep infected with benzimidazole-resistant *H. contortus*.

Fecal egg output has no direct relationship with the actual numbers of adult nematodes that may be found in the digestive tract postmortem. It has been well documented that the egg-laying capacity of different nematode species may camouflage the presence of a particular species or a change in another. Hall *et al.* (1978) have shown that egg counts in feces may be reduced by more than 90% in mixed infections of resistant *H. contortus* and *T. colubriformis* treated with benzimidazole drugs. However, when total worm counts are performed on the same animals, it is found that the decrease in fecal egg counts is due to a partial reduction in the number of *H. contortus* adults, with relatively little change in *T. colubriformis* (see Table V).

B. Egg Embryonation

The benzimidazole anthelmintics prevent egg embryonation or hatching and, hence, the production of free-living larvae. Eggs of benzimidazole-resistant *H. contortus* and *T. colubriformis* are resistant to the ovicidal activity of these drugs, and Coles and Simpkin (1977) and Le Jambre (1977) have described methods for using this feature as a simple screen for detection of resistance in nematodes. Such a procedure offers considerable advantages over the costly and time-consuming technique of dosing and following egg counts or performing postmortems.

Resistance factors, based on percent inhibition of egg embryonation have been determined for a wide range of benzimidazole anthelmintics (see Table XI). We postulate that the differences in resistance factors may be related to the type of compound, e.g., benzimidazoles vs. carbamated benzimidazoles, or to its degree of use in the field (the higher the factor the more the compound has been used and the greater the selection against the compound). There is no quantitative relationship between resistance levels and stage of development of the parasite, e.g., with the sheep blowfly *Lucilia cuprina,* the RF factors for the adult and first instar larval stages are 8 and 55, respectively.

C. Larval Culture

Methods of testing new compounds for anthelmintic efficiency have used feces containing nematode eggs, impregnated with serial doses of active ingredient. After culturing the mixture for 8 days, larval counts have been made to assess the compound's suitability (in terms of larvicidal activity) for further development.

Parnell (1964) devised a similar test and showed that it was possible to grade existing anthelmintics and demonstrate activity for potential new compounds. The test has not, to our knowledge, been developed nor is it in use at the present time. N. J. Campbell and C. A. Hall (personal communication) reviewed the test in 1974, as a possible technique to monitor the presence or otherwise of benzimidazole resistance in nematodes. It has a great potential when dealing with single experimental infections, but in mixed infections where only a single strain of nematode was resistant (one of many present in the feces) difficulty was experienced in interpretation.

TABLE XI

LC$_{50}$ CONCENTRATIONS OF BENZIMIDAZOLE ANTHELMINTICS IN PREVENTING EGG EMBRYONATION AND HATCHING: DETERMINATION OF RESISTANCE FACTORS

Compound	LC$_{50}$[a]			Resistance factor (RF)[b]	
	Susceptible	CFS strain	Selected strain	CFS strain	Selected strain
		H. contortus			
Thiabendazole	0.023	0.42	1.15	18.0	50.0
Cambendazole	0.470	0.90	4.25	1.9	8.0
Parbendazole	0.070	0.50	37.00	7.1	529.0
Mebendazole	2.300	12.00	30.00	5.2	13.0
Fenbendazole	500.000	3500.00	5100.00	7.0	10.2
Oxibendazole	0.015	0.62	1.20	4.1	8.0
Albendazole	0.034	0.22	0.40	6.5	11.8
		T. colubriformis			
Thiabendazole	0.015	0.85	0.86	56.0	56.0
Cambendazole	1.000	2.70	2.70	2.7	2.7
Parbendazole	0.041	1.50	1.50	37.0	37.0
Mebendazole	1500.000	7600.00	7600.00	5.0	5.0
Fenbendazole	4250	5000.00	5000.00	1.2	1.2
Oxibendazole	0.030	0.155	0.155	5.1	5.1
Albendazole	0.045	0.20	0.20	4.4	4.4

[a] LC$_{50}$ = concentration of anthelmintic (parts per million) required to prevent 50% of incubating eggs hatching.
[b] See Section II,B of text.

This type of test is limiting, since it is dependent on the compound having an effect on the eggs or on free-living larvae as they emerge. A candidate compound could fail this test, yet *in vivo* it may have a high efficiency in removing the adult or larval stages of the parasites.

D. Critical Tests

Estimation of total worm burdens in treated and nontreated animals infected with resistant nematodes is the most accurate and reliable method of assessing anthelmintic resistance. The use of graded doses against susceptible and potentially resistant strains enables the use of dose–response lines (e.g., Fig. 4) to detect or predict changes in drug performance and, hence, alterations in the degree of resistance of the parasite; for example, we can calculate the RF$_{50}$ factors for thiabendazole and fenbendazole against the VRSG strains of *H. contortus* and *T. colubriformis* (see Table XII).

TABLE XII

RESISTANCE FACTORS FOR THIABENDAZOLE AND FENBENDAZOLE AGAINST *Haemonchus contortus* AND *Trichostrongylus colubriformis*

Anthelmintic	Resistance status	Dose required to kill 50% adult worms (mg/kg)			
		H. contortus	RF_{50}	*T. colubriformis*	RF_{50}
Thiabendazole	Res	80.0	6.4	48.0	2.4
	Sus	12.5		20.0	
Fenbendazole	Res	5.0	10.0	12.0	24.0
	Sus	0.5[a]		0.5[a]	

[a] The 0.5 mg/kg removes approximately 85% adult *H. contortus* and *T. colubriformis;* precise figures for LD_{50} are not available.

VII. Control of Resistant Helminths

A. Recommendations for Use of Anthelmintics

Anthelmintics available at present for the treatment of gastrointestinal helminthiasis may be categorized as shown in Table XIII.

Given the present state of knowledge on resistance, it would be inadvisable completely to withdraw benzimidazole-type compounds from use and to switch to levamisole, morantel, or some of the nonbenzimidazoles (see Table VI) since continuous high-level use could result in the selection of resistant strains.

In cases where broad-spectrum drenches are required continuously, it would be possible to remove the resistant individuals with either levamisole or morantel for several treatments and then follow with a benzimidazole-type drench until the resistant individuals have again built up in numbers. Thus alternation of drenches could be utilized as frequently as was required.

TABLE XIII

CATEGORIZATION OF ANTHELMINTICS

Compound	Activity	Resistance status
Levamisole	Broad-spectrum	Resistance to *O. circumcincta* and *T. colubriformis*
Morantel	Broad-spectrum	Resistance to *O. circumcincta* and *T. colubriformis*
9 Benzimidazoles	Broad-spectrum	Resistance in *Haemonchus contortus*, *O. circumcincta*, and *Trichostrongylus colubriformis*
Several nonbenzimidazoles	Narrow-spectrum	No resistance in *Haemonchus contortus*. Ineffective against susceptible *Trichostrongylus colubriformis*

In other cases where a specific pathogen, e.g., *H. contortus,* is a major problem only at certain periods of the year, a suitable nonbenzimidazole drug could be used to remove the resistant worms, followed by broad-spectrum drenches of levamisole or morantel.

It is reasonable to assume that populations of eggs and infective larvae on pasture carry the same frequency of benzimidazole-resistant individuals as the adult population from which they were derived. In many summer rainfall zones, the maximum longevity of *H. contortus* eggs and larvae does not exceed 30 weeks. In fact, under practical field conditions, the majority of eggs and larvae do not survive longer than 12 weeks. This means that *H. contortus* will have a population turnover of approximately three complete generations of the parasite. Therefore, the use of a chemically unrelated anthelmintic over three generations would select the free-living population on pasture toward one with a normal frequency of benzimidazole-susceptible individuals.

In the future, if more than one chemically unrelated anthelmintic becomes available at the same time, the question of how to ensure their maximum value becomes important. Should one chemical be allowed to be used alone until resistance to it develops and then hopefully change to another and repeat? What assurance is there that, when resistance to the first anthelmintic develops, there will be no cross-resistance to the other?

It may be more practical to allow both or several drugs to be used at the same time, but to recommend that neither one nor the other is ever used in a continuous or repetitive program. This method has a potential for delaying or hindering the appearance of resistance. It must be stressed, however, that there are no long-term critical field experiments available to show the effectiveness or otherwise of any of the foregoing schemes, and it is, therefore, difficult to make firm recommendations for planned anthelmintic use.

The optimum strategy for alternation of anthelmintic treatments depends to some extent on the genetic basis for resistance to each one as well as on the problem of cross-resistance. Suppose a population of worms has been subjected to selection for resistance to a particular drug over many generations, so that resistance was nearly 100%. If this drug was then withdrawn from use, if the resistance was polygenic, if some loci were still segregating, and if alleles for susceptibility had higher fitness than alleles for resistance in the absence of the drug, the level of resistance measured on the population would decrease, but not hypothetically to the original value because of fixation of some alleles for resistance. On the other hand, if resistance were due to a single allele at one (or each of very few) loci, the frequency of the gene(s) for resistance would be high. In the absence of selection pressure due to drug use, the initial decrease in resistance level would be expected to be slow, because of the low frequency of the now favored allele(s) for susceptibility, but the resistance level should hypothetically decrease to the initial level. In either case, the time scale of the reversion cannot be predicted without knowledge of the relative fitnesses of the genotypes.

With shorter-term selection for resistance (i.e., fewer generations of worms exposed to the drug), so that the resistance level is increased only to some intermediate value, each of the problems just mentioned should be avoided. Thus, if control of resistance were polygenic, the population should revert to a resistance level closer to the original, because fewer loci will be homozygous. If control were due to one or a few loci, then reversion would be more rapid because the alleles would be at intermediate frequencies. Rapid alternation of anthelmintic treatments therefore would seem to be indicated.

B. Standards for Anthelmintic Activity

The level and number of resistant individuals occurring within a helminth population will determine: (*a*) whether an anthelmintic is still of value in field use; (*b*) whether to continue use of the drug at the normal dose but with a lowered efficiency; and (*c*) whether the normal therapeutic dose needs to be increased to maintain efficiency. These and related questions pose important problems for drug-registering authorities.

Test methods used in establishing activity profiles for anthelmintics should be standardized—and these should include critical tests against known resistant populations. Resistance factors should be determined for all existing and new anthelmintics. Anthelmintics should be pressured at discriminating doses over a minimum of ten parasite generations to determine possible changes in RF. Dose–response lines should be available for all anthelmintics against known susceptible and resistant strains of parasites (both immature and adult stages).

In summary, in the field, resistance is usually reported to the most frequently used compound. This resistant strain then becomes the standard against which existing and new compounds are tested.

Consideration should be given to changes in levels of resistance that may be brought about following use of other compounds with a similar action and side-resistance. It may be that the level of resistance will be increased, resulting in all compounds with a similar action becoming totally ineffective. At the same time, an adverse effect may be shown to compounds with dissimilar action showing a cross-resistance that was not evident to the primary cause of resistance.

VIII. Conclusions

The presence of an increasing number of nematode species in domestic livestock resistant to anthelmintics is of major concern.

Side-resistance among all known benzimidazole anthelmintics for *H. contortus* and *T. colubriformis* indicates a limit to their potential usefulness.

The laboratory evidence of a cross-resistance to thiabendazole, levamisole, and morantel, at present only a laboratory phenomenon, may well emerge as a field problem in the near future.

In general, it does not appear that reversion offers any practical hope of control at least in the short term. The development of newer anthelmintics for use in sheep, cattle, and other domestic livestock is essential for the continuing development of animal industries. Parasitologists with the responsibility for developing these compounds will need to pay attention to the question of resistance.

The dose rate at which these anthelmintics will be administered will need to be critically evaluated. Should they be administered at dose rates in excess of the LD_{99} to produce an overkill? It may be reasoned that with no survivors to produce an F_1 generation, there cannot be any development toward resistance.

Should they be used at levels for efficiency in the intermediate range (say LD_{70})? Then a sufficient number of hybrid resistant individuals would survive for mating inter se to take place so that the buildup to a 100% resistant population is statistically impossible.

The most successful delaying tactic would be the use of management strategies that, when combined with highly efficient anthelmintics, will limit their use to a minimum and reduce the selection pressures toward drug resistance. The use of immunological methods of control for nematode infections should be encouraged so that minimal reliance is placed on routine chemotherapy.

Biological control for nematode parasites may be possible if a suitable organism can be found that kills the parasite without interfering with the functions of the host.

Nematode parasites are adapted to live and survive in a wide range of host organs and tissues. It may be possible to use chemicals that for a short period of time change these conditions adversely, rendering the microenvironment of the parasite unsuitable for its continued survival. An example of this type of approach is the use of nonspecific mediators of inflammation, such as prostaglandins (Kelly and Dineen, 1976) to remove thiabendazole-resistant *T. colubriformis* from the gastrointestinal tract of infected sheep (Kelly *et al.*, 1976). This work is of a preliminary nature but does indicate that nonanthelmintic technology may be of value in the future control of anthelmintic-resistant strains of helminths.

Acknowledgments

The authors wish to thank Ms. Janet Bullard for her generous and efficient help in the preparation of this manuscript. Associate Professor J. S. F. Barker and Dr. L. F. Le Jambre provided constructive criticism, and Mr. C. Porter assisted in the artwork.

References

Allen, R. W., Schad, G. A., and Samson, K. S. (1958). *J. Parasitol.* **44,** 26.
Armour, J., and Bruce, R. G. (1974). *Parasitology* **69,** 161.
Arundel, J. H. (1963). *Aust. Vet. J.* **39,** 214.
Bennett, D. G., and Todd, A. C. (1964). *Am. J. Vet. Res.* **25,** 456.
Bennett, D. G., and Todd, A. C. (1966). *Am. J. Vet. Res.* **27,** 136.
Berger, J. (1975). *J. S. Afr. Vet. Assoc.* **46,** 369.
Byerly, T. C. (1977). *Science* **195,** 450.
Campbell, N. J., Hall, C. A., Kelly, J. D., and Martin, I. C. A. (1978). *Aust. Vet. J.* **54,** 23.
Clarkson, M. J., and Begg, M. K. (1970). *Ann. Trop. Med. Parasitol.* **65,** 87.
Coles, G. C., and Simpkin, K. G. (1977), *Res. Vet. Sci.* **22,** 386.
Colglazier, M. L., Enzie, F. D., and Lehmann, R. P. (1967). *Am. J. Vet. Res.* **28,** 1711.
Colglazier, M. L., Kates, K. C., and Enzie, F. D. (1969). *Proc. Helminthol. Soc. Wash.* **36,** 68.
Colglazier, M. L., Kates, K. C., and Enzie, F. D. (1970). *J. Parasitol.* **56,** 768.
Colglazier, M. L., Kates, K. C., and Enzie, F. D. (1972). *Proc. Helminthol. Soc. Wash.* **39,** 28.
Colglazier, M. L., Kates, K. C., and Enzie, F. D. (1974). *J. Parasitol.* **60,** 289.
Colglazier, M. L., Kates, K. C., and Enzie, F. D. (1975). *J. Parasitol.* **61,** 778.
Commey, J. O., and Haddock, D. K. (1970). *Ghana Med. J.* **9,** 94.
Conway, D. P. (1964). *Am. J. Vet. Res.* **25,** 844.
Das, K. M., and Whitlock, J. H. (1960). *Cornell Vet.* **50,** 182.
Dos Santos, V. T., and Franco, E. B. (1967). *Proc. Congr. Lat.-Am. Parasitol.* p. 105.
Douglas, J. R., and Baker, N. F. (1968). *Annu. Rev. Pharmacol.* **8,** 223.
Drudge, J. H. (1965). *Vet. Med. & Small Anim. Clin.*, 243.
Drudge, J. H., and Elam, G. (1961). *J. Parasitol.* **47,** 38.
Drudge, J. H., and Lyons, E. T. (1965). *Proc. Annu. Meet. Am. Assoc. Equine Pract.* **11,** 381.
Drudge, J. H., Leland, S. E., Wyant Z., and Elam, G. W. (1954). *Ky., Agric. Exp. Stn., Annu. Rep.* p. 56.
Drudge, J. H., Leland, S. E., and Wyant, Z. N. (1957a). *Am. J. Vet. Res.* **18,** 133.
Drudge, J. H., Leland, S. E., and Wyant, Z. N. (1957b). *Am. J. Vet. Res.* **18,** 317.
Drudge, J. H., Leland, S. E., Wyant, Z. N., Elam, G. N., and Hutzler, L. B. (1959). *Am. J. Vet. Res.* **44,** 670.
Drudge, J. H., Wyant, Z. N., and Elam, G. (1964). *Am. J. Vet. Res.* **25,** 1512.
Drudge, J. H., Lyons, E. T., and Tolliver, S. C. (1974). *Am. J. Vet. Res.* **35,** 1409.
Gibson, T. E. (1960). *Vet. Rec.* **72,** 37.

Gilles, H. M., Watson-Williams, E. J., and Worlledge, S. M. (1961). *Ann. Trop. Med. Parasitol.* **55,** 70.

Gordon, H. McL. (1935). *Aust. Vet. J.* **11,** 109.

Gordon, H. McL. (1957). *Aust. Vet. J.* **33,** 39.

Gordon, H. McL. (1962). *Aust. Vet. J.* **38,** 170.

Gordon, H. McL., and Clunies-Ross, I. G. (1936). *Aust. Vet. J.* **12,** 111.

Hall, C. A., Kelly, J. D., Campbell, N. J., and Martin, I. C. A. (1978). *Res. Vet. Sci.* (in press).

Hall, C. A., Campbell, N. J., and Carroll, S. N. (1979). *Aust. Vet. J.* **55** (in press).

Hasche, M. R., and Todd, A. C. (1963). *Am. J. Vet. Res.* **24,** 670.

Herlich, H. (1973). *Proc. Helminthol. Soc. Wash.* **40,** 165.

Hogarth-Scott, R. S., Kelly, J. D., Whitlock, H. V., Ng, B. K. Y., Thompson, H. G., James, R. E., and Mears, F. A. (1976). *Res. Vet. Sci.* **21,** 232.

Hotson, I. K., Campbell, N. J., and Smeal, M. G. (1970). *Aust. Vet. J.* **46,** 356.

Kates, K. C., Colglazier, M. L., Enzie, F. D., Lindahl, I. L., and Samuelson, G. (1971). *J. Parasitol.* **57,** 356.

Kates, K. C., Colglazier, M. L., and Enzie, F. D. (1973). *J. Parasitol.* **59,** 169.

Katz, N. (1973). *Rev. Soc. Bras. Med. Trop.* **7,** 381.

Kelly, J. D., and Dineen, J. K. (1976). *Aust. Vet. J.* **52,** 391.

Kelly, J. D., Whitlock, H. V., Hogarth-Scott, R. S., and Mears, F. A. (1975). *Res. Vet. Sci.* **19,** 105.

Kelly, J. D., Gordon, H. McL., and Whitlock, H. V. (1976). *N. S. W., Vet. Proc.* **12,** 18.

Kelly, J. D., Hall, C. A., Whitlock, H. V., Thompson, H. G., Campbell, N. J., and Martin, I. C. A. (1977). *Res. Vet. Sci.* **22,** 161.

Kelly, J. D., Thompson, H. G., Hall, C. A., Martin, I. C. A., and Whitlock, H. V. (1978). *Res. Vet. Sci.* **25,** 376.

Knight, R. A., Morrison, E. G., and McGuire, J. A. (1967). *J. Am. Vet. Med. Assoc.* **151,** 1438.

Lee, H. G., Cheeven, A. W., and Fairweather, W. R. (1971). *Bull. W. H. O.* **45,** 147.

Le Jambre, L. F. (1974). *CSIRO Div. Anim. Health Rep.* p. 82.

Le Jambre, L. F. (1977). *Proc. Int. Conf. World Assoc. Adv. Vet. Parasitol., 8th, 1977* p. 5.

Le Jambre, L. F., Southcott, W. H., and Dash, K. M. (1976). *Int. J. Parasitol.* **6,** 217.

Le Jambre, L. F., Royal, W. M., and Martin, P. J. (1978). *Int. J. Parasitol.* (in press).

Leland, S. E., Drudge, J. H., Wyant, Z. N., and Elam, G. W. (1957). *Am. J. Vet. Res.* **18,** 851.

Levine, N. D., and Garrigus, V. S. (1962). *Am. J. Vet. Res.* **23,** 489.

McKenna, P. B. (1973). *Res. Vet. Sci.* **14,** 312.

Malkin, M. F., and Camacho, R. H. (1972). *J. Parasitol.* **58,** 845.

Mazzotti, L., and Hewitt, R. (1948). *Medicina (Mexico City)* **28,** 39.

Parnell, I. W. (1964). *J. Helminthol.* **38,** 47.

Partosoedjono, S., Drudge, J. H., Lyons, E. T., and Knapp, F. W. (1969). *Am. J. Vet. Res.* **30,** 81.

Poynter, D., and Hughes, D. L. (1958). *Vet. Rec.* **70,** 1183.

Prichard, R. K. (1970). *Nature (London)* **228,** 684.

Prichard, R. K. (1973). *Int. J. Parasitol.* **3,** 409.

Prichard, R. K., Kelly, J. D., and Thompson, H. G. (1978). *Vet. Parasitol.* **4,** 243.

Rogers, S. H., and Bueding, E. (1971). *Science* **172,** 1057.

Romanowski, R. D., Rhoads, M. C., Colglazier, M. L., and Kates, K. C. (1975). *J. Parasitol.* **61,** 777.

Round, M. C. (1976). *Vet. Annu.* **16,** 143.

Round, M. C., Simpson, D. J., Haselden, C. S., Glendinning, E. S. A., and Baskerville, R. E. (1974). *Vet. Rec.* **95,** 517.
Rowland, H. A. K. (1966). *Trans. R. Soc. Trop. Med. Hyg.* **60,** 313.
Silangwa, S. M., and Todd, A. C. (1964). *Am. J. Vet. Res.* **25,** 914.
Silangwa, S. M., and Todd, A. C. (1966). *J. Parasitol.* **52,** 141.
Sinclair, D. P. (1953). *Aust. Vet. J.* **29,** 13.
Smeal, M. G., Gough, P. A., Jackson, A. R., and Hotson, I. K. (1968). *Aust. Vet. J.* **44,** 108.
Southcott, W. H., and Barger, I. A. (1973). *Proc. World Conf. Anim. Prod., 3rd, 1973* p. 246.
Theodorides, V. J., Scott, G. C., and Laderman, M. (1970). *Am. J. Vet. Res.* **31,** 859.
Vargas, L., and Tovar, J. (1957). *Bull. W. H. O.* **16,** 682.
Watson, R. H. (1944). *Aust., Commonw. Counc. Sci. Ind. Res., Bull.* **180,** 1.
Zelentsov, A. G. (1970). *Tr. Vscs. Inst. Gel'mintol.* **16,** 87.

ADVANCES IN PHARMACOLOGY AND CHEMOTHERAPY, VOL. 16

Diethylcarbamazine and New Compounds for the Treatment of Filariasis

FRANK HAWKING

Commonwealth Institute of Helminthology, St. Albans, England

I. Chemistry 130
- A. Chemical Name 130
- B. Relation of Structure to Activity 130
- C. Other Compounds like Diethylcarbamazine 132
- D. Chemical Estimation of Diethylcarbamazine 135

II. Absorption, Excretion, Distribution, and Metabolism 135
- A. Absorption, Distribution, and Excretion 135
- B. Metabolism 136
- C. Local Absorption into Eye 138
- D. Absorption through Skin 138

III. Pharmacology 138
- A. General 138
- B. Anti-inflammatory Effect 140
- C. Bronchial Asthma 145

IV. Antifilarial Activity 145
- A. Action on Microfilariae 145
- B. Action on Adult Worms 156
- C. Action on Forms in the Insect Vector 158
- D. Action on Infective Larvae and Immature Worms 158
- E. Development of Drug Resistance 161
- F. Action on Other Worms 161

V. Toxicity 164
- A. Animals 164
- B. Man—Uninfected 164
- C. Man—Infected with Filariae 165
- D. Deaths Reported as Due to Diethylcarbamazine Treatment 169

VI. Clinical Use 171
- A. Single Patients 171
- B. Mass Therapy 174
- C. Treatment of Tropical Eosinophilia 180

VII. Review of Other Antifilarial Compounds 180
- A. Older Compounds 180
- B. Arsenical Compounds 181
- C. Organophosphorus Compounds 181
- D. Broad-Spectrum Anthelmintics 184
- E. Miscellaneous Drugs 186

VIII. Conclusion 187

References 188

Addendum 194

ISBN 0-12-032916-6

Diethylcarbamazine (DEC) (I) is the most important compound for the treatment of filarial infections. It was discovered by Hewitt *et al.* (1947).

I. Chemistry

A. Chemical Name

Diethylcarbamazine is 1-diethylcarbamyl-4-methylpiperazine; it is also known as Hetrazan, Banocide, Notézine, Caricide, Carbilazine, Supatonin, and R.P. 3799.

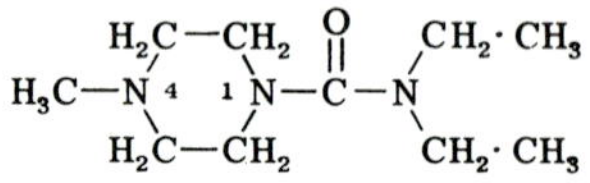

$$\begin{array}{ccccc} & H_2C-CH_2 & O & CH_2\cdot CH_3 \\ & / \quad \backslash & \| & / \\ H_3C-N & 4 \quad\quad 1 & N-C-N & \\ & \backslash \quad / & & \backslash \\ & H_2C-CH_2 & & CH_2\cdot CH_3 \end{array}$$

(I)

It was first put out as the chloride, but is now issued as the dihydrogen citrate, which contains only half its weight as base. In reports, it should be indicated whether the doses refer to a specific salt or to the base; unless otherwise stated, it can usually be assumed that the dose refers to the citrate. Diethylcarbamazine is a white powder, freely soluble in water, and has a slightly unpleasant sweetish taste. It is stable under all ordinary laboratory conditions. Furthermore, it is fully stable to autoclaving, even if mixed with diet (simulating cooking procedure).

B. Relation of Structure to Activity

The piperazine ring is of fundamental importance, as was shown during the original investigations of Hewitt and his colleagues, although piperazine itself has no antifilarial activity. (However, piperazine is active against *Ascaris* and other round worms in the intestine, and perhaps this ring has specific action on parasite nematodes in general.) Various compounds with slightly different rings, e.g., *N,N*-diethyl-4-methyl-1,4-diazacycloheptane-1-carbamaxide hydrochloride (JGS-110) have some antifilarial activity, but not so great as diethylcarbamazine (Reinertson and Thompson, 1955). In the piperazine series, a carbethoxy radical in position 1 of the ring with various substitutions in position 4 produces compounds with high antimicrofilarial activity; but as the alkyl chain is increased the toxicity becomes greater and the activity less. If the alkyl group is greater than $—C_4H_9$, activity is lost. However, the alkyl group in position 4 is not very important since high activity is still retained after it is removed.

The only compounds lacking the carbethoxy group that show marked activity against microfilariae contain an ethyl-, diisopropyl-, dimethyl-, or diethylcarbamyl group in position 1. A compound with formula II is also

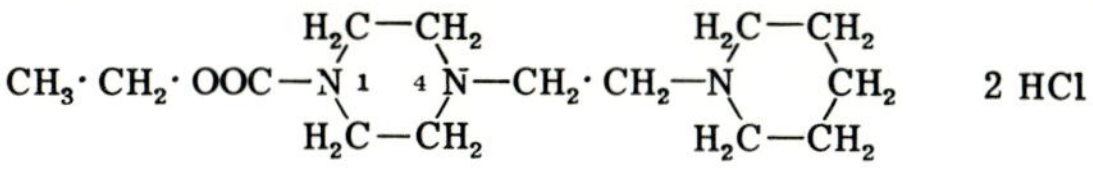

$$CH_3\cdot CH_2\cdot OOC-\overset{H_2C-CH_2}{\underset{H_2C-CH_2}{N^1\quad ^4N}}-CH_2\cdot CH_2-\overset{H_2C-CH_2}{\underset{H_2C-CH_2}{N\qquad CH_2}}\quad 2\,HCl$$

(II)

active (Patra *et al.*, 1969). Apparently there are two aliphatic amines connected by a saturated carbon framework; one amine must be basic and the other must be modified by some type of carbonyl function. The spatial separation of these amines in diethylcarbamazine is optimal, and compounds with wider separation are less active.

A modification of the diethylcarbamazine structure has been described by Saxena *et al.* (1970) and studied further by Thompson *et al.* (1973) and by Sturm *et al.* (1974). It is named Compound II (or Centperazine) for convenience and is described in more detail in Section I,C. In this compound the terminal carbon of one ethyl group has been bent round and attached to the piperazine ring at carbon 2 (see formula III). The essential

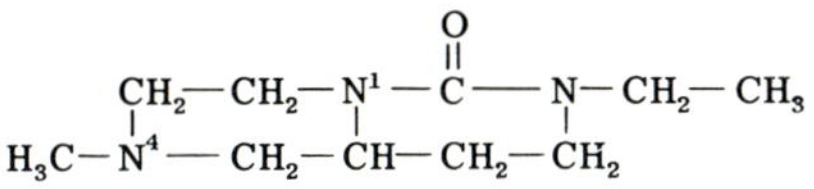

$$\begin{array}{l} \quad\;\; CH_2-CH_2-N^1-\overset{O}{\overset{\|}{C}}-N-CH_2-CH_3 \\ H_3C-N^4-CH_2-CH-CH_2-CH_2 \end{array}$$

(III)

structure is similar to that of diethylcarbamazine but the change makes the molecular structure rigid and locks the urea moiety into a single rotational conformation. By contrast, in diethylcarbamazine the diethylcarbamyl group can rotate on all its single bonds. The new compound is approximately planar with the C=O bond of the carbamyl and all the nitrogens lying in the same plane. The distance between N-1 and N-4 of the piperazine ring is 2.8 Å and between N-1 and the other N, 2.3 Å (see Fig. 1). Since the compound is as active or perhaps more active than diethylcarbamazine, this configuration is apparently optimum.

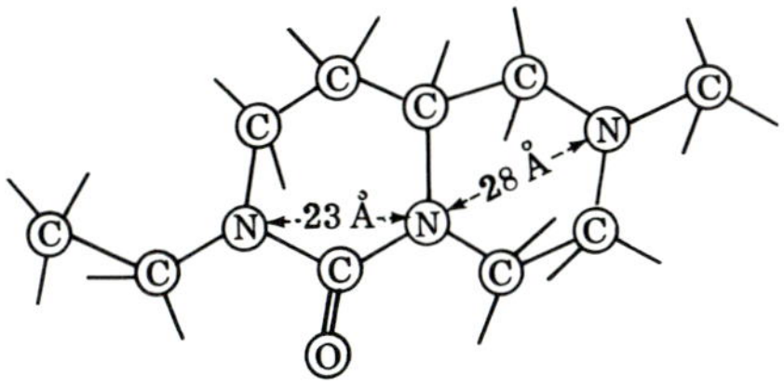

FIG. 1. The interatomic distances in Compound II (Centperazine; 3-ethyl-8-methyl-1,3,8-triazabicyclo[4.4.0]decan-2-one.) (From Saxena *et al.*, 1971.)

In addition to this modification, various linkages across the piperazine ring by —CH_2—CH_2— have been investigated by Sturm *et al.* (1974). Linkage across 3 and 5 does not diminish activity; other linkages, 2–5 and 2–6, diminish activity moderately.

C. Other Compounds like Diethylcarbamazine

1. *Compound II* (*Centperazine*)

The action of Compound II is almost identical with that of diethylcarbamazine. When tested by Saxena *et al.* (1970) and by Thompson *et al.* (1973) in cotton rats and jirds infected with *Litomosoides carinii* the antifilarial response was not closely proportional to the dose so that accurate comparison was difficult. Saxena *et al.* claimed it was 5 times more active than diethylcarbamazine and Thompson *et al.* agreed that it was as active or slightly more active (on the microfilariae). Like diethylcarbamazine it had no action on the adult worms of *L. carinii*. The acute toxicity in mice was slightly less than diethylcarbamazine. This compound ought to be investigated further and tested in man against *Wuchereria bancrofti* and against *Onchocerca volvulus*. Although closely similar to diethylcarbamazine in cotton rats and jirds, it is possible that in man it might present some advantages of greater activity on adult worms or of diminished toxicity. It had no action against *Hymenolepis nana* or *Nippostrongylus* or against *Chandlerella hawkingi* in crows. Like diethylcarbamazine it showed anti-inflammatory action in rats and inhibited passive cutaneous anaphylaxis (Saxena *et al.*, 1970, 1971).

2. *Hoechst 33258*

2-[2-(4-Hydroxyphenyl)-6-benzimidazolyl]-6-(1-methyl-4-piperazyl)-benzimidazole–3 HCl (see formula IV) was described by Raether and

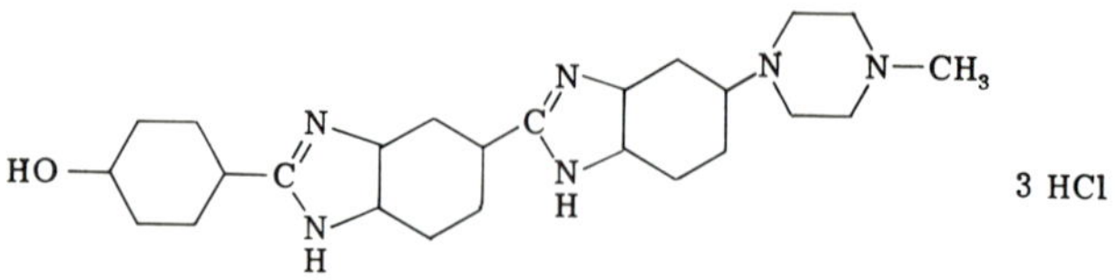

(IV)

Lämmler (1971). It is fluorescent. The hydrochloride is water soluble but the diphosphate is sparingly soluble and so it is only slowly absorbed after oral and parenteral administration. In cotton rats infected with *L. carinii*, its action resembled that of diethylcarbamazine but was slower, more complete, and more prolonged. The phosphate given as 8 mg/kg, i.p., on five consecutive days caused all the microfilariae to disappear within 14–67 days, and only very few had returned after 111–297 days. In half of the rats the adult female worms were dead, but in the other half, females were alive and producing microfilariae. The compound is active against all the larval stages of *L. carinii* (Lämmler and Wolf, 1977).

The maximum tolerated dose of the hydrochloride for mice was 250 mg/kg, i.p., or 625 mg/kg, s.c. The prolonged action is probably due to a depot effect since the compound stays in the tissues a long time. After administration to mice, the nuclei of the liver and kidney still showed fluorescence after 37 days (Lämmler *et al.,* 1971b). The compound binds to DNA, but it seems to the reviewer that whether such binding would be a danger or a merit would depend on whether nuclei of the host or of the parasite are preferentially involved.

Hoechst 33258 has been tested by B. O. L. Duke (unpublished) on chimpanzees infected with human *O. volvulus*. One animal was given 5 mg/kg, i.m., on five consecutive days. Four weeks later the skin had been completely cleared of microfilariae, but 10 days after this the chimpanzee was found dead. There were large sterile abscesses at the sites of injection. Adult worms were alive and contained both live and moribund microfilariae. Two other chimpanzees were treated with an improved pharmaceutical preparation, 4 mg/kg, i.m., twice weekly for 2–4 weeks. This preparation did not cause abscesses. One lightly infected animal was completely cleared of microfilariae for over 10 months (? cure). In the other case the microfilariae were reduced to near zero but after the sixth dose the animal became very weak, relapsed into coma, and died. Most of the adult worms were dead, but a few were still alive although the microfilariae in them were deformed and mostly immobile. (These worms were probably moribund.) It appears that the compound kills the microfilariae of *O. volvulus* and many of the adult worms, but it may be dangerously toxic. Unless the danger of toxicity can be removed, further trials seem inadvisable.

A further modification of this compound named Compound E has been introduced by Friedheim (1974) in which 2 molecules of Hoechst 33258 are combined with 1 molecule of an arsenical compound (F151) closely similar to melarsoprol. When Compound E was given intramuscularly to dogs infected with *Dirofilaria immitis* (dose: 3–41.5 mg/kg, 1–4 doses at 2–4 day intervals), it killed the microfilariae and the adult worms. This combination was tested against *O. volvulus* by B. O. L. Duke (unpublished experiments). One infected chimpanzee was given 4 intramuscular doses of 6 mg/kg at 3–4 day intervals and another was given 3 mg/kg weekly. Both animals showed anorexia, lassitude, and loss of weight. In both, the microfilariae and the macrofilariae appeared to have been killed.

One heavily infected man was then given 4 weekly doses of 1 mg/kg. The treatment was well tolerated; but the microfilarial count was little altered, and 3 weeks after the last dose an excised nodule showed healthy adult worms. Six weeks after the last dose, the patient developed a large vitreous hemorrhage in his right eye producing blindness in that eye. After some months the hemorrhage cleared and a degree of useful vision was restored. Another patient received 4 doses of 2 mg/kg/week and suffered anorexia, lassitude, and pain in knee joints after the last injection. His microfilaria count fell dramatically during the 4 weeks to 3% of its initial value, and an excised nodule showed no living worms. However, about 6 weeks later he died suddenly in what appeared to be a diabetic coma. In view of these two mishaps further trials were discontinued. In any case, arsenical compounds are always liable to produce dangerous symptoms (encephalopathy or acute atrophy of the liver) in occasional persons who have an idiosyncrasy to them.

3. *Hoechst 28637a*

Cyclohexane carboxylic acid–*N*-methylpiperazine citrate (see formula V) was closely similar in structure and activity to diethylcarbamazine

O
‖
C—N N—CH_3· citrate

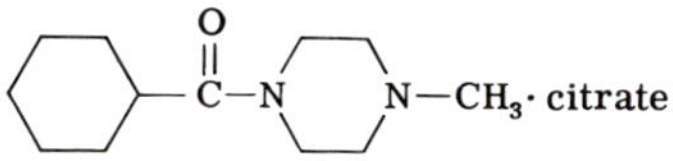

(V)

when tested on *L. carinii* in *Mastomys natalensis,* but its toxicity was lower (Lämmler *et al.,* 1971b).

4. *Hoechst 26961a*

Tetrahydropyrane carboxylic acid–*N*-methylpiperazide citrate (see formula VI) is another compound closely related to diethylcarbamazine. It is

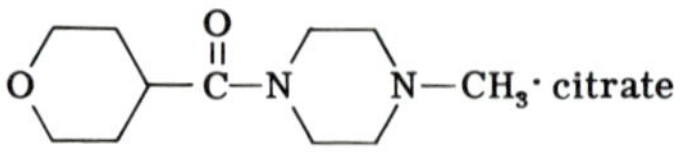

O
‖
O C—N N—CH_3· citrate

(VI)

a little more active than diethylcarbamazine against the microfilariae of *L. carinii* in *M. natalensis* and a little less toxic (Lämmler *et al.,* 1971b).

5. *Hoechst 37598*

This compound belongs to the bisbenzimidazole series and has a long-acting repository effect. It was given by B. O. L. Duke (unpublished experiments) to a chimpanzee infected with *O. volvulus,* at a dose of 6 mg/kg, i.m., daily for 5 days. There was a temporary diminution of microfilariae, but they built up again in 2 months. The animal was then treated with 10 mg/kg twice weekly for 7 doses, but there was no change in the microfilaria count during the next 12 weeks. However, at 24 weeks after treatment there were two enormous abscesses at the sites of injection.

D. Chemical Estimation of Diethylcarbamazine

Estimation in blood and urine can be made by a colorimetric method using bromthymol blue described by Lubran (1950). Amounts can be measured as low as the normal blank value, which is about 1 μg/ml for serum, and 3–10 μg/ml for urine. A similar technique has been described by Hujimaki (1958). A modification using bromophenol blue has been described by Rao and Subrahmanyam (1970). Another method of estimation by picric acid has been reported by Ramachandram (1973). Recently, a new method of estimation by gas–liquid chromatography has been described by Rée *et al.* (1978). Methods for pharmaceutical estimation based on reineckates have been described by Sheng *et al.* (1963), and based on bromocresol green by Vadodaria *et al.* (1968). When diethylcarbamazine has been added to the food of animals, its concentration can be measured by colorimetry or by gas–liquid chromatography but not by polarography (Allen and Beckman, 1964). Diethylcarbamazine has also been estimated with radioactive techniques by Bangham (1955), using samples labeled with ^{14}C in the piperazine ring or in the methyl group, and by Faulkner and Smith (1972).

II. Absorption, Excretion, Distribution, and Metabolism

A. Absorption, Distribution, and Excretion

When diethylcarbamazine is given by mouth to either animals or man, it is rapidly absorbed from the alimentary canal. One dose of 10 mg base/kg produces a peak blood level of 4–5 μg/ml in 3 hours (when toxic symptoms are most prominent); the level gradually falls to zero within about 48 hours. Most of the excretion in the urine occurs in the first 24 hours during which time 10–26% of the dose may be recovered as diethylcarbamazine. When 3 mg base/kg is taken twice daily for 4½ days the blood concentration reaches 4–5 μg/ml by the third day and then falls, even though the dosage is continued. According to the estimations of Rée *et al.* (1978) made by gas–liquid chromatography, after a single oral dose of 200–400 mg to man the concentration in the plasma reached a peak in 1 to 2 hours and then it died away; after 200 mg the half-life was 8.1 ± 3.5 hours, and after 800 mg, it was 11.7 ± 2.3 hours. Repeated doses of 900 mg daily produced a sustained level of about 3 μg/ml, with no tendency to accumulate. Diethylcarbamazine apparently penetrates readily into hydrocele fluid (and presumably into other body fluids) (Hawking, 1950; Lubran, 1950).

The distribution of tritium-labeled diethylcarbamazine in mice after intraperitoneal injection has been studied by radioautography (Sakuma *et al.*, 1967). The compound was rapidly distributed, and 20 minutes after injection the radioactivity in the liver, kidney, adrenal gland, muscle, and gastrointestinal tract reached its highest density; by 6 hours it had diminished rapidly. It accumulated in the brain at 20 minutes and diminished after 1 hour. Specially high accumulations occurred (at 1–3 hours) in the salivary gland, medulla of the adrenal, pituitary gland, and lymph nodes. The compound was accumulated and excreted from the kidney, from the glandular portion of the stomach wall, and from the liver into the bile.

The relations among dosage, blood levels, and microfilaricidal effect have been studied in patients infected with *Wuchereria bancrofti* by Hujimaki (1958). Treatment lasted 10–14 days. With daily oral doses (divided into 3) of 0.3–0.6 mg/kg citrate, the morning blood level was less than 0.65 μg/ml, and there was no therapeutic effect. With 1.5 mg/kg daily, the blood level was 0.5–1.1 μg/ml in the morning and over 1.0 μg/ml during the day, and microfilariae were eventually all exterminated. After a single daily dose, e.g., 6 mg/kg, there was a peak blood level of 3.0 μg/ml that rapidly fell within several hours. On the other hand, if the same amount was divided into 3 or 6 doses, the blood level remained steady throughout the day. The minimum effective concentration in the blood seemed to be 0.8–1.0 μg/ml. For the treatment of bancroftian filariasis, Hujimaki recommended a daily dose of 6 mg/kg, divided into 6, for 14 days; this should give a blood level of 1.8–2.6 (average 2.1) μg/ml in the morning and probably a higher level during the day.

B. Metabolism

A more specific analysis of the metabolism and the distribution in rats and monkeys was made by Bangham (1955), who worked with drug labeled with ^{14}C in the piperazine ring. An oral dose is rapidly absorbed, and about 70% of the piperazine metabolites is excreted in the urine in 24 hours. After an intravenous dose of 2.25 mg/kg, 95% is excreted in 30 hours, 10–20% appearing as unchanged drug depending on the dose level given. Metabolism is very rapid, and the drug is excreted in four different forms in all of which the piperazine ring remains intact. Diethylcarbamylpiperazine accounts for 5–15%; methylpiperazine for 2–5%, and piperazine for 1–6%. The fourth form was an unstable basic compound that was not identified by Bangham. This metabolite could be demonstrated in the blood within 2 minutes of an intravenous injection.

The metabolism has been further investigated in rats by Faulkner and Smith (1972) using diethylcarbamazine labeled with ^{14}C in the 3,5-positions of the piperazine ring. They found that the main metabolite (not identified by Bangham) was diethylcarbamazine-*N*-oxide (see formula in Fig. 2). A second major metabolite is 1-ethylcarbamyl-4-methylpiperazine accounting for 23% of the compound excreted in the urine, whereas unchanged drug accounted for 15% of the urinary radioactivity. Thus when 20 mg/kg was given by mouth to rats, the radioactivity was excreted in the urine as follows (Fig. 2): unchanged drug, 10–20% of dose; methylpiperazine, 2–5%; piperazine, 1–6%; diethylcarbamylpiperazine, i.e., the methyl group is split off, 5–10%; 1-ethylcarbamyl-4-methylpiperazine, i.e., one ethyl group is split off, 23%; diethylcarbamazine-*N*-oxide, 50%.

Although metabolism is rapid and extensive, no metabolite so far isolated appears to have a sufficiently profound effect to account for the extraordinary speed of action on the circulating microfilariae. Accordingly, this action is probably due to diethylcarbamazine itself. Studies of the distribu-

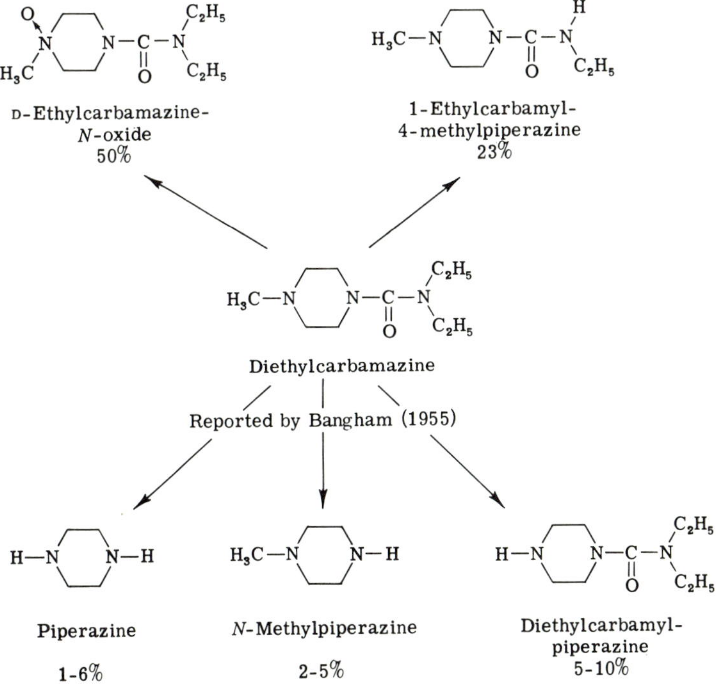

FIG. 2. The metabolic products of diethylcarbamazine (Faulkner and Smith, 1972).

tion of the radioactive preparation show that diethylcarbamazine soon equilibrates with all organs, blood cells, and tissues (except fat) and that neither the microfilariae nor the adult worms (of *Dirofilaria immitis*) concentrate it to any pronounced extent as compared with the surrounding tissues or fluids. Excretion takes place almost entirely by the urine. The feces contain only small amounts of piperazine metabolites.

C. Local Absorption into Eye

When diethylcarbamazine solutions are applied locally to the eyes of rabbits, the compound enters the aqueous humor in high concentration, and there is no toxic effect after an 8-week trial (Lazar *et al.*, 1968). The matter is discussed further in Section 6,A,3,b. A general account of the penetration of many types of drugs into the eye after local application is given by Benson (1974).

D. Absorption through Skin

Apparently diethylcarbamazine is also absorbed readily through the skin. According to a preliminary report by Langham *et al.* (1978), complete elimination of microfilariae from the skin of onchocerciasis patients has been achieved by such local application. They state that virtual cures of patients have been maintained for long periods by the self-application of diethylcarbamazine lotion once a week. No further details are available at present.

III. Pharmacology

A. General

When examined by the techniques of classical pharmacology, diethylcarbamazine is not very active. Reactions vary somewhat with different species and they cannot be assumed to be necessarily the same in man.

1. *Smooth Muscle*

On rabbit intestine, 10 μg/ml diethylcarbamazine produces relaxation. On the isolated uterus of rabbit and rat, there was no action at 1/100,000 (10 μg/ml), but with virgin guinea pig uterus this concentration caused weak contractions (Harned *et al.*, 1948). Subbu and Biswas (1971) reported that 20 μg/ml caused contraction of the uterus of guinea pig and rat and concluded that diethylcarbamazine might cause abortion in women (although this has not otherwise been reported clinically in spite of very wide use of diethylcarbamazine all over the world). The question was extensively investigated by Fraser (1972) who found that large doses (100–200 mg/kg) given by mouth daily to pregnant rats and rabbits had no abortifacient action and no harmful effect on the fetuses. Sareen *et al.* (1961), while testing many substances as antifertility agents, found that diethylcarbamazine given to breeding mice at 200 mg/kg daily for 10 days produced 50% infertility, but many other compounds were more active.

2. *Blood Pressure*

When injected intravenously into anesthetized dogs (2.5–10 mg/kg) diethylcarbamazine causes a rapid rise of blood pressure, followed after about 1 minute by a moderate fall. Both these reactions are blocked by hexamethonium (which blocks action on ganglia). The action of diethylcarbamazine is similar to that of nicotine. Apparently diethylcarbamazine stimulates sympathetic ganglia (causing vasoconstriction), stimulates the adrenal medulla to release adrenaline, and stimulates the respiratory chemoreceptors in the aortic and carotid bodies (Forbes, 1972). These effects are of no clinical significance. In rats and calves, the intravenous injection of diethylcarbamazine, 20 mg/kg, causes changes in the arterial blood pressure similar to those produced by the injection of histamine; and in rats, diethylcarbamazine causes the release of histamine from the lungs, probably from the mast cells (Deline *et al.*, 1973).

3. *Respiration*

Intravenous injection into anesthetized dogs produces deeper and more rapid respiration. Probably this is due to direct action on the respiratory center and also to action on the chemoreceptors just mentioned (Harned *et al.*, 1948; Forbes, 1972).

4. *Central Nervous System*

Parenteral injection (25 mg/kg) into cats and dogs often causes vomiting apparently by stimulation of the vomiting center. [Oral administration to dogs (50 mg/kg) also causes vomiting, probably by direct action on the stomach.] Larger doses may cause sleepiness (Harned *et al.*, 1948). Toxic doses, 560 mg/kg orally in mice, cause convulsions. This convulsive action is probably due to stimulation of the cerebral cortex since the same convulsions have been seen in cases of piperazine citrate poisoning in children (Savage, 1967; Miller and Carpenter, 1967; Martindale, 1967). These children suffered from headache, incoordination, myoclonic jerks, and coma but recovered within 24 hours. The dose required is very large

(1.5 gm daily for 2–3 days to small children) and such convulsions have never been seen with normal doses of diethylcarbamazine. Nevertheless, the headache, sleepiness, and vomiting that may occur after clinical doses of diethylcarbamazine are probably due to the action of the compound on the central nervous system and on the stomach.

B. Anti-inflammatory Effect

Diethylcarbamazine has an anti-inflammatory or blocking action in many anaphylactic reactions. These reactions are very complex, and during the last 10 years they have been studied by many workers in a great variety of animals and organs. The usual procedure has been to provoke some systemic or localized anaphylactic reaction and to see whether the reaction is inhibited by a long series of blocking agents of which diethylcarbamazine is one. Thus diethylcarbamazine has been used as a tool, imperfectly understood, to elucidate reactions that are also not yet understood. Further, the results obtained by one worker in one set of experimental conditions do not agree with those of other workers in other conditions; and results with one species of animal often differ from those with another species. Consequently, it is difficult or almost impossible to give a coherent account of these actions of diethylcarbamazine or to relate them to a logical system of underlying physiological events.

Briefly, however, during anaphylaxis and other reactions in sensitized tissues, antibodies (mainly IgE) adhere to sites on tissue mast cells, basophil leukocytes, and similar cells, and thus sensitize them to the antigen. When antigen comes into contact with them and reacts with them, these cells release various pharmacological agents called mediators, e.g., histamine, serotonin, slowly reacting substance of anaphylaxis (SRS-A), prostaglandins, kinins, and others still unknown. The release of these mediators from the cells requires enzymes, calcium ions, and probably also the breakdown of cyclic adenosine monophosphate. When the mediators have been released they then stimulate smooth muscles (arterioles or bronchioles) to contract, capillaries to dilate and to become more permeable, leukocytes of various kinds to congregate. Thus the phenomena of anaphylaxis and/or of localized inflammation are produced. These anaphylactic reactions may be partially inhibited by a great variety of blocking compounds that act in one of two ways. They may directly antagonize the pharmacological reaction of histamine or serotonin or one of the other active substances, perhaps by blocking the receptor sites on the muscle or other cells sensitive to the substances; this is called direct neutralization of histamine, etc. Alternatively, they may act on the cells (e.g., mast cells) that release histamine or other substances, inhibiting one or more of the several stages leading to such release, so that one or more of the mediators are not liberated. In the case of diethylcarbamazine, it is believed that it usually does not neutralize histamine or serotonin directly but that its main action is to block the release of SRS-A [SRS-A is an unsaturated hydroxy acid of low molecular weight (?400) with biological activity at 1 ng or less]. Sometimes, however, the action of diethylcarbamazine seems to be nonspecific and in some circumstances it may antagonize the effects of histamine and serotonin directly (Burka and Eyre, 1974a). Furthermore, diethylcarbamazine usually has to be supplied in extremely high concentrations to produce its effects. Thus, during *in vitro* experiments, concentrations of 0.4 or 4.0 mg/ml have been employed (Burka and Eyre, 1974b), and *in vivo* experiments on anaphylaxis of calves, intravenous doses of 20 mg/kg supplemented by constant infusion were used to maintain the blood level. These concentrations are much higher than those of other inhibitory compounds and much higher than would be obtained by therapeutic doses in man.

The more important other inhibitory compounds with which diethylcarbamazine is compared are as follows:

a. Cromoglycate (FPL 670, INTAL). A complex molecule, it is believed to inhibit the *release* of histamine from cells, especially mast cells, started by reagin-type antibodies (Cox, 1967); possibly it stabilizes the membranes of the mast cells.

b. Meclofenamate. An "anti-inflammatory agent," it inhibits the action of SRS-A and antigenic bronchospasm of guinea pigs. It also inhibits prostaglandin synthesis.

c. Methysergide, which is an antagonist for serotonin (5-hydroxytryptamine, 5-HT).

d. Isoproterenol (Isoprenaline). A sympathomimetic amine; it acts exclusively on beta receptors. It inhibits the *in vitro* allergic response in which antigen acts on sensitized leukocytes to cause a release of histamine (Lichtenstein and De Bernardo, 1971).

These compounds have no structural similarity to diethylcarbamazine. Since the reactions involved are manifold, highly complex, and still imperfectly understood, it is impossible at this stage to present a clear consistent picture, but the main pieces of experimental evidence are summarized in the following.

1. *Anaphylaxis*

a. In Calves. Calves are sensitized by injections of horse serum and then anaphylactic shock is produced by later intravenous injection of the same antigen. In calves the main reaction takes place in the lungs where both the arterioles and the bronchioles are stimulated to contract. As already described, the combination of antigen with antibody stimulates the release of both histamine, serotonin, and SRS-A (Eyre, 1971). Eyre *et al.* (1973) studied agents that inhibited this anaphylactic shock in the intact animal when administered previously. They found that the most effective inhibition was given by meclofenamate (1.3 mg/kg) or by a combination of cromoglycate and diethylcarbamazine (20 mg/kg). These together inhibited almost all the symptoms of anaphylaxis (contraction of bronchioles and pulmonary arterioles, hemoconcentration, and hyperkalemia, but not the leukopenia). Diethylcarbamazine alone produced 50% inhibition of the changes in systemic arterial blood pressure, but it did not inhibit changes in pulmonary arterial blood pressure or in respiration (Burka and Eyre, 1974a). Cromoglycate alone was inactive. It is concluded that in calves anaphylactic shock is due mainly to the release of SRS-A and that diethylcarbamazine blocks the release of SRS-A or antagonizes its action (it might also block the release of histamine or serotonin or prostaglandins) (Wells *et al.,* 1973; Eyre *et al.,* 1973; Wray and Tomlinson, 1974); Burka and Eyre, 1974a).

If strips of pulmonary vein from sensitized calves are studied *in vitro,* they contract when brought into contact with antigens. This reaction is inhibited by antihistamines and by methysergide (antiserotonin); also there is 50% inhibition by diethylcarbamazine or by cromoglycate separately, but 100% inhibition by the two combined (Eyre, 1971). It is concluded therefore that the reaction of sensitized calf pulmonary vein is a complex one of histamine, serotonin, SRS-A, prostaglandins, and possibly other agents.

b. In Rats and Monkeys. In rats that were first sensitized by chick ovalbumin and then shocked with albumin given intravenously, diethylcarbamazine up to 40 mg/kg did not modify the cardiovascular collapse caused by the shock. These findings indicate that rats differ from calves and that in rats the shock is *not* due to liberation of SRS-A (Lecomte and Salmon, 1972).

When serotonin or histamine were perfused through rat lungs, spasmogens (e.g. prostaglandins, SRS-A, etc.) were released; but this release was blocked by diethylcarbamazine (1 mg/ml) or indomethacin (10 μg/ml). There is a marked difference in lungs from different species of animal (Bakhle and Smith, 1972).

If sensitized monkey lung is exposed to antigen *in vitro,* diethylcarbamazine inhibits the release of SRS-A and also of histamine (Ishizaka *et al.,* 1971); in this reaction it is synergic with isoproterenol.

c. Cutaneous Anaphylaxis. Many studies have been made on cutaneous anaphylaxis in rats and other animals. The results vary according to the technique by which the reaction is provoked and also the species of animal used. Active cutaneous anaphylaxis is produced by immunizing the rat with antigen (albumin) and later injecting the same antigen intradermally. Passive cutaneous anaphylaxis is produced by intradermal injection of antiserum from an immunized animal and by injecting the antigen intravenously hours later (or some other period). Both these reactions are inhibited by diethylcarbamazine and by antihistamines but not by colchicine (Harada *et al.,* 1971). Passive cutaneous anaphylaxis in calves was inhibited by diethylcarbamazine (20 mg/kg), and this inhibition was increased by cromoglycate (Eyre, 1971; Wells and Eyre, 1972). Harada *et al.* (1971) found that diethylcarbamazine (250 mg/kg, i.p.) also inhibited the reactions to intradermal injections of histamine or serotonin in rats, i.e., in this experimental model, diethylcarbamazine neutralized histamine and serotonin directly. However, Pelczarska (1974) reported that in her experiments the direct neutralization did not occur. In mice, passive cutaneous anaphylaxis was not prevented by diethylcarbamazine or cromoglycate, but specific antagonists for serotonin or histamine did prevent it (Casey and Tokuda, 1973).

2. *Rat Peritoneal Cells*

When peritoneal cells from sensitized rats are stimulated *in vitro* by antigen, SRS-A is released from the polymorphs and this release is inhibited by diethylcarbamazine. (By contrast, histamine is released from mast cells and the release caused by antigen is *not* inhibited by diethylcarbamazine; Orange *et al.,* 1968.) On the other hand, if the basophil cells are stimulated by concanavalin A, so that they release histamine, then this histamine release *is* inhibited by diethylcarbamazine (Siraganian and Siraganian, 1974). As a further complication, if rat peritoneal cells are stimulated by corticotropin or compound 48/80 to release histamine from the mast cells granules, then this release is inhibited by diethylcarbamazine citrate (which is used by most experimenters) but not by diethylcarbamazine HCl. Thus some of the observed effects might be due to citrate rather than to diethylcarbamazine base (Ruegg and Jaques, 1974).

3. *Experimental Eosinophilia*

Repeated injection of *Trichinella* antigen into the footpads of guinea pigs provokes eosinophilia in the corresponding lymph nodes. This effect is inhibited by diethylcarbamazine, provided it is given 5–180 minutes *before* the injection of antigen (Thevathasan and Litt, 1971). Probably this is due, once again, to inhibition of release of SRS-A. Diethylcarbamazine does not modify the eosinophilia occurring during anaphylaxis in rats or that produced in guinea pigs or rats by repeated injections of histamine or 48/80; but it does prevent the rise of eosinophils that takes place between 3 to 7 days after feeding guinea pigs with ova or larvae of *Ascaris*. Perhaps this action may be due to removal of the parasites (Sanyal, 1961; Sanyal and Sinha, 1962). Diethylcarbamazine is effective in the treatment of tropical eosinophilia, which is discussed in Section VI,C.

4. *Prostaglandins*

Other substances that are formed and released locally by enzymes during inflammation include prostaglandins, which are highly active unsaturated fatty acids with a 20 carbon atom structure, and many different pharmacological reactions according to the particular compound (Leopold, 1974). Their stimulatory or relaxant actions on ox pulmonary vein strips *in vitro* may be antagonized by diethylcarbamazine in high concentration (0.4 and 4 mg/ml) and also more powerfully by phloretin or by SC-19220. This action of diethylcarbamazine seems to be nonspecific (Burka and Eyre, 1974b).

5. *Effect on Skin Tests*

If patients were given diethylcarbamazine 1.5 gm/day for 5 days and then skin tests were performed by intradermal injection of antigen from infective larvae of *Wuchereria bancrofti,* the resultant reaction was much diminished or even suppressed (Katiyar *et al.,* 1974). This is probably another example of the anti-inflammatory reaction described above.

6. *Summary of Anti-inflammatory Action*

The liberation of pharmacologically active agents, such as histamine and SRS-A, during inflammation and during antigen–antibody reactions is still poorly understood and it differs in different experimental models and in different species of animal. Diethylcarbamazine is only one of a dozen compounds that interfere in these series of reactions. It is obvious that diethylcarbamazine has a general tendency to inhibit the release of SRS-A (and sometimes other agents) that takes place following antigen–antibody reaction or in inflammation and this may explain the palliative action in bronchial asthma. Unfortunately, the exact details differ greatly under different experimental circumstances. Usually the concentration required *in vitro* (up to 1 mg/ml) is much higher than that of other inhibitors. It is not clear whether this anti-inflammatory reaction is always due to the same basic mechanism or whether multiple mechanisms are involved. Similarly, it is not clear whether this action is due to the same structural configuration as the antifilarial action or whether piperazine might not have a somewhat similar action; or even whether the action sometimes depends on the citrate part of the molecule (Ruegg and Jaques, 1974).

The chief clinical effect of diethylcarbamazine in onchocerciasis is to cause inflammatory reactions in the skin (presumably due to release of microfilarial antigens in sensitized tissues), and this contrasts sharply with the anti-inflammatory actions that have been reported in the foregoing. As will be described later the action of diethylcarbamazine on microfilariae seems to be to cause them to release or to expose antigens inside a sensitized host. The relation between this action and the anti-inflammatory action reported in the preceding is not clear. Perhaps the two reactions are not related to one another.

C. Bronchial Asthma

Bronchial asthma is a complicated anaphylactic-like reaction in which some antigen–antibody reaction takes place releasing active substances, including SRS-A, which then provoke the characteristic symptoms. Probably there are multiple causes and reactions (see review by Orange, 1973). In 1965 Salazar-Mallén reported that diethylcarbamazine in a daily dose of 10 mg/kg was effective in the treatment of asthma and this was confirmed by many workers, e.g., Srinivas and Antani (1971), Sly (1974), Thiruvengadam *et al.* (1974), and others. Relief of subjective symptoms was usually greater than objective change in vital measurements. On the other hand, Benner and Lowell (1970) and Rantanen (1971) found no significant improvement in their patients. Good reports tend to come from geographical areas where human parasites are common and this may explain the differences reported (Koivikko, 1973).

IV. Antifilarial Activity

The action on microfilariae and that on adult worms must be described separately. Moreover, the effectiveness differs according to the different species of worms involved.

A. Action on Microfilariae

1. *In Vitro*

In contrast to its powerful action *in vivo,* diethylcarbamazine has no action *in vitro* on either microfilariae or adult worms of *Litomosoides carinii,* and they can live in relatively high concentrations of this drug for several days. Furthermore, serum from animals treated with diethylcarbamazine is not microfilaricidal *in vitro,* i.e., there is no conversion into an active metabolite (Hawking *et al.,* 1950; Kobayashi *et al.,* 1969).

Cavier *et al.* (1971) have stated that diethylcarbamazine, 1/1000, at 28° immobilized the microfilariae of *Dipetalonema witeae* in 24 hours. (Apparently the pH was not controlled, and, in any case, diethylcarbamazine does not act on the microfilariae of *Dip. witeae in vivo.*) Gonzalez Barranco *et al.* (1962) reported that the compound, 1/100,000–1/1,000, at room temperature immobilized (killed) 82% of the microfilariae of *Onchocerca volvulus* in 1 day, but, since 50% of the controls were also immobilized, pH was not controlled, and there was no correlation between the concentration of drug and the percent immobilized, this work probably has little relevance to what happens in the body. Natarajan *et al.* (1973b) state that the microfilariae of *Breinlia sergenti* from the slow loris are immobilized after 12 hours by 1/1000 or 1/10,000 at 28° or at 37°C. In their experiments, the pH was stabilized at 7.2, and nonspecific substances of similar structure, namely sodium benzoate, and methylpiperazine HCl, had no effect. All the same, the concentrations that they used are far higher than are reached *in vivo,* and the whole course of the reaction is so different *in vivo* that this weak *in vitro* action is probably not significant.

Hewitt *et al.* (1947) studied microfilariae in the frog filaria *Folyella dolichoptera,* placed in solutions of diethylcarbamazine HCl, 1/100–1/10,000 (which may have been acid). These are very large microfilariae with a narrow whiplike anterior end and a thicker posterior one. Immediately when they came into contact with the drug the anterior end contracted into a tight coil and violent jerky movements occurred. Then the microfilariae straightened out and became motionless in 5–15 minutes. This behavior has probably nothing to do with the way diethylcarbamazine kills microfilariae *in vivo,* but it may be a manifestation of its action on acetylcholine and choline esterase in the microfilariae (see Section IV,A,3,b).

2. *In Vivo*

When diethylcarbamazine is administered to infected animals or men by any of the usual routes, microfilariae rapidly disappear from the circulation. Single intraperitoneal doses of 50 mg (citrate)/kg given to cotton rats usually cause marked diminution of the microfilariae count, which passes off after 4–8 days. Daily doses as low as 1–5 mg/kg (for 6 days) exert a recognizable action. Large doses (up to 1100 mg/kg in 9 hours) do not remove all microfilariae from the blood. After all these treatments, numerous living microfilariae can be found postmortem in the pleural cavities (Hawking *et al.,* 1950).

If diethylcarbamazine (60 mg/kg) is injected intravenously into cotton rats (so as to avoid delay of absorption), 80% of the microfilariae disappear in 1 minute (which is an astonishingly rapid disappearance), and the same occurs with *Wuchereria bancrofti* in man. By contrast, however, a few microfilariae often persist in cotton rats or in man for days even if large doses have been given (Hawking *et al.,* 1950). In cats, infected with *Brugia malayi* and *Brugia pahangi* and treated with adequate doses of diethylcarbamazine that killed all the adult worms (as shown by autopsy), some microfilariae still persisted in the blood (Edeson and Laing, 1959). The reason for this persistence has not been elucidated. It may be that persistent microfilariae are biologically different from the others (either newborn or very old) or that there is some reservoir outside the circulation from which the microfilariae continually enter the blood. The latter is a probable explanation, since diethylcarbamazine does *not* affect microfilariae that are outside the circulation, e.g., those of *L. carinii* in the pleural cavity of a cotton rat, those of *W. bancrofti* in a hydrocele, or those of *O. volvulus* in a fibrous nodule (Hawking, 1950, 1952). Another plausible explanation is that the microfilariae that persist are in a different immunological state from the others (see Section IV,A,3,b). The microfilariae of *W. bancrofti* that persist in the blood of patients treated with diethylcarbamazine are still capable of developing in *Culex p. fatigans* mosquitoes (Chen and Fan, 1977).

As regards the sensitivity of the different species, diethylcarbamazine is effective against most species of microfilariae (including those of *O. volvulus* and *Dipetalonema streptocerca* when they are in the skin). There is surprisingly little information about *Manzonella ozzardi.* Mazzotti (1948b) reported that it had no effect in Mexico. Montestruc *et al.* (1950) treated 5 patients in Martinique with 400 mg daily for 10 days and stated that the microfilariae disappeared from the blood in a few days. Botero *et al.* (1965) refer to 1 patient who was treated previously by Restrepo *et al.* (1962) without any effect on the microfilariae. F. Biagi (personal communication) states that Mazzotti made extensive trials in Yucatan; he found that 10 mg/kg per day was ineffective but that 30 mg/kg per day for 15 days easily achieved total cure; this treatment was used successfully as mass chemotherapy in heavily infected areas of Yucatan but, unfortunately, Mazzotti died before writing a final report on the subject (see also Biagi, 1974). Diethylcarbamazine is less effective, or even inactive, against the microfilariae of *Dipetalonema perstans* (Hawking, 1950), of *Dip. witeae* of jirds, and of *Edesonfilaria malayensis* from Thailand. It has little action on the microfilariae of *Dirofilaria repens* (Dalip Singh, 1962): 2 dogs were treated with 3.8 and 5.6 mg/kg, respectively, daily for 5 days, but there was no reduction of the microfilaria count and the microfilariae developed normally in mosquitoes that were allowed to feed during this treatment. The compound acts on the microfilariae of *Icosiella neglecta* of frogs (Minning and Ding, 1951) and on those of *Setaria equina* in horses (Lapeyrad, 1970) and of *Setaria cervi* transplanted into rats or dogs (Singhal *et al.,* 1972a,b).

3. *Mode of Action on Microfilariae*

a. Experimental Evidence. If search is made for the microfilariae of *Litomosoides carinii* that disappear from the circulation of cotton rats after treatment with diethylcarbamazine, they can be found in the liver, and to a lesser extent in the spleen and bone marrow. Within an hour after the administration of drug, phagocytes congregate round these trapped microfilariae and within 18 hours most of them have been destroyed (Hawking *et al.,* 1950). This trapping of microfilariae has been studied in the living liver by Taylor (1960) and with the electron microscope by Schardein *et al.* (1968). Before diethylcarbamazine, the microfilariae could be seen in the living liver circulating freely through the capillaries. Within 5 minutes of intravenous injection of diethylcarbamazine, most of the microfilariae had become adherent to the walls of the capillaries, usually by their tails. They remained like this wriggling for 4–60 minutes. Sometimes a leukocyte became attached to the tail of a stationary microfilaria; occasionally, the microfilariae became so numerous that they blocked the capillary. In the electron microscope studies, before diethylcarbamazine the liver contained only a few microfilariae, which were normal and enclosed in a sheath, 20 minutes after the drug, there were many microfilariae in the liver. Some were free in the sinusoids (an attachment by the tail would not be seen under the electron microscope) and they appeared similar to untreated ones except that *no sheath was visible.* The microfilariae were surrounded by a clear space. There were occasional microfilariae *inside* hepatocytes that otherwise showed no localized cellular reaction or destruction; the microfilariae were partitioned from the cytoplasm by a clear space. Four hours after diethylcarbamazine the microfilariae were less numerous in the liver, and many of those in the sinusoids were undergoing lysis. The adjacent Kupffer cells and hepatocytes contained many lysosomes, and there were foci of inflammatory cells, mostly polymorphs, around the microfilariae that were undergoing lysis. The collection and destruction of the microfilariae in the liver is probably a function of the reticuloendothelial system, which is concentrated in the liver of rodents more than in other organs; it seems to depend on the large fixed macrophage of the tissues. Destruction of the microfilariae of *Loa loa* has been shown to occur in the liver of man also (Woodruff, 1951). In a drill, infected with *L. loa,* which was treated with diethylcarbamazine and then killed after 6 hours, many microfilariae were found to be undergoing destruction by the reticuloendothelial cells of the liver but few or none were being destroyed in the spleen (Duke, 1960) (although in the spontaneous immune reaction of the drill against *L. loa,* most of the microfilariae are destroyed in special nodules in the spleen, and none in the liver). The part played by the bone marrow has not been properly investigated. Presumably the microfilariae of *W. bancrofti* are destroyed in the same way as those of *Loa loa* and *Litomosoides carinii.*

According to Kobayashi *et al.* (1969), who studied *L. carinii* in cotton rats, diethylcarbamazine is not effective in removing microfilariae from the blood unless antibodies are present. Thus, if microfilariae or adult worms are transplanted into a clean host that is then treated with diethylcarbamazine, the microfilaricidal action of the drug is almost or completely absent. If microfilariae are soaked in diethylcarbamazine (1500 μg/ml) *in vitro* and then transfused into a clean host, they are not destroyed. If cotton rats containing inoculated microfilariae had been passively immunized by injecting serum of infected cotton rats, then diethylcarbamazine had an immediate but transient effect in reducing the number of microfilariae in the blood (see also Tanaka *et al.,* 1970). Kobayashi's conclusions have been disputed by Zahner *et al.* (1977). They reported (without giving full experimental details) that if microfilariae from the blood of *Mastomys* were injected intravenously into another animal, oral administration of diethylcarbamazine, 500 mg/kg, 1 hour later (or 1, 3, or 14 days later) led to a quick and sustained reduction in the microfilaremia. Similar results were seen if the microfilariae were taken from the blood of cotton rats and the diethylcarbamazine was given 3 days later. On the other hand, if the microfilariae injected had been collected from the pleural cavity, the reduction of microfilaremia was diminished if the treatment was given 1 hour later, but it was increased if given 3 days later. The workers concluded that microfilariae recovered from the pleural cavity are less sensitive to diethylcarbamazine (and to Haloxan) if no antibodies are present, but that microfilariae taken from the blood and injected into a clean animal are sensitive to both these compounds even without antibodies. Perhaps the results depend on differences in technique, about which information is at present incomplete. More investigations on this important question are desirable.

Tanaka *et al.* (1977) have found that if infected cotton rats were treated repeatedly with antilymphocytic or antithymic serum and were then given diethylcarbamazine intravenously the expected fall of microfilaraemia was much diminished and was not sustained. This finding shows that lymphocytes (also T-cells) are important for the microfilaricidal action of the compound.

b. Theoretical Conclusions. In view of all this evidence, the mode of action of diethylcarbamazine on microfilariae is probably as follows:

1. In the first place, since the action of diethylcarbamazine depends on a specific chemical configuration, it would seem that this must be an attachment to the microfilaria. No such fixation of the compound on microfilariae has yet been demonstrated but it would be desirable to reinvestigate the subject with radioactive labeled compound.

2. After fixation, diethylcarbamazine modifies the microfilariae in two ways, which may be independent of one another.

Effect on neuromuscular system. Microfilariae are in a constant state of muscular activity (wriggling), waves of contraction passing down them from head to tail producing forward movement, and less frequently from tail to head producing backward movement. By this means, microfilariae can move toward more favorable locations or back away from unfavorable ones. Most important in the case of *W. bancrofti, Loa loa,* and other periodic microfilariae in the blood, these reverse movements enable the microfilariae in the blood to hold themselves in the small arterioles of the lungs (Hawking, 1967). Microfilariae contain acetylcholine (Mellanby, 1955) and choline esterase (Bueding, 1952) that doubtless play a part in their neuromuscular activity. Diethylcarbamazine potentiates the action of acetylcholine in causing the contraction of nerve muscle preparations of *Ascaris,* such potentiation being shown in as high dilutions as those of eserine (i.e., about 50 nmol/ml at 27°) (Natarajan *et al.,* 1973a). Such interference with the acetylcholine mechanism might well disturb the normal waves of contraction in microfilariae (perhaps blocking the power to reverse). Clinically this would explain (1) the liberation of microfilariae of *W. bancrofti* from the lungs into the blood during the daytime by provocative doses of diethylcarbamazine (see Section IV,A,4,a); (2) the reaction of the microfilariae of *O. volvulus* to the compound by passing from the dermis into the epidermis, which is an unfavorable environment and in which they are not normally found; (3) similarly, an increase in the number of onchocercal microfilariae in the urine, blood, and sputum; and (4) after administration of diethylcarbamazine, the penetration of some microfilariae of *Litomosoides carinii* into the hepatocytes of the liver, where they are never found normally (Schardein *et al.,* 1968). Admittedly no obvious effect of diethylcarbamazine on the mobility of microfilariae *in vitro* has yet been reported, but the usual technique of inspection under a cover slip would not reveal the more subtle changes of reversal of waves of contraction. These should be studied by cinematographic technique with the microfilariae compressed on an agar pad (Hawking and Clark, 1967).

This action of diethylcarbamazine in deranging the muscular activity of microfilariae might depend on the piperazine ring part of the molecule rather than on the microfilaricidal structure (see Section IV,B,3). It would be interesting to investigate whether piperazine alone can liberate microfilariae into the bloodstream. In any case, this deranging action, although interesting, may not contribute much to the ultimate destruction of the microfilariae (see also Section IV,A,4).

Apparently organophosphorus compounds, particularly Haloxan, have a microfilaricidal action very similar to that of diethylcarbamazine, i.e., when tested on *L. carinii* in *Mastomys* they cause a rapid reduction in the number of microfilariae in the blood, which does not last more than 3 days. [Reduction by 86% takes 1 hour after an oral dose of Haloxan, 100 mg/kg, or 10 minutes after diethylcarbamazine 500 mg/kg (Lämmler and Grüner, 1975).] Organophosphorus compounds are well known to inhibit cholinesterases of worms and of mammals, but such inhibition has not been demonstrated for diethylcarbamazine (except as discussed in the preceding lines).

The actions of diethylcarbamazine and of Haloxan upon microfilariae in *Mastomys natalensis* have recently been compared in detail by Zahner *et al.* (1976). In many respects they are closely similar. Both of these compounds tend to immobilize the microfilariae in the blood and to cause adherence of phagocytic cells; but there are minor differences in that diethylcarbamazine immobilizes particularly the microfilariae in the lungs and Haloxan immobilizes particularly those in the pleural cavity. Also diethylcarbamazine causes cell adhesion predominantly in the liver, and Haloxan predominantly in the spleen. It may be doubted however whether the technique employed (study of living microfilariae in dab smears from the different organs) can give reliable quantitative measurements about the true position in the organs; thus, those microfilariae which were really adherent to the cells of the organ would not appear in the dab smears at all.

This similarity between diethylcarbamazine and Haloxan should certainly be investigated further, particularly to answer the following questions:

i. Does Haloxan cause microfilariae of *L. carinii* to be accumulated and destroyed in the liver, as diethylcarbamazine does?

ii. Does the microfilaricidal action of Haloxan require the presence of antibodies in the host? [cf. Kobayashi *et al.,* 1969; Zahner *et al.,* 1977; see also the following discussion].

iii. Do Haloxan (and diethylcarbamazine) alter the waves of contraction/relaxation that pass down and up microfilariae (to be examined by cinematography on an agar pad; see the preceding).

Effect on the surface layers of microfilariae. As already described, after diethylcarbamazine is given *in vivo,* microfilariae are seized by phagocytes and destroyed—but the finer mechanism of this reaction is not yet completely known. Within 5 minutes of injecting diethylcarbamazine, microfilariae of *L. carinii* begin to adhere by their tails to the walls of liver sinusoids (Taylor, 1960). According to electron microscopy the microfilariae of *L. carinii* had lost their sheath in less than 20 minutes (Schardein *et al.,* 1968). In the case of the microfilariae of *O. volvulus* (which do not have a sheath but which have a five-layer cuticle), Rougemont *et al.* (1974) reported that when examined after 12 hours the cuticle had disappeared and the layers could no longer be differentiated. In more recent work, Gibson *et al.* (1976) report that the earliest change (3.5–18 hours) consists of an irregular enlargement of the middle layer of the cuticle (called by them the "electrolucent" zone) and this is confirmed by A. Rougemont (personal letter). They also describe deposits of granular substance on the surface of the cuticle, which could be antigen–antibody complexes; but Rougemont has not seen these.

When the surface coat of the microfilariae has been removed or deranged by diethylcarbamazine, antigens would become exposed. The exposed antigens would immediately react with the antibodies present in the plasma forming antigen–antibody complexes. Such complexes are known to attract and activate eosinophils. The eosinophils and other phagocytes would then attach themselves and destroy the microfilariae as described in the foregoing. [If there were no antibodies present, as contrived experimentally by Kobayashi *et al.* (1969), there should be no destruction of microfilariae; see earlier.]

4. *Mobilization of Microfilariae by Diethylcarbamazine*

a. Wuchereria bancrofti. When diethylcarbamazine is injected intravenously into dogs infected with *D. immitis* or into patients infected with *W. bancrofti* during the daytime, at which time the microfilariae count is relatively or absolutely low, the microfilariae count is much increased with a peak after 2 minutes and a return to normal by 30 minutes (Fukamachi, 1960; Hawking and Adams, 1964). (This is in apparent contrast to the rapid fall that results when the compound is injected intravenously into patients with *W. bancrofti* at night, or into cotton rats with *L. carinii,* as described previously). The initial rise of the count is presumably due to liberation of microfilariae from the capillaries of the lung where they accumulate in the daytime. Probably the compound interferes with the mechanism by which the microfilariae hold themselves in the lungs, although they appear quite motile when examined microscopically under a cover slip at this time (Section IV,A,3,b). The subsequent fall of the count is presumably due to the capture of the microfilariae by fixed phagocytes under the influence of the drug. If the intravenous injection is repeated on successive days, the rise of the microfilariae count becomes less on each occasion, probably because many microfilariae have been destroyed by previous injections. Fukamachi (1960) reported that this rise of the count of *D. immitis* was inhibited by the previous administration of atropine (which would implicate acetylcholine in the reaction); but Hawking and Adams (1964), working with *W. bancrofti,* found that atropine made no difference.

This action of diethylcarbamazine has recently been investigated by many workers as a possible means of conducting filarial surveys by daytime collection of blood samples rather than by night ones. The general procedure has been to give a dose of diethylcarbamazine by mouth about 10 A.M. and then to take blood slides 30–60 minutes later to examine for microfilariae (e.g., Sullivan and Hembree, 1970).

Iwamoto (1971) found that, if 0.1 mg/kg was given by day, microfilariae often appeared in the circulation within 5 minutes and were maximum after 15 minutes. Manson-Bahr and Wijers (1972) reported that a dose of 100 mg by mouth during the day increases the microfilaria count to one-third of that found by night. Katiyar *et al.* (1974) gave 4 mg/kg by mouth to 10 carriers at 6:00 P.M. (when the count was negligible); 2 hours later the average microfilaria count had risen to 6.7% of the midnight "maximum." Rajapakse (1974) gave 5 mg/kg by mouth at 10:00 A.M.; before diethylcarbamazine only 2.5% of the night-positive persons were positive, but 20 minutes later 40% of the night positives could be detected by this method. Russel *et al.* (1975) gave the compound to carriers of *W. bancrofti* and *B. malayi* and found that 60–93% of the night positives could be detected by day sampling. For *W. bancrofti* they recommended that the dose should be 4–6 mg/kg with examination at 30–60 minutes later, and for *B. malayi* the dose should be 2 mg/kg with examination after 90 minutes.

To summarize it may be said that this provocative administration of diethylcarbamazine would be sufficient to distinguish villages heavily infected with *W. bancrofti* from those lightly infected, but it would not detect a high enough percentage of carriers if treatment was later to be confined to carriers only. If daytime surveys for *W. bancrofti* are desired, the membrane filtration method of Desowitz and Southgate (1973) might be more accurate if it were acceptable (it requires venous blood instead of finger blood). It would be best if the two methods were combined.

b. Onchocerca volvulus. A somewhat similar effect occurs in onchocerciasis. When this is first treated with diethylcarbamazine, microfilariae become more common in the blood, urine, sputum, and cerebrospinal fluid.

The occasional presence of microfilariae in the urine of untreated onchocerciasis patients was first emphasized by Buck *et al.* (1969) who found that in the Chad area this might happen in 11.4% of patients; in later work (Buck *et al.*, 1971), they showed that the microfilariae probably came alive from the kidney or renal pelvis but they died during their transit of the bladder. In patients treated with diethylcarbamazine, however, microfilariae are found more often (Mazzotti and Osorio, 1949). Roux and Picq (1974) found microfilariae in the urine of 40 out of 42 patients during a course of diethylcarbamazine. Fuglsang and Anderson (1973) found that treatment caused a twelve-fold increase in the number of microfilariae in the urine within 24 hours of the first treatment; some of their patients showed respiratory distress after the first tablet and microfilariae were found in their sputum. Mazzotti (1959) has shown that, after diethylcarbamazine, onchocercal microfilariae are more commonly found in the blood and in the cerebrospinal fluid; and other workers reported that diethylcarbamazine causes mobilization of microfilariae in the epidermis (Rougemont *et al.*, 1974) and in the cornea (Anderson and Fuglsang, 1973).

Estimations of the total number of microfilariae in the various body fluids during treatment with diethylcarbamazine and suramin have been made by Duke *et al.* (1976b). Naturally these estimations can only be approximate ones. Microfilariae are thought to pass from the skin through the lymphatics into the bloodstream. From the blood some of them pass through the capillary walls of the glomeruli (not readily) into the urine, through the pulmonary alveoli (not readily) into the sputum, and through the choroid plexuses (fairly easily) into the cerebrospinal fluid. Microfilariae in the anterior chamber of the eye appear to come, not from the blood, but from uveal tissues; when diethylcarbamazine is given, they are not destroyed *in situ,* but their numbers fall because their source of replenishment has been cut off. After diethylcarbamazine has been given the number in the blood and the urine rises rapidly on the second and third days of treatment and may remain high for 1–2 weeks. In 5 heavily infected patients, studied by Duke *et al.* (1976a), the mean total number of microfilariae in the skin was about 28×10^6 the total number in the blood was about 40×10^3 (i.e., 0.14% of those in the skin), and the total number excreted in the urine during the first week of treatment was 460, i.e., 1.2% of the total blood load. The total number passing from the blood into the urine, sputum, and cerebrospinal fluid was relatively small so that apparently over 97% of those in the blood, killed by diethylcarbamazine treatment, were destroyed elsewhere (presumably in the liver).

This mobilization of onchocercal microfilariae is interesting but as regards the blood, urine, and sputum, it does not seem to have much practical significance. Mobilization of microfilariae into the cerebrospinal fluid is more dangerous, however, and, if the number in the fluid exceeds 3 microfilariae/ml, diethylcarbamazine treatment may provoke vertigo and other neurological symptoms (Duke *et al.,* 1976a; see Section V,C,1,a).

With both *W. bancrofti* and *O. volvulus* this early provocative action of diethylcarbamazine may be interpreted as a disturbance (probably partial paralysis) of the muscular mechanisms by which microfilariae normally hold themselves in their preferred positions in the lung capillaries (*W. bancrofti*) or in the skin (*O. volvulus*) (see Section IV,A,3,b).

5. *Other Actions of Diethylcarbamazine on Microfilariae*

Attempts to interfere with the *in vivo* action of diethylcarbamazine by previous treatment with compounds of somewhat similar chemical structure, e.g., diethylurea, nicotinamide, nicotinic acid, nikethamide, quinine, or lucanthone, were unsuccessful (Hawking *et al.,* 1950).

If microfilariae of *L. carinii* (but not of *W. bancrofti* or *D. immitis*) are placed in an electrophoretic field, they orientate their head toward the anode and then their wriggling gradually carries them in that direction; there is no true electrophoretic transportation of these or other microfilariae by the electrophoretic force. Addition of diethylcarbamazine to the medium does not alter this state of affairs; consequently, there is no sign that the compound affects the electric charges of microfilariae.

Ortiz y Ortiz *et al.* (1962) reported that microfilariae of *O. volvulus* had a proteolytic action on human serum *in vitro,* setting free amino acids, and that this action was increased by diethylcarbamazine 1/6250 at 37°; but this observation has never been confirmed or extended.

Jaffe and Doremus (1970) made an exhaustive study of the metabolism of glucose by microfilariae. They found considerable utilization of radioactive glucose and incorporation into many vital compounds. This metabolism was not affected by diethylcarbamazine apart from slight inhibition of incorporation of glucose into the lipid fraction. The significance of this work is that it shows that the compound has no direct toxic action on microfilariae.

Mohan (1973, 1974) report that in the white rat infected with *L. carinii* and treated with diethylcarbamazine, he did not find that phagocytes destroyed microfilariae in the liver; he considers that the main action of diethylcarbamazine was stimulation of eosinophils that showed excess lobation of the nucleus. This view, however, seems to be based on a single infected rat treated with diethylcarbamazine and killed 6 hours later, and more evidence is required before his conclusion can be properly evaluated.

B. Action on Adult Worms

1. *In Vitro*

Diethylcarbamazine has no action at 37° *in vitro* on the adult worms of *L. carinii* or *Dip. witeae* in concentrations 10 times greater than those obtainable *in vivo*. (But it does not act on these species *in vivo* either.) When adult worms of *Breinlia sergenti* (from slow loris) were exposed to 1/1000 for 7 hours at 28° they became elongated and sluggish. When they were examined *in vitro* attached to a recording lever, 0.3 μmole (approximately 1/9000) caused a reduction of tone and of spontaneous contractions, and 1.0 μmole (1/3000) caused loss of tone and paralysis (Natarajan *et al.*, 1973b). But it is doubtful if this action has any significance for the therapeutic action *in vivo*.

2. *In Vivo*

In experimental animals, the action on adult worms can easily be observed by inspection at postmortem examination. In man, on the other hand, it must usually be inferred from indirect evidence. Different species of worm vary greatly in their susceptibility. The adult worms of *L. carinii* are not susceptible both *in vitro* and *in vivo:* after prolonged treatment of cotton rats, e.g., 250 mg/kg, i.p., twice daily for twenty-eight doses, most of the adult worms can be found alive and they contain active microfilariae (Taylor and Terry, 1960). Similarly, the adult worms of *D. immitis* or *Dip. repens* of dogs and of *Dip. witeae* of the jirds are also resistant. The adult worms of *O. volvulus* are also not susceptible, and, after intensive treatment of man with diethylcarbamazine, live worms can be found in the nodules. (These nodules even in untreated patients usually contain some dead worms, so that it is impossible to say whether a few may or may not have been damaged by the drug.)

On the other hand, with *Loa loa* the compound almost certainly kills the adult worms. Soon after treatment, small elongated wheals may appear under the skin, and on biopsy, these wheals are found to contain a dead worm. Furthermore, the microfilariae disappear from the blood and do not reappear even during prolonged follow-up observations.

In the same way the adult worms of *Dip. streptocerca* (which live under the skin) are killed by diethylcarbamazine. When it was given to a patient, papules 1.0–2.5 cm appeared in the skin; and if these were excised 24 hours after the first dose of diethylcarbamazine, dead worms were found. The worms were coiled up and were sometimes surrounded by exudate containing degenerating eosinophils and a few polymorphs; there might be fractures in the cuticle of the worms (Meyers *et al.*, 1972).

With *W. bancrofti* and *Brugia malayi*, it has seldom been possible to excise and examine the adult worms, but there is indirect evidence as follows:

1. After adequate treatment the microfilariae of most patients disappear (quickly) and do not reappear even after 12 months, by which time any surviving worms could presumably have recovered from their temporary damage.
2. In some patients, perhaps 5%, there are small areas of acute inflammation persisting for about a week in the groin, spermatic cord, etc., where adult worms are probably situated.

Moreover, direct evidence on the subject has been supplied by Ch'en (1964). When patients with bancroftian or malayan filariasis are treated in China with single, large doses of diethylcarbamazine, it has been found that small nodules often develop on the lymphatics of the thigh, spermatic cord, or axilla; if these nodules are excised they have been found to contain dying or dead adult worms surrounded by degenerated cells. From all this evidence it is concluded that the adult female worms are killed or permanently sterilized by adequate treatment with diethylcarbamazine.

In cats infected with *B. malayi* or *Brugia pahangi*, adequate doses of diethylcarbamazine (e.g. more than 5 mg base/kg, i.p., daily for 7 days) killed all the adult worms as was shown by subsequent autopsy (Edeson and Laing, 1959). Curiously, microfilariae still persisted in diminished numbers in the blood of these cats after the adult worms had been killed.

In the case of *Setaria digitata* in the anterior chamber of the eye of horses, diethylcarbamazine, given orally as 80 mg/kg body weight, was apparently successful in removing the worms in 2 out of 4 horses (Ahmed and Gupta, 1965).

The foregoing discussion may be summarized by saying that diethylcarbamazine kills the adult worms of *L. loa, W. bancrofti, B. malayi, Dip. streptocerca,* and *S. digitata,* but not those of *O. volvulus, D. immitis, D. repens, L. carinii,* or *Dip. witeae*. There is possibly a slight lethal or sterilizing action on *Dip. perstans* (McGregor *et al.*, 1952).

The mechanism by which diethylcarbamazine kills adult worms of *Loa*, etc., is not clear, and it is difficult to investigate since the adults of experimental infections (*Litosomoides, Dirofilaria*) are not affected by it *in vitro* or *in vivo*. It is probable that phagocytes are concerned, and certainly dead worms of *Loa* are surrounded by such cells, but it is not clear whether the phagocytosis is the cause of the worms' death or the result.

3. *Action of Piperazine on Ascaris*

Piperazine and derivatives of piperazine including diethylcarbamazine cause paralysis of the muscles of intestinal nematodes such as *Ascaris lumbricoides,* and this action often leads to the expulsion of the *Ascaris* through the anus.

In vitro the stimulating action of acetylcholine on fragments of *Ascaris* is blocked by piperazine (Norton and De Beer, 1957). The action of piperazine on muscle cells of *Ascaris* has been further studied by Del Castillo *et al.* (1964) by electrophysiological techniques. They found that piperazine produces hyperpolarization of the cell membrane of the muscle cells around the neuromuscular synapse leading to inhibition of the muscle cell. The hyperpolarization depends on an increase in the permeability of the membrane to chloride ions and to those of volatile fatty acids. In this way, piperazine acts as a pharmacological analog of a natural inhibitory neurohormone. In view of all this, it is possible that the action of diethylcarbamazine interfering with the neuromuscular activity of microfilariae (see Section IV,A,3,b) might be due to the piperazine ring part of the molecule rather than to the specific filaricidal configuration. Incubation of *Ascaris* with piperazine greatly reduces the production of succinic acid (Bueding *et al.,* 1959) which might have something to do with the increase of cell permeability to volatile fatty acids previously mentioned.

C. Action on Forms in the Insect Vector

The developing forms of *Dirofilaria repens* in the mosquito are resistant to diethylcarbamazine (Hawking *et al.,* 1950).

Microfilariae of *L. carinii* are not prevented from developing in the mites if the host has been treated with diethylcarbamazine just before the vectors suck blood; and, similarly, *W. bancrofti* and *D. immitis* are not prevented from developing in mosquitoes (Kanda *et al.,* 1967b). Apparently, diethylcarbamazine is *not* active in the arthropod vector. Microfilariae of *W. bancrofti* in patients, who have been treated with diethylcarbamazine more than 46 days earlier, are still capable of developing normally in *Culex p. fatigans* (Chen and Fan, 1977).

D. Action of Infective Larvae and Immature Worms

1. The infective larvae of *L. carinii* seem to be destroyed by diethylcarbamazine if given as 500 mg/kg daily for 12 days during exposure to infec-

tive mites, since the subsequent development of microfilariae is prevented. Given for 6 days, 1 week or 2 weeks later, the compound is much less effective. It certainly seems able to prevent the male infective larvae developing, but whether it also kills the female ones is less clear (Hawking *et al.*, 1950). According to Lämmler and Wolf (1977) working with *Mastomys natalensis,* the greatest effect is obtained against the fifth-stage larvae (i.e., treatment given from the twenty-fifth to the thirty-second day after infection). The pure third-stage larvae are not affected (by treatment given from the second to the sixth day), but they become more sensitive at the moulting period a few days later (seventh to eleventh day).

2. There is no action on infective larvae of *W. bancrofti in vitro* (Moreau and Pichon, 1972); Jordan, 1958); the action *in vivo* is not known.

3. The prophylactic action on *B. malayi* in cats has been investigated by Ewert and Emerson (1975). Cats were infected by the injection of infective larvae and the compound was given from the day of infection and for 7 successive days. The cats were killed 14 days after infection and a search was made in the appropriate tissues for developing larvae. In 37 control cats, larvae were found in all. Diethylcarbamazine (citrate) at 1 mg/kg had no prophylactic action. After 2 mg/kg, a few moribund larvae were found in 8 out of 10 cats; after 5 mg/kg in 2 out of 5 cats; after 10 mg/kg in 1 out of 5 cats; and after 25–100 mg/kg, they were found in only 1 out of 17 cats. Apparently diethylcarbamazine at 25 mg/kg is effective in preventing the development of the infective larvae of *B. malayi* and *B. pahangi.*

4. Extensive studies of early forms of *Loa* have been carried out by Duke (1961, 1963). Infective stages of *Loa loa* were obtained from the insect vector (*Chrysops*), and infected subcutaneously into young monkeys (drills); these were killed 3 to 6 months later and the number of adult worms that had developed under the skin was counted. In untreated controls about a third of the injected worms established themselves. Other groups of monkeys were treated with diethylcarbamazine given as 4–20 oral doses of 150 mg/kg or of various smaller amounts. The minimum dose to produce complete prophylaxis in 90% of the animals was 5 mg/kg given from 2 days before, until 14 days after, infection. The work was then extended to human volunteers, and it was found that the minimum effective dose was 5 mg/kg given for at least 3 days; this was effective if given within 1 month after infection. When the invading worms were killed by this treatment they caused small papules in the skin at the sites of their destruction; consequently, by infecting a man and then administering treatment after a suitable number of days, a picture could be obtained of the migration of the worms from their portal of entry. The infective early forms of *Loa* are more susceptible than are the adult worms. For practical

prophylaxis of man against infection by *Loa,* a regimen of 200 mg per person twice daily for 3 days every month is recommended. Possibly the same procedure might be effective as prophylaxis against *B. malayi* or *W. bancrofti,* but this needs further investigation. In the case of *W. bancrofti* infections, it might be simpler to administer a curative course once yearly, rather than monthly prophylactic ones. As a public health measure, it would be better if all the population could be treated and the reservoir of microfilariae for reinfection would then be removed.

5. Prolonged studies of early forms of *D. immitis* have been carried out by Kume and his colleagues (1962, 1964, 1967). With this worm the early stages develop under the skin, but after 85–120 days they migrate to the right ventricle of the heart; their environment is obviously quite different during these two phases. Infective larvae were injected subcutaneously into dogs; 130–165 days later the dogs were killed and the number of worms in the heart was counted. Diethylcarbamazine was given to the dogs according to various schedules. When given by mouth at 220 mg/kg daily for 5 consecutive days beginning 1, 30, or 60 days after inoculation, it did not prevent infection (Kume *et al.,* 1962a), but when 11 mg/kg was given daily, beginning 2 months before and 7 months after inoculation, diethylcarbamazine prevented infection completely. It is now recommended by Kume that dogs exposed to infection should be given 5.5 mg/kg daily beginning just before the season of infection and continued for 4 weeks afterward. This dosage is nontoxic, and it will completely prevent infection. Apparently diethylcarbamazine (45 mg/kg for 3 days every 3 months) has been used successfully for prophylaxis in Northern Australia by Aubrey (1964). This action of diethylcarbamazine on the immature forms of *D. immitis* is interesting because the compound has little action on the adult worms in the heart; perhaps the subcutaneous position of the worms makes them more susceptible, although this is not the case with *Dip. witeae* which is not susceptible (either microfilariae or adults) to diethylcarbamazine. More likely the metabolism or cuticle of immature *D. immitis* differs from that of the adult.

6. The prophylactic action on *O. volvulus* has been investigated by Duke (1968) in two chimpanzees given, respectively, 5 and 23 mg/kg daily for 18–24 days following inoculation of infective larvae and in 2 human volunteers given, respectively, 10 mg/kg daily for 5 and 16 days. No prophylactic action against the development of the infective larvae could be found.

Thus diethylcarbamazine prevents the development of infective larvae and immature worms in the case of *B. malayi, B. pahangi, Loa loa, D. immitis,* and *Litomosoides carinii* but not in the case of *O. volvulus*. The action on developing *W. bancrofti* is not known.

E. Development of Drug Resistance

According to modern conceptions, drug resistance develops from mutants that appear during the reproduction of an organism and which are then selected out for propagation by exposure to drug. The reproductive cycle of filariae (3 months to several years) is so long compared with that of bacteria or protozoa, that it seems theoretically unlikely that acquired drug resistance to diethylcarbamazine or to any other drug will become important in connection with these worms. This conclusion is supported by some investigations by Hawking *et al.* (1950) on the effect of prolonged treatment. Two groups of cotton rats infected with *L. carinii* were treated with diethylcarbamazine 10 or 100 mg/kg, respectively, by mouth, daily for 108 days. This treatment caused most (but not all) of the microfilariae to disappear from the blood, but they gradually reappeared when treatment stopped. There was no evidence of drug resistance during this period.

In onchocerciasis, Vargas and Tovar (1957) noted that not all microfilariae were destroyed by diethylcarbamazine, and they speculated about the development of drug-resistant strains. However, their forebodings seem to be completely misplaced since with this infection further microfilariae are always being produced by adult onchocercae (which are unaffected by the drug) and since mass treatments are never likely to be undertaken because the effects of treating onchocerciasis with diethylcarbamazine are so short-lived.

F. Action on Other Worms

Diethylcarbamazine is also active against various other worms, which fact might give some clue to the nature of its action on filariae.

1. *Setaria*

When adult worms of *Setaria* are taken from the peritoneum of cattle at the slaughterhouse and transplanted intraperitoneally into rats or dogs, microfilariae appear in the blood of the new host and persist for many days. These microfilariae are sensitive to doses of diethylcarbamazine and such artificially infected animals can be used for screening antifilarial drugs (Singhal *et al.*, 1972a,b).

Four horses with *S. digitata* (*Filaria oculi*) in the anterior chamber of the eye were treated by oral doses of diethylcarbamazine 80 mg/kg, and the worms were destroyed in 2 of them (Ahmed and Gupta, 1965). During *in vivo* tests on *S. digitata* (host not stated), Kono (1965) found that diethylcarbamazine reduced the number of microfilariae in the blood, but had no obvious effect on the adult worms.

Four horses near Seville infected with *S. equina* were treated with diethylcarbamazine 200 mg/kg for 3 days repeated after 15 days; the microfilariae disappeared from 3 of them (Lapeyra, 1970). Sheep in Iran, suffering from lumbar paralysis probably due to infection of the spinal cord by *Setaria,* were successfully treated with diethylcarbamazine (Baharsefat *et al.,* 1973).

2. *Guinea Worm—Dracunculus medinensis*

It was reported by Rousett (1952) that diethylcarbamazine had a prophylactic action in man preventing the development of immature worms and killing the adult ones. But this treatment for guinea worm has now been replaced by niridazole, metronidazole, and thiabendazole.

3. *Lung Worms—Dictyocaulus viviparus in Calves*

Diethylcarbamazine is most active against the adult forms in the bronchi. Accordingly, treatment should be started at the first sign of respiratory distress that might be "husk." The dose is 22 mg/kg given i.m. on 3 successive days. Diethylcarbamazine is also active against *Dict. filaria* in sheep. It has been recommended for the cat lung worms *Aleurostrongylus abstrusus* (Connan and Zurborg, 1966) and for *Metastrongylus apri* of pigs (Kashinskii, 1963). Nishimura (1965) tested it on the rat lung worm, *Angiostrongylus cantonensis,* a worm that sometimes causes eosinophilic meningitis in man in South East Asia and the Pacific. He found that diethylcarbamazine was *not* effective.

4. *Toxocara canis*

Several workers have reported that diethylcarbamazine is active against *Toxocara canis* infections in mice. It is most effective if given while the larvae are migrating through the viscera and before they have established themselves in the brain and skeletal muscle (Burren, 1968; Pike, 1960; Wiseman *et al.,* 1971).

5. *Strongyloidiasis*

Nwokolo and Imohiosen (1973) reported a human case of strongyloidiasis of the respiratory tract resembling asthma, but there were larvae and ova in the sputum. The patient improved when diethylcarbamazine was given at 12 mg/kg daily for 18 days, but relapsed 8 weeks later and was treated with thiabendazole. This action may be due to the piperazine ring.

6. *Ascaris*

Diethylcarbamazine is active in removing *Ascaris lumbricoides* in man. This action is due to the piperazine ring and it is exerted more powerfully by piperazine citrate and similar compounds. The activity appears to depend on temporarily paralyzing of the muscular movements of the *Ascaris* by which it maintains its normal position in the human intestine and, consequently, the worm is expelled by anus. Diethylcarbamazine has also been found active in the treatment of dog ascarids and of dog hookworm (often in combination with styryl pyridinium) (Berger *et al.*, 1969; Casey *et al.*, 1971) and in the treatment of *Cooperia* infections in calves (Cornwell *et al.*, 1972).

7. *Other Infections*

Diethylcarbamazine in full doses has been recommended to kill the larvae of *Ancylostoma caninum,* which cause creeping eruption in the skin of man, but the drug is probably inferior to thiabendazole.

Thelazia gulosa and *Thelazia skrjabin* infections of cattle are said to be cured by subcutaneous injection of 14 mg/kg in the upper third of the body (Gorodovich, 1971).

In large doses, diethylcarbamazine can kill the adult worms of *Trichinella spiralis* when they develop in the intestine during experimental infections, but it has little effect on encysted larvae.

Against *Cysticercus cellulosae* in young pigs, subtoxic doses of diethylcarbamazine (10–25 mg/kg daily) gave promising results (Baretto and de Siqueira, 1963); but Urquhart (1960) found no action in 4 steers infected with *Cysticercus bovis*. In 13 patients in Iran, diethylcarbamazine seemed to be successful in suppressing epileptic seizures (Tumada and Margono, 1973); but this action might be an anti-inflammatory one rather than an anthelmintic one.

Paragonimus westermani infections in children have been treated with diethylcarbamazine by Gutman *et al.* (1969); this caused a reduction of egg output but did not produce a radical cure as did bithionol.

In experimental infections of rabbits with *Fasciola hepatica,* diethylcarbamazine plus bis(2-hydroxy-3,5-dichlorophenyl) sulfoxide was effective against the immature flukes (Kimura and Ono, 1971).

8. *Summary*

The action of diethylcarbamazine on worms in the alimentary canal seems to be due more to the piperazine ring rather than to the specific diethylcarbamazine structure; it apparently depends on paralysis of the muscles of the worms. The other actions, e.g., on lung worms, seem to be more specific, but they give little indication of the mechanism by which this helminticidal action is produced.

Sharma *et al.* (1976) have recently claimed that diethylcarbamazine (50 mg/kg single dose) is effective in the treatment of buffalo calves with acute infections of *Theileria annulata*.

V. Toxicity

A. Animals

The toxicity of diethylcarbamazine is very low. In mice, the acute LD_{50} by intraperitoneal injection is 240 mg/kg and by oral administration 560 mg/kg. In rats the oral LD_{50} is 395 mg/kg. There is little accumulation of the compound in albino rats given repeated doses (Harned *et al.,* 1948). Chronic toxicity does not occur even if high doses such as 170 mg/kg are given intraperitoneally to cotton rats twice daily for over 12 doses (all doses as base). Young rats fed for 9 weeks on a diet yielding them 9 mg/kg body weight per day gained weight practically as fast as the controls. Breeding pairs of mice placed for 4 months on a diet yielding 15 mg/kg body weight per day bore as many (or slightly more) baby mice than the controls on a normal diet and all the offspring were normal. There was no sterility, male or female, and no teratogenic effect (Hawking and Marques, 1967). Fraser (1972) found that large doses (100–200 mg/kg) given daily to pregnant rats and rabbits had no abortifacient action and no harmful effects on the fetuses (see Section III,A,1).

B. Man—Uninfected

When given to man, the compound is remarkably safe. Although hundreds of thousands of people have been treated, no case of death proved to be due to diethylcarbamazine has been reported. (Deaths that have been *attributed* to diethylcarbamazine are discussed in Sections V,C and D. The untoward reactions in man (when they do occur) may be annoying but they are seldom dangerous.

In uninfected persons, large oral doses of the compound, e.g., 10–20 mg base/kg, may cause gastrointestinal disturbances, that is anorexia, nausea, and vomiting, which come on in 2–4 hours. Headache and sleepiness have also been noted. These symptoms are probably due to the direct action of the drug on the patient. In China, single doses of 1.0–1.5 gm per person have been given to large numbers of people during mass campaigns. Apparently many persons vomited, and it is recommended that the dose is best administered in the evening; but otherwise no ill effects were reported (Ch'en, 1964).

C. Man—Infected with Filariae

With infected persons, however, different and more severe reactions may occur that vary according to the type of infection, being most marked with *Onchocerca volvulus* and less with *Wuchereria bancrofti*.

1. *Onchocerca*

a. Clinical. In patients with onchocerciasis, a specific reaction (Mazzotti's reaction) occurs; it is so constant that it can be used as a convenient diagnostic test. Obviously, the reaction is due to the destruction of many microfilariae in a sensitized subject. There is often premonitory itching, which begins 15–30 minutes after the first dose and which may not last very long. After a few hours there is usually a strong reaction that is well marked in 16 hours. It includes swelling and edema of the skin, especially of the buttocks, thighs, and genitals (these being the areas where there are most microfilariae), intense pruritus, enlargement and tenderness of the inguinal lymph nodes, sometimes a fine papular rash, hyperpyrexia up to 39°, tachycardia, and headache. There may occasionally be a fall of blood pressure and there may be respiratory distress. These symptoms persist for 3–7 days and then subside, after which quite high doses (12 mg/kg/day) can be tolerated without further reaction. The severity of the reaction is proportional to the number of microfilariae initially present in the skin and only partially to the size of the initial doses. Particularly severe symptoms have been reported by Fuglsang and Anderson (1974) after the administration of 50 mg to 15 heavily infected patients in north Cameroon: 2–4 hours later most of them were prostrated. One man of 30 years collapsed and seemed unconscious for 10 minutes; breathing was shallow and rapid with scanty frothy sputum; pulse 135/min, weak. After 2 hours, he recovered somewhat, and after 2 days he was normal again. Six other patients also developed severe or moderate respiratory distress. Similar severe reactions have been reported by Rougemont *et al.* (1975) who treated 290 persons in Bamako, Mali. The dose was 25 mg twice daily rising to 200 mg. Children were free from reactions except for pruritus, but some of the older people (15–45 years old) were severely affected. Thirty-six hours after the first dose, 20 people were prostrated. In particular, 3 women who tried to keep on working were found lying on the ground semiconscious, polypneic, and with a systolic blood pressure of 70–80 mm Hg; they were treated with 60 mg methylprednisolone, i.v. or i.m., and improved in a few hours. In heavily infected patients in Nigeria, treated by Bryceson *et al.* (1977), there was an acute fall of systolic blood pressure a few hours after the first dose of diethylcarbamazine, the number of circulating eosinophils fell profoundly and so did the level of complement (C3) in the serum. The reactions to diethylcarbamazine (and to suramin) seem to be much more severe in the savanna zone of West Africa than in other parts of Africa or America.

Many heavily infected patients complain of vertigo during the first week of diethylcarbamazine treatment, and Duke *et al.* (1976a) have shown that this is probably due to passage of increased numbers of microfilariae into the cerebrospinal fluid under the stimulation of the compound (see Section IV,A,4,b). Such vertigo usually begins on the second or third day of treatment and may continue for 5 to 16 days; sometimes it stops before the treatment stops. The vertigo often causes prostration and incapacitation. It may be accompanied by headache, nausea, and vomiting. In one of Duke's patients, there was a syndrome like Parkinsonism, which lasted for 7 days. The vertigo is believed to be due to the action (? allergic) of microfilariae on the cerebellum rather than on the labyrinth. It occurs when the microfilariae in the cerebrospinal fluid exceed 3 microfilariae/ml. Usually the smptoms disappear without leaving permanent damage, and a second course of treatment can be given without incident. One case has been reported however in the Ivory Coast in which a heavily infected woman of 52 years was being treated with diethylcarbamazine; on the eighth day she quickly relapsed into a coma; many microfilariae were found in the cerebrospinal fluid (which was otherwise normal); and she died inspite of the administration of hydrocortisone (Bureau *et al.*, 1976). Fuglsang and Anderson (1974) emphasize that with patients in heavily infected foci of onchoncerciasis, great care is needed in the administration of diethylcarbamazine and that corticosteroids should be given to prevent or diminish the reactions.

b. Histology of Diethylcarbamazine Reaction in Onchocerciasis. The histology of the cutaneous reaction in onchocerciasis has been described by Hawking (1952), Martinez Baez (1960), Rodger (1962), Connor *et al.* (1970), and more recently and in greater detail by Rougemont *et al.* (1974). According to the last named, before treatment with diethylcarbamazine there is usually a mild and variable inflammation of both epidermis and dermis; microfilariae are present but there is usually no reaction around them. When teatment is given, changes begin in a few hours and are maximal on the second and third days. The epidermis becomes swollen with fluid and infiltrated by some eosinophils; microfilariae actively penetrate the epidermis, head to surface, but their structure in this position is not altered; apparently the normal reactions of the microfilariae have been deranged by the compound. In the papillary dermis, there is inflammation, and lymphocytes and polymorphs especially eosinophils accumulate in foci, the eosinophils often causing microabscesses. The microfilariae first stain more faintly and then disappear in small granulomata. In some patients the reaction is intense with fibrinoid necrosis of collagen fibers and of the walls of blood vessels, together with infiltration by eosinophils. In the middle dermis the pilosebaceous follicles are surrounded with inflammatory cells especially polymorphs; microfilariae are few and are often located between the fibers of the erector muscles and they are lysed. The deep dermis is relatively unaffected. Conner *et al.* (1970) reported that 1 hour after giving diethylcarbamazine, microfilariae penetrated into the epidermis and simultaneously other microfilariae began disintegrating in the dermis, and eosinophils collected around them. Rougemont *et al.* (1974) did not find eosinophils numerous in the dermis until after 1–2 days. After the fourth to eighth day of treatment the inflammation subsides; eosinophils become fewer and lymphocytes and plasma cells predominate; microfilariae disappear.

When preliminary examinations were made by electron microscopy, it was seen that before treatment the microfilariae (*Onchocerca*) have a cuticle consisting of three dense layers and two clear zones under which there is a fibrillar locomotor system. Twelve hours after the first dose of diethylcarbamazine the cuticle had disappeared and the different layers could not be differentiated (Rougemont *et al.*, 1974) (cf. the action of diethylcarbamazine on microfilariae in the liver, Section IV,A,3,b). More electron microscope studies are desirable.

c. Causes and Treatment of therapeutic Shock. This response to treatment (which has been named "therapeutic shock" by Salazar Mallén) is obviously a kind of allergic reaction to the sudden destruction of microfilariae and the liberation of filarial antigens in the skin and other sensitized tissues. It differs from anaphylactic shock in various ways, since true urticaria or angioneurotic edema are not seen, blood pressure usually remains normal, there is usually no respiratory obstruction, and pyrexia and prostration are marked (Salazar Mallén *et al.*, 1962). Blood histamine and complement are not changed during the reaction (in Mexico), but serotonin increases significantly in the venous (jugular) blood and a "reactive protein C" also appears in the blood. During therapeutic shock the mast cells of the conjunctiva become degranulated (? liberation of histamine or serotonin) with diffusion of a fluorescent substance (Salazar Mallén and Chévez Zamon, 1965). Salazar Mallén and colleagues (1962) suggested that an endopeptidase is liberated from the disintegrating microfilariae and acts as a toxic factor; but no further support has come for this hypothesis. It has recently been shown by Saxena *et al.* (1977) that microfilariae of *Litomosoides carinii* (and presumably of other filariae also) contain relatively high concentrations of serotonin, histamine, and norepinephrine; presumably these are liberated into the blood when large numbers of microfilariae are destroyed by diethylcarbamazine and they might account for part of the therapeutic shock.

Much work has been devoted to finding drugs that diminish the reaction both for practical purposes and for investigating the causation of the reaction. The results have been reviewed by Aranda-Villamayor (1970). Antihistamine drugs have usually proved to be valueless. Antagonists of serotonin, such as methysergide and cyproheptadine, have been recommended but they have been disappointing. Salazar Mallén *et al.* (1962) found that cyproheptadine alone was ineffective although cyproheptadine and dexamethasone reduced all the reactions (pruritus reduced least). Lagraulet *et al.* (1964) found that the effect of methysergide in Upper Volta was barely significant and not worthwhile. Aranda-Villamayor (1970) in a study of 200 patients (treated with methysergide and indomethacin) in Mexico found that although methysergide might alter the relative frequency of symptoms somewhat, the total number of reactions was not diminished; moreover, there were some harmful side effects and the antimicrofilarial action was reduced somewhat. He concluded that methysergide should be banned from field use.

On the other hand, corticosteroids in some form have usually been found to be beneficial, although some of them may be too expensive for field use, or they may weaken the antifilarial action. Prednisone was used by Schofield and Rowley (1961) for patients with *W. bancrofti* in Papua; they found that 3-4 times more microfilariae persisted in patients after prednisone than in patients with diethylcarbamazine alone. Sasa *et al.* (1963) found that the febrile reaction (to *W. bancrofti*) was diminished by paramethasone and chlorpromazine. Triamcinolone plus methdilazine was found beneficial in *Onchocerca* patients by Torroella (1964). Bernhard *et al.* (1964) found that triamcinolone given before starting diethylcarbamazine reduced the reactions (*Onchocerca*) significantly. This treatment was expensive, however, and the same authors (Garcia Manzo *et al.*, 1965) later recommended betamethasone beginning 12 hours before the first dose of diethylcarbamazine. This reduced most of the symptoms except the pruritus. Duke and Anderson (1972) recommend betamethasone if severe reactions are expected.

In summary, specific antagonists of histamine, or of serotonin, have proved disappointing for onchocercal reactions and should be avoided. Corticosteroids especially betamethasone diminish most of the reactions that occur in patients with *Onchocerca* or other filariae; presumably this is due to a general anti-inflammatory action. It must be remembered that corticosteroids and serotonin antagonists may also diminish the antifilarial action slightly.

2. *Other Filariae*

In patients infected with *Brugia malayi* (Wilson, 1950) or with *Loa loa,* there are often similar but milder general symptoms, without the local swelling and inflammation of the skin. In patients infected with *W. bancrofti,* symptoms are often absent but some patients (25%) may suffer from headaches, nausea, vomiting, anorexia, cough and pain in the chest, pains in muscles or joints, general malaise and pyrexia, or rarely a papular rash. The reactions are proportional to the number of microfilariae originally present in the blood. They are more common in older persons than in younger persons. After a few days, these symptoms (including those of onchocerciasis patients) subside, and then treatment can be continued, the same or a higher dose being given without any reaction occurring. In the absence of heavy onchocerciasis or of encephalitis due to *L. loa,* none of these symptoms are ever so severe as to endanger life or to cause anxiety; but they are of great practical importance because they often render mass administration of the compound unpopular and unacceptable, and thus prevent the use of diethylcarbamazine to eradicate filariasis on a community basis.

3. *Local Reactions*

In addition to the general symptoms already described, small focal reactions of pain, tenderness, and inflammation sometimes occur in the groins or thighs of persons infected with *W. bancrofti* or *B. malayi,* and small nodules may develop at these sites. They subside in a few days. They are probably due to a local reaction around a dying adult worm (Ch'en, 1964). In patients with *L. loa,* small wheals may appear in the skin due to dying worms, and in patients with *Dipetalonema streptocerca* there may be flat papules in the skin due to the same cause. In onchocerciasis, severe pain in the hip may be caused by the death of adult worms in the capsule of this joint.

D. Deaths Reported as Due to Diethylcarbamazine Treatment

Although deaths during diethylcarbamazine treatment have been reported, the evidence that they were in fact due to such treatment is usually slight. Oomen (1969) reported that he had treated 327 hospital patients for onchocerciasis and 7 had died. All were in poor condition before treatment (but so were 49 other patients who took the treatment well). There had been no clinical reaction to the diethylcarbamazine (but this had also happened in 65 other patients). All relapsed into coma after taking 225–900 mg during 3–8 days. Death occurred in 4–12 days after taking the first dose. The evidence that these deaths were really due to diethylcarbamazine is slight, but, nevertheless, if patients are in poor general condition it would be well to give the compound cautiously.

Jones (1970) reported the case of a woman in Nepal who had many microfilariae of *W. bancrofti* in her blood and who was given 2 doses of 100 mg diethylcarbamazine at $4\frac{1}{2}$ hour intervals: 1 hour after the second dose she was found pulseless and dying. Although the cause of death is obscure, there is little evidence that it was due to the compound, in view of the fact that almost a million other people have taken similar doses without serious reaction.

Encephalitis

Encephalitis occurring during infection with *L. loa* with microfilariae present in the central nervous system and in the cerebrospinal fluid is a very grave condition. Over 20 cases have been reported in the literature. Cauchie *et al.* (1965) give a good review of the literature and report a case which was apparently aggravated by treatment with diethylcarbamazine in spite of prednisone given prophylactically: the patient went into a coma and died (see also microfilariae of *O. volvulus,* Section V,C,1,a). Downie (1966) reviewed 12 cases of encephalitis said to have been due to filariasis, especially *Loa,* although no microfilariae were found in the cerebrospinal fluid of many of these patients. Five were treated with diethylcarbamazine alone of whom 4 died; 4 were treated with diethylcarbamazine plus steroids and all recovered, often with neurological lesions. Apparently, encephalitis believed to be due to loiasis should certainly be treated with corticosteroids, but the decision about diethylcarbamazine treatment is more difficult. Since the condition of encephalitis indicates inflammatory (allergic) reactions already proceeding in the brain and since these allergic reactions will certainly be exacerbated by diethylcarbamazine, it would seem advisable to postpone diethylcarbamazine treatment in the hope that the encephalitis will subside under corticosteroid therapy. If this happens, diethylcarbamazine may be given with great caution at a later date. The compound per se is certainly not toxic but if a dangerous allergic condition is already present it might exacerbate it.

Since so many filarial patients all over the world have been given diethylcarbamazine, it is not surprising if some deaths occurred during such treatment. Nevertheless, it has not been possible to find any specific case (apart possibly from encephalitis) in which the death could be clearly proved to have been due to diethylcarbamazine.

VI. Clinical Use

In describing the clinical use of diethylcarbamazine, a distinction must be made as to whether the aim is to improve the condition of single patients, or whether it is to suppress (or eradicate) the infection in a whole community.

A. Single Patients

In the case of individual patients, microfilariae and adult worms of *Wuchereria bancrofti, Brugia malayi,* and *Loa loa* can certainly be destroyed by adequate courses of treatment. After the worms have been removed, further damage due to them will cease (once the reaction to the disintegration products has subsided); but the damage already caused, e.g., lymph stasis or elephantiasis, is not reversed. In the case of *Onchocerca volvulus* the microfilariae can be destroyed but not the adult worms, so that after a few months the microfilariae gradually reaccumulate in the skin.

1. *Patients with W. bancrofti*

With *W. bancrofti,* a patient of average weight (60–70 kg) should be given 100 mg of the citrate salt by mouth, 3 times a day for 10 days. If preferred the course can be extended to 21 days, but it is really better to examine the blood a few nights after the end of the first course; then, if the microfilariae have not completely disappeared, a second course can be given after an interval of several weeks. The drug can also be given as a single dose of 200–300 mg daily; this is simpler to administer, but it is more likely to cause gastrointestinal disturbance. Hujimaki (1958) recommends 6 mg/kg per day, divided into 6 doses, for 14 days, in order to maintain a constant high level of drug in the blood (see Section II,A). There is no evidence as to whether a constant high level is more, or less, effective than a succession of high peaks.

Patients may be classified into several categories.

1. The symptomless carrier with microfilariae in the blood. Although the worms may seem to be causing no harm, they are certainly doing no good; moreover, they are a source of infection to others. Therefore he should be treated.

2. The patient with attacks of lymphangitis, with or without microfi-

lariae. He should be treated, preferably in a quiescent period between attacks. Although the treatment may not immediately stop all further attacks, it will probably diminish their number and severity.

3. The patient with advanced hydrocele, elephantiasis, chyluria, etc. Unless microfilariae are present, treatment is hardly worthwhile, since it cannot reverse these chronic lesions.

4. The patient with tropical eosinophilia (see Section VI,C).

2. *Patients with B. malayi and L. loa*

They should be treated in the same way as those with *W. bancrofti.* Treatment is usually very effective; but "allergic" reactions are often greater than with *W. bancrofti,* and dosage should be reduced to 50 mg of the citrate salt by mouth, 3 times a day for 3 days, and then 100 mg, 3 times a day for 7 days. In patients infected with *Loa loa,* wheals may appear under the skin, which mark the sites of dead or dying adult worms.

3. *Patients with Onchocerca*

Duke and Anderson (1972) recommend that light or moderate infections should be treated first with diethylcarbamazine to kill the existing load of microfilariae. On the first day, 50 mg (citrate) by mouth; on the second day 100 mg after morning and evening meals, and on the next 5 days, 200 mg twice daily. For persons under 40 kg, these doses should be reduced in proportion to their weight. The authors consider that symptomatic relief of the reaction may be obtained with antihistamines, e.g., 100 mg antazoline HCl (Antistin) every 6 hours for an adult, and antipyretics or analgesics. If the reaction is expected to be very severe, it may be damped by betamethasone without interfering greatly with the destruction of microfilariae. One milligram betamethasone 3 times daily should be given orally from 1 day before starting diethylcarbamazine to 3–5 days later; after that the dose is gradually reduced to zero in the next 4 days. Later a course of suramin should be given to kill the adult worms since radical cure of onchocerciasis is never obtained with diethylcarbamazine alone. If treatment with suramin is not acceptable, the treatment with diethylcarbamazine may be repeated at 3 to 6 monthly intervals, or 100 mg may be taken weekly to maintain the suppression of the microfilariae. During these subsequent treatments, the allergic reactions will probably be smaller and may be absent.

a. Treatment of Ocular Onchocerciasis. Anderson *et al.* (1976) treated 39 patients with ocular lesions in north Cameroon. The dose regimen was as follows: 50 mg twice daily for the first day; 100 mg × 2 on the second day; 150–200 mg × 2 for 10 days; also betamethasone 1.0–1.5 mg × 2 on the day before treatment and continued for 5 days. General reactions were severe and acceptability was low. Patients could not be persuaded to take weekly suppressive doses afterward. The numbers of microfilariae in the eye were temporarily reduced and the lesions of the anterior segment were temporarily improved, but both soon relapsed when treatment ceased. Lesions in the posterior segment were not improved. These authors concluded that in heavily infected cases with ocular involvement, the administration of diethylcarbamazine should be handled with care. Its main use would be as an emergency drug together with betamethasone in acute onchocerciasis of the anterior segment, or to reduce the microfilariae in the eye before giving suramin. There is not sufficient benefit for it to be given *after* suramin. Possibly it might also be used to supplement the excision of all head nodules.

b. Local Application for Ocular Onchocerciasis. The local application of diethylcarbamazine to the conjunctiva was first suggested by Lazar *et al.* (1968, 1970). They showed that if the compound was instilled into the conjunctival sac of rabbits, high concentrations appeared in the aqueous humor; no local irritation occurred. Lazar *et al.* (1969) produced experimental uveitis in the eyes of rabbits by injection of bovine serum albumin and found that the local application of diethylcarbamazine had no anti-inflammatory action (although 6-mercaptopurine, chloromycetin, and antilymphatic serum were anti-inflammatory). Ben-Sira *et al.* (1970) treated 10 blind patients in Malawi with 5% diethylcarbamazine citrate neutralized to pH 7, 2 drops 4 times daily for 2 weeks. The treatment was well tolerated but there was a small reaction due to death of microfilariae; it consisted of moderate edema of eyelids and slight congestion of the conjunctiva that subsided during the second week of treatment and disappeared when treatment ceased. The microfilariae (as studied by slit lamp) disappeared from the anterior chamber within 48 hours from the beginning of treatment but reappeared in the original numbers 48 hours after the cessation of treatment. Anderson and Fuglsang (1973) treated 8 patients in Cameroon, instilling 3% diethylcarbamazine into the conjunctival sac at a dosage of 2 drops 4 times daily for 9 days. This was well tolerated by a control patient without microfilariae in the eye, but in heavily infected patients, it provoked severe anterior uveitis, causing treatment to be stopped in 3 out of 6 such subjects. In the anterior chamber, microfilariae were somewhat reduced in number but they were not eliminated and reappeared quickly when treatment stopped. In the cornea, microfilariae were initially stimulated to invade the cornea (cf. Section IV,A,4,b) but afterward most of them died; microfilariae reappeared quickly when treatment stopped. These workers consider that in heavily infected patients there is no subjective improvement following the local application of diethylcarbamazine to eyes, and the reactions that may occur require adequate ophthalmological supervision. The suppression of microfilariae in the anterior chamber is only temporary. Accordingly, local therapy was not recommended for general use.

Treatment by local application has recently been reinvestigated by Anderson *et al.* (1977) with particular reference to the possible prolonged liberation of drug under the eyelid by a device known as an "ocusert." They conclude that ideally topical applications should comprise three formulations: a low concentration (e.g., 0.02%, 1 drop 3 times daily) for the preliminary reduction of the microfilariae in the periorbital tissues; then a high concentration (up to 3.0%) to eliminate microfilariae inside the orbit; and finally an intermediate concentration to keep fresh microfilariae out of the eye. The whole subject clearly deserves further investigation.

c. Local Application for Cutaneous Onchocerciasis. Recently, Langham *et al.* (1978) have applied an oil–water emulsion containing 2% diethylcarbamazine once daily to the whole body of 6 patients with onchocerciasis in Liberia. Microfilariae disappeared from the skin in about 6 days. Itching and pruritus occurred after 3–6 hours, but they subsided by the third day. Twenty-seven patients were then treated with 1 or 2% lotion daily for 7 days. The mean microfilaria count as originally 5.5 per patient (4 skin snips) and, after 4–12 days from the beginning of treatment, it fell to 0.49 microfilaria. Later 93 patients were treated with 2% lotion for 1 week and then they were asked to treat themselves once weekly. The mean microfilaria count was initially 12.8 but after 12 weeks it fell to 0.70 (in 35 patients).

B. Mass Therapy

1. *Bancroftian and Malayan Filariasis*

Although diethylcarbamazine is very effective and satisfactory for the treatment of individual patients, the most promising use lies in its administration to all the infected persons in a district so as to suppress the infection on a public health basis. There is no animal reservoir of infection for *W. bancrofti,* and even with *B. malayi* such a reservoir (in monkeys) occurs only in limited parts of Malaya. The only important source of infection for man is man himself. Therefore, in theory, if all persons infected with *W. bancrofti* (or *B. malayi* or *L. loa*) were adequately treated, all the worms would be destroyed, there would be no microfilariae left to be transmitted by mosquitoes to new patients, and the disease would die out. Such a procedure would have the advantage over the public health alternative, namely, suppression of the mosquito vectors or *Chrysops* by insecticides, in that the destruction of the worms would be immediate, whereas with vector control it would be 10 years or more before the worms die out. Moverover, control of culicine mosquitoes by insecticides is usually difficult, and eradication has been impossible. In practice, however, the procedure is not so easy, and mass therapy has encountered many difficulties. These difficulties are proportional to the size of the population to be treated. Where the procedure was adequately applied, as was first done in Tahiti by Kessel (1957) and his colleagues, or in pilot trials in single villages and small islands, the results have been good and filarial infection has been redued to an insignificant level; but elsewhere the minor toxic and allergic reactions described in the foregoing have often made treatment unpopular and unacceptable to the populations who have to be treated. There is a large literature on the subject.

Briefly, four main types of dosage schedule have been employed. The first three are administered to all the population without blood examination.

1. One dose (e.g., 4 mg citrate/kg) daily for 5–7 days. This is the easiest schedule to administer, and it is the minimum that is likely to have any effect. It has been used in India and also in Japan, Africa, and Brazil.

2. An interrupted dose of 5 mg/kg monthly or weekly for 6–12 doses. The total dose should be 72 mg/kg for *W. bancrofti* and 40 mg/kg for *B. malayi*. This is more effective and less toxic than other schedules, but it is more laborious to administer. If administrative problems can be overcome, it is probably the best to employ. It has been employed particularly in the Pacific and Malaya.

3. A large single dose, e.g., 1.0–1.5 gm. This is somewhat heroic since many patients vomit; but if the population can be persuaded or compelled to accept it, the simplicity of administration makes it attractive (employed in China; Ch'en, 1964).

4. Treatment of microfilariae carriers, detected by systematic surveys, e.g., 100 mg per person, thrice daily for 7 days. This is usually acceptable and may reduce the level of infection considerably; but it involves laborious blood surveys and, theoretically, it cannot eradicate the infection, since many latent cases will be missed. In practice, moreover, the procedure is often vitiated further by taking too small samples of blood for examination, so that only the carriers with large numbers of microfilariae are detected. This method has been used in Sri Lanka and northeast Brazil.

Experience has shown that all these schedules have been effective in greatly reducing the level of infection provided that people can be persuaded to take them. Unfortunately, there is often difficulty over this point. Persuasion is more easy if the incidence of elephantiasis is high so that people are afraid of infection, and if the population is small so that personal influence is easier. Thus it has been successful in Tahiti with a population of 20,000, and in many pilot trials involving some hundreds of persons. On the other hand, it has proved impossible in India where populations amounting to millions have to be treated.

Review of Mass Therapy. The attempts to control filariasis (bancroftian and malayan) have differed in their success in different parts of the world.

In the Pacific area, treatment has been usually given to the whole population of an island once weekly or monthly for 12 doses. It has usually been possible to obtain the cooperation of the population concerned and the results have been very successful in reducing the microfilaria rate (as measured by blood films) to a low level, even though little or no mosquito control has been carried out. In fact, except for Tonga, in which a mass campaign is in process of being planned, filariasis has been greatly reduced over most of the area. Thus in American Samoa, in which mass treatments began in 1963 the microfilaria rate before 1963 was 21%, in 1965 it was 3.1% and in 1967 it was 0.36% (Kessel *et al.*, 1970).

It has recently been shown, however, by Desowitz and Southgate (1973) using filtration technique methods for detecting very low levels of microfilariemia (e.g., 1 microfilaria in 5 ml blood) that a few microfilariae still persist in many (23%) of the previous carriers after such mass therapy. Furthermore, such microfilariae are capable of developing in mosquitoes and of being transmitted. This finding might seem to cast doubt on the permanent value of such control measures, but the doubt is unjustified. The aim of these mass campaigns is control and not eradication. If the reservoir of infection is reduced to a small fraction of its original level, it will take a long time for a slowly multiplying parasite such as filaria to build up to its previous level, and it might even die out from the difficulty of the two sexes of worm meeting each other in sufficient quantities to maintain the next generation. In any case, the practical results of chemotherapeutic control in Tahiti and Samoa are most striking. In Tahiti in 1955, before control started, the microfilaria rate was high (over 40%), and filarial fever and elephantiasis were common. Now, after 20 years of control, the microfilaria rate has been reduced to a low level (5.6% in 1967) and clinical symptoms of filariasis are negligible.

In Western Samoa there was mass administration of diethylcarbamazine during 1965–1966. Before treatment, the infective rate among *Aedes polynesiensis* mosquitoes (the main vector) was 2.95%; After treatment only three infective mosquitoes could be found during 4 years, the rate being 0.071% (Suzuki and Sone, 1975). In these instances, filariasis may not have been eradicated but it has been reduced to a level where it is no longer a serious health problem.

In Japan and the adjacent islands, a national filariasis control program has been conducted since 1962, mainly by examination of the population at risk and treatment of detected microfilaria carriers. As a result the mean microfilaria rate in the infected areas fell from 2.8% in 1962 to 0.5% in 1969 (Ishimaru, 1972; Sasa, 1974). In South-East Asia and in Indonesia including New Guinea, no large-scale control programs have yet been possible.

In India a big National Filariasis Control Programme was started in 1955, based particularly on a 5–7 day course of 4 mg/kg per day for all at risk. Unfortunately, there was insufficient popular cooperation, and it proved impossible to persuade the vast populations concerned to accept and swallow the tablets that were offered them. Consequently, the campaign had to be abandoned. Since then, antifilarial measures have been restricted to a few pilot trials of diethylcarbamazine and to attempted mosquito control.

In Malaya, diethylcarbamazine was given weekly for 6 weeks, and between 1956 and 1958, 112,700 persons were treated. In one typical area (Burkit Meriam in Kedah) infected with *B. malayi,* the microfilaria rate fell from 26% in 1957 to 0.7% in 1966.

In Ceylon (Sri Lanka) mosquito control and treatment of carriers with diethylcarbamazine has been applied; since 1969 mass treatment has been given in some area. A great reduction has been effected in the microfilaria rate.

In Brazil, control has been attempted by the detection and treatment of carriers with 6 mg/kg daily for 7 days. In Belem, the microfilariae rate fell from 9.8% in 1952 to 2.0% in 1966 and in Recife, from 6.9 to 1.8% in the same period.

In summary, mass chemotherapy often with little or no effort at mosquito control has reduced bancroftian and malayan filariasis to a low level over most of the Pacific area, Malay peninsula, and Japan. In Ceylon there has been great reduction, with recent recrudescence. In Brazil there has been reduction in many parts but filariasis was less intense here than in Asia. Elsewhere the level of filariasis has probably remained unchanged except for small pilot trials.

2. *Diethylcarbamazine in Cooking Salt*

Since most of the difficulties of mass administration of diethylcarbamazine are due to the difficulties of persuasion, it has been suggested that these might be circumvented by incorporating diethylcarbamazine in some article of common diet such as cooking salt. Alternatively, it might be incorporated in some popular food such as the Japanese miso soup or orangeade (Kanda *et al.,* 1967a). Incorporation of a drug in salt has been widely employed with chloroquine in Brazil in order to prevent malaria. Thus the technical and administrative problems involved are well understood. The conditions for diethylcarbamazine in salt against filariasis are much more favorable than they were for chloroquine against malaria. Further, diethylcarbamazine is stable to cooking with food; it is not destroyed during cooking and it does not develop harmful by-products. It is well tolerated by growing rats and pregnant mice. Furthermore, this procedure of incorporating diethylcarbamazine in the food has been employed in veterinary practice to protect dogs against infection with *D. immitis;* e.g., Abadie *et al.* (1969) used diethylcarbamazine in dog food to protect 33 dogs for 31 months.

As regards human therapy, a number of pilot trials have now been conducted. In Brazil, it was given to two closed communities totalling 2300 adults. Diethylcarbamazine was added to the salt in concentrations of 0.2 or 0.4% (w/w) giving a calculated intake of 40 or 80 mg per head per day. Administration was continued at a lower level (0.1%) for a whole year. These concentrations were completely acceptable to the men and no adverse comments about taste were received. There were no untoward reactions. After the first 6 weeks, 70% of the carriers no longer showed microfilariae in the blood and the others showed only single ones in 40-cmm samples (Hawking and Marques, 1967).

In another trial carried out in East Africa by Davis and Bailey (1969), medicated salt containing 0.1% diethylcarbamazine was supplied to a closed community of 700 adult men for 6 months. Tolerance of the drug–salt mixture was extremely good. The mean microfilarial densities fell steadily, being reduced by 90% after 6 months. In this trial 0.1% was too low; and a concentration of 0.2 or 0.3% would have been better.

Several trials have been carried out in India under village conditions by Raghavan *et al.* (1968) and by Basu *et al.* (1970a,b) employing 0.1% diethylcarbamazine for 8–12 weeks, by Krishna Rao *et al.* (1976) employing 0.1% drug for 45 weeks, and, more recently, by Sen *et al.* (1974) who gave 0.26% diethylcarbamazine for 11 weeks. In all these trials acceptance was good, there were no significant allergic reactions, and the microfilaria counts were greatly reduced although not always to zero. Judging by these Indian trials the drug concentration should be 0.25–0.3%, and the medication should be continued for 4 months or more to obtain optimal results.

A very successful trial has been carried out in the Kinmen (Quemoy) Islands, Taiwan, by Fan *et al.* (1975). Medicated salt containing 0.33% diethylcarbamazine was supplied to 7128 persons in 26 villages for 6 months. This is equivalent to 42 mg, 3 times daily. The salt was completely acceptable and no side effects were recorded. The microfilaria rate fell from 9.6 to 0.4%, the mean microfilaremia fell from 14.4 microfilariae per 20 cmm to 1.9, and the infective rate among *Culex fatigans* mosquitoes fell from 3.7 to 0.2%. These workers concluded that diethylcarbamazine medicated salt was a very rapid and efficient agent for the control of filariasis, and it was probably also the cheapest and most practical method for use in the future.

Note. In all campaigns for public health control, including diethylcarbamazine by whatever method of administration, it is essential to obtain the enthusiastic cooperation of the people concerned by suitable approach and propaganda. The public health work in the Peoples Republic of China is a striking illustration of the great results that can be obtained by enlisting the active cooperation of the people themselves.

3. *Mass Therapy of Other Filarial Infections*

Diethylcarbamazine can be used against *B. malayi* in the same way as against *W. bancrofti,* but the doses should be reduced, since the worms are more susceptible to treatment and allergic reactions are more severe. Single doses of 1.5 gm once yearly for several years have been recommended in China (Ch'en, 1964).

As regards *L. loa,* a trial was carried out by Duke and Moore (1961) on 50,000 persons living on a rubber estate in Nigeria. All who contained microfilariae in the blood were offered treatment at 200 mg (citrate), 3 times a day for 20 days. This treatment was well tolerated and the microfilarial reservoir of infection was reduced to 2–12% of its previous level in the persons who were treated. Unfortunately, one-third of the people did not cooperate (probably on account of apathy). This failure to cooperate is a serious handicap to the control of filariasis by means of drug.

Against *O. volvulus,* mass administration of diethylcarbamazine has not been acceptable (because of reactions) or efficacious (because the adult worms are not killed). In Mexico and Guatemala, the Public Health Service endeavors to detect infected persons and to treat them, either by excision of nodules or by chemotherapy. The use of diethylcarbamazine is handicapped by the reactions that it produces. However, Torroella (1964) recommends a course consisting of 8 mg metdilazine alone on the first day; this is repeated on the second, third, and fourth days, half an hour before giving treatment with diethylcarbamazine, 600 mg/day, plus triamcinoline, 24 mg/day (combined as Filaricort); on the fifth to eleventh days, only diethylcarbamazine (with or without triamcinoline) is given. It should be given 2 or 3 times a year to persons exposed to infection.

In Ghana, Sowa and Sowa (1978) treated 88 onchocercal children with 12.5 or 25 mg diethylcarbamazine daily for 5 months. There were some severe reactions with 25 mg, and, accordingly, it is better to start with 12.5 mg. The acceptability was poor owing to the adverse reactions but the clinical results were very good. At the end of the 5 months, 45 nodules were excised from ten of the children and almost all the female worms contained only degenerate microfilariae. These results are promising and further study is desirable.

C. Treatment of Tropical Eosinophilia

Tropical eosinophilia is a condition characterized by eosinophilia, patches of consolidation in the lungs, and raised erythrocytic sedimentation rate. It occurs in many warm, moist parts of the world. There has been much speculation as to its etiology but work by Beaver, Danaraj, and their associates make it highly probable that it is a hypersensitive state due to infection with some filarial worm, usually *W. bancrofti*. Accordingly, the treatment consists of diethylcarbamazine. This has been described in detail by Danaraj (1958). He recommends large doses, i.e., 6 mg/kg, 3 times daily for 5 days. Marked improvement in the symptoms occurs in 2–4, days, and cure should be completed in 2 weeks. In about 10% of his patients, severe bronchial spasm occurred; this should be treated with antispasmodics. Before giving treatment the night blood should be examined for microfilariae. If these are present, smaller doses (3–4 mg/kg) should be given. In the rare cases in which there is no response to diethylcarbamazine, oxophenarsine or neoarsphenamine should be given intravenously in the usual doses as for syphilis, weekly for 6–8 weeks. The possibility of dangerous idiosyncrasy should, however, be remembered.

VII. Review of Other Antifilarial Compounds

In order to supplement the preceding review of diethylcarbamazine and a previous one of suramin (Hawking, 1978), a brief survey will be given of other antifilarial compounds. This subject has previously been covered by Lämmler (1974, 1977) and by Lämmler *et al.* (1975) whose reviews have been used extensively in the present work.

A. Older Compounds

1. Antimonial compounds
2. Cyanines
3. Methylene violet
4. Bisisoquinolinium compounds

5. Proguanil, amethopterin, 6-mercaptopurine, Cytoxan, and 6-azauridine (slight effects on *Litomosoides carinii*).

All the compounds listed here have been reviewed by Hawking (1963, 1973). Their antifilarial action is too small or their toxicity is too great for them to be of practical importance.

B. Arsenical Compounds

It has been shown repeatedly that trivalent arsenical compounds are very active in killing adult filarial worms. For animal filariasis, e.g., *Dirofilaria immitis* in dogs, these compounds are excellent. Unfortunately for human use, a small number of persons (perhaps 1% or less) have an idiosyncrasy for organic arsenicals and may die from encephalopathy or acute yellow atrophy of the liver after receiving doses much smaller than those easily tolerated by many other patients. This renders all arsenical compounds inacceptable for the treatment of nonfatal infections such as onchocerciasis or bancroftian filariasis, even though they may be valuable for otherwise incurable fatal infections such as trypanosomiasis. If some test could be discovered, such as a skin test that would detect patients with this idiosyncrasy in order to exclude them from treatment, arsenicals might become a valuable antifilarial remedy. Research for such a test would be well worthwhile. The arsenical compounds used for filariasis include arsenamide (thiacetarsamide, etc.), melarsoprol (Mel B, Arsobal), Mel W (Trimelarsan) and dichlorophenarsine. These have been reviewed by Hawking (1963, 1973) and Lämmler *et al.* (1975). A combination (named Compound E) of an arsenical F151 (similar to Mel W) and Hoechst 33258 has been described in Section I,C,2 (Friedheim, 1974).

Until the idiosyncrasy can be detected and avoided, arsenical compounds are too dangerous for the treatment of human filarial infections, although they may be valuable for infections of dogs.

C. Organophosphorus Compounds

1. *Metriphonate* (*Trichlorphor*)

This drug, dimethyl-(2,2,2-trichloro-1-hydroxyethyl)-phosphonate, is water soluble. It was reported by Salazar Mallén *et al.* (1970) to have promising action against micro- and macrofilariae in human onchocerciasis. The oral dosage under investigation was 10 mg/kg daily, given 3–6 times on consecutive days or at varying intervals. Experimental studies have shown the substance to be highly effective against microfilariae of *L. carinii* in *Mastomys natalensis* (Lämmler *et al.*, 1971b; Thomas, 1972). The extremely rapid decrease in the microfilaria count in the circulating blood (i.e., more than 98%, during treatment with 5 × 75 mg/kg, p.o., and higher doses) was followed by a steep increase within the following week. No action against adult parasites was seen. Metriphonate also proved to be effective against both the micro- and macrofilariae of *Dipetalonema witeae* in *M. natalensis,* although its microfilaricidal activity against this parasite was less pronounced than against *L. carinii*. In contrast to these results, the drug was found to be completely ineffective against micro- and macrofilariae of *Dip. witeae* when the same parasite strain was kept in *Meriones persicus* (Thomas, 1971). In further experimental trials the compound showed both macro- and microfilaricidal activity against *Brugia pahangi* in cats after the administration of oral doses of 25 mg/kg daily on 5 consecutive or alternate days; but the principal effect of metriphonate in mature infections seemed to be to kill the adult parasites (Denham *et al.*, 1971).

Studies on the prophylactic activity of metriphonate, given orally in daily doses or 15 mg/kg for 6 days a week during 6 months, did not show any efficacy in preventing infection with *D. immitis* (Warne *et al.*, 1969).

Duke (1974a) tested metriphonate on a chimpanzee infected with human *Onchocerca volvulus*. The dose was 31 mg/kg twice weekly by mouth for 6 doses. After this treatment the microfilariae in the skin fell from 40 microfilariae/mg of skin to 0.6 microfilariae/mg, but they returned in 2 weeks and reached their original level in 10 weeks. The chimpanzee was then given 22 mg/kg daily for 6 days. This dose produced toxic symptoms (listlessness). The microfilariae in the skin fell as before but came up again. The action upon *O. volvulus* seemed to be exerted on the microfilariae rather than on the macrofilariae.

In Mexico, metriphonate is routinely given to patients who can be kept under supervision. The dose is 10 mg/kg daily for 6 days with atropine to minimize the muscarinic effects (Salazar Mallén, 1974). The action on onchocerciasis in West Africa has recently been studied by Fuglsang and Anderson (1977). They gave a single oral dose of 10 mg/kg to 15 fairly heavily infected patients in the Cameroon rain forest. The effects on microfilariae were similar to those of diethylcarbamazine, but somewhat less marked. At 48 hours the mean number of microfilariae in the skin fell to 49% of the initial value, and at 2 weeks it was still only 54%; microfilariae were mobilized into the urine, blood, and cornea; and there were limbal infiltrates in the eyes and reactions around microfilariae in the cornea. The side effects (itching and edema of skin, fever, etc.) were similar to those after diethylcarbamazine, but they were less intense and were better tolerated by the patients. In view of the obvious effect on the microfilariae without severe inflammatory reactions in the eye, it was concluded that metriphonate deserved further investigations for the treatment of ocular onchocerciasis in West Africa.

2. *Fenthion*

o,o-Dimethyl-*O*-(4-methylthic-*m*-tolyl)phosphorothioate is an organophosphorus compound insoluble in water. It has been used for the treatment of *D. immitis* infection in dogs. The administration in a single intramuscular dose of 0.15 ml/kg body weight (100 mg active ingredient per milliliter) showed high activity against microfilariae (McCarthy, 1970; Wallace, 1970). The drug was used as a microfilaricide 3 weeks after a 2-day treatment with sodium thiacetarsamide (Merrit, 1970). Experimental trials in *M. natalensis* infected with *L. carinii* revealed high activity against microfilariae (Lämmler and Grüner, 1975), but not against the larval stages (Lämmler and Wolf, 1977).

Fenthion was given to dogs inoculated with larvae of *D. immitis*. The dose was 5.5 mg/kg, 6 days of the week for 160 days. It completely prevented the development of the worms (Fowler *et al.*, 1971).

3. *Haloxan* (*Enstidil*)

This drug has been used extensively for 10 years in veterinary practice as an anthelminthic (on gastrointestinal worms). It was tested against *L. carinii* in *M. natalensis* by Lämmler and Grüner (1975) and found to be the organophosphorus compound with the best chemotherapeutic index. The maximum tolerated dose by month (on 5 successive days) was greater than 2000 mg/kg. The minimum effective dose (5 successive days) was 12.5 mg/kg. This dose reduced the microfilariae in the blood by 88% in 3 days but they increased again 3–10 days after treatment. There was no action on adult worms of *L. carinii* or on the larval stages (Lämmler and Wolf, 1977). B. O. L. Duke (unpublished experiments) tested Haloxan on 1 chimpanzee infected with *O. volvulus*. The dose was 20 mg/kg by mouth daily for 5 days, but there was no change in the microfilariae of the skin (95 microfilariae before treatment, and 115 microfilariae after treatment). The 5-day course was then repeated at 100 mg/kg. The microfilariae in the skin were reduced slightly (127 before, 68 after), a result that may be just significant. There was no evidence for action upon adult worms. This trial in a chimpanzee is not very encouraging, but since Haloxan in *Mastomys* is more active and less toxic than metriphonate, further small trials would be interesting, perhaps in Mexico as an alternative to metriphonate which is already being used there.

4. *Tiguvon*

Tiguvon is another organophosphorus compound that can be absorbed through the skin. It was tested (by B. O. L. Duke, unpublished) in a chimpanzee infected with *O. volvulus*. The compound was applied to the skin as a 5% oily solution. After 5 days the microfilariae were reduced to about 30% of their initial numbers, not only at the application sites but all over the body. Nevertheless, when treatment was stopped the microfilariae returned to their original numbers within a month and subsequent tests with diethylcarbamazine showed that Tiguvon had no action on the adult worms.

4. *Other Compounds*

Dichlorvos resembles metriphonate; it is 10 times as active and 10 times as toxic so that the chemotherapeutic index remains the same. Chlorpyrifos, Abate, and Coumafos are microfilaricidal but their ratios of activity to toxicity are less favorable than those of metriphonate (Lämmler, 1977).

5. *Further Research on Organophosphorus Compounds*

Haloxan and the other compounds superficially resemble diethylcarbamazine in their action (namely, transient reduction in the microfilaria count but no action on adult worms). They are also known to inhibit cholinesterases of mammals and of worms. Such action on cholinesterase has not been demonstrated so clearly for diethylcarbamazine (see review of diethylcarbamazine action in Section IV). It would be interesting further to investigate the analogy between these two types of compounds with *L. carinii* in *M. natalensis* by studying whether (a) Haloxan causes microfilariae to be accumulated in the liver and later destroyed there (b) Haloxan fails to remove microfilariae if no antibodies are present in the host (c) Haloxan alters the waves of contraction that pass down (or up) microfilariae (see Section IV,A,3,b).

D. Broad-Spectrum Anthelmintics

1. *Levamisole*

Levamisole (L-2,3,5,6-tetrahydro-6-phenylimidazole[2,1*b*]thiazole HCl) is the levorotatory isomer of tetramisole. It is active against the microfilariae of *L. carinii* in *M. natalensis* when given as 10–25 mg/kg orally for 5 days, but the microfilariae soon return (Lämmler *et al.*, 1971b). It is also active against the microfilariae and adult worms of *Breinlia sergenti* in the slow loris (Zaman and Natarajan, 1973; Natarajan *et al.*, 1974). The third-stage larvae of *L. carinii* are very sensitive, and the fourth- and fifth-stage larvae are somewhat less sensitive (Lämmler and Wolf, 1977).

Levamisole showed high activity in three dogs infected with *D. immitis*.

After daily doses of 2 and 4 mg/kg orally for 3 weeks each, followed by a single dose of 4.5 mg/kg, the microfilaria counts fell to zero and the adult heartworms in the pulmonary arteries were killed (Tulloch and Anderson, 1972). The use of the drug in oral doses of 11 mg/kg daily for 6–9 days revealed high microfilaricidal activity in *D. immitis* infection in dogs. A lower dose of 6.6 mg/kg given daily for various periods was not uniformly effective in killing the microfilariae (Jackson, 1972). The activity against adult worms proved to be unsatisfactory. Although the compound in daily oral doses of 2.2 mg/kg body weight was effective in preventing the development of the third-stage larvae to adult worms, the side effects produced were such that it cannot be recommended as a satisfactory prophylactic drug for *D. immitis* infection in dogs.

Following such work Duke (1974b) tested levamisole on *O. volvulus*. One chimpanzee was given 10 mg/kg, i.m., daily for 15 days; this dosage was micro- and macrofilaricidal, but it produced unacceptable toxic effects. A second chimpanzee was given 2.5 mg/kg, i.m., daily for 15 days; this dosage was nontoxic but it had no discernible effects on the micro- or macrofilariae. One human patient was given 2.5 mg/kg. This dose produced transient giddiness and slight disorientation and had to be reduced to 2 mg/kg before it could be tolerated for 14 days. There was no discernible effect on microfilariae or adult worms. It was concluded that the maximum tolerated doses of levamisole in man are not effective against *O. volvulus*.

As regards *W. bancrofti*, levamisole was given orally to 10 infected persons in Tahiti as 6 mg/kg daily for 3 days (Merlin *et al.*, 1977). One man (who had previously reacted badly to diethylcarbamazine) had severe reactions and could not complete the course. Five patients had moderate reactions, 2 had mild ones, and 2 had none. When the blood was examined after 7 days, the microfilariae had disappeared in 6 patients and they were much reduced in the other 3. They began to reappear, however, after 30 days; and after 90 days they had returned to 52% of their original mean number. No signs of death of adult worms were seen.

2. *Other Broad Action Anthelmintics*

Methyridine [2-(2-methoxyethyl)pyridine], pyrantel, morantel, thiabendazole [2-(4-thiazolyl)benzimidazole], and fenbendazole showed no activity against microfilariae or adults of *L. carinii* (Lämmler *et al.*, 1971b, 1975). Slight activity against both was shown by parbendazole. Mebendazole shows remarkable activity against macrofilariae (*L. carinii* in *M. natalensis*), fair activity against the third- and fifth-stage larvae, and a pronounced but delayed action against microfilariae (Lämmler, 1977). On the other hand, it had no effect on adult worms or microfilariae when given by mouth to a chimpanzee infected with *O. volvulus* (Duke, 1974c).

E. Miscellaneous Drugs

The antimalarial drug amodiaquin exhibited strong antifilarial activity against adult *L. carinii* in Mongolian jirds, *Meriones unguiculatus* (Thompson *et al.,* 1968), and in *M. natalensis* (Lämmler *et al.,* 1971b). Comparable oral doses of 100 mg/kg for 5 consecutive days had only feeble activity against the same strain of *L. carinii* in cotton rats (Thompson *et al.,* 1968).

In further investigations using *L. carinii*-infected gerbils, azacrine 5-oxide dihydrochloride was lethal to adult parasites at daily oral doses of 25 or 50 mg/kg and was roughly comparable in potency to amodiaquin, azacrine, quinacrine, and quinacrine 10-oxide (Elslager *et al.,* 1970).

Dithiazanine iodide (3,3′-diethylthiadicarbocyanine iodide) has been described as a microfilaricidal agent against *D. immitis* in dogs. Elimination of microfilariae within 4–6 days could be accomplished with the oral administration of 50–100 mg/kg body weight, but these doses produced considerable side effects (Wallace and Screws, 1972). By using an oral dose of 55 mg/kg for 1 day, Chapman and Smith (1971) observed good microfilaricidal activity, but there was no effect against adult worms or migrating larvae of *D. immitis*. The authors stated that at this dose rate intoxication did not appear to be an important factor. Dithiazanine proved to be of no value for preventive medication when given in oral doses of 2.5 mg/kg body weight over a period of several months (Kume, 1970). Experimental studies with dithiazanine iodide in *L. carinii* infection of *M. natalensis* did not reveal any micro- or macrofilaricidal activity even when toxic doses were used (G. Lämmler and D. Grüner, unpublished data, 1973).

Nitrofurantoin (1-[5-nitrofurfurylideneamino]hydantoin) well known for the therapy of microbial infections in man, has been shown to have antifilarial properties. Intragastric (150 mg/kg) and intraperitoneal doses (40 mg/kg) given daily on 5 consecutive days showed high activity against adult parasites, but no action was noted against microfilariae of *L. carinii* in *M. natalensis* (Foster *et al.,* 1969). It is active against all the larval stages (Lämmler and Wolf, 1977). Further studies of this compound on *L. carinii* in *M. natalensis* revealed pronounced and differential activity against male and female parasites. In addition, there was considerable action against microfilariae, but because of the very low chemotherapeutic index the drug cannot be considered for further evaluation (Lämmler *et al.,* 1974).

Nifurtimox (Lampit) has been tested by B. O. L. Duke (unpublished) on two chimpanzees infected with *O. volvulus*. The first (an adolescent female) tolerated 40 mg/kg by mouth for 10 days well; there was only a slight temporary reduction in the microfilariae. A second adult chimpanzee was started on the same dosage but after 3 days it became semicomatose. After a week's rest, treatment was started again at 10 mg/kg for 10 days which was well tolerated. There was no effect on the microfilariae. Nifurtimox is active against the fourth- and fifth-stage larvae of *L. carinii* (Lämmler and Wolf, 1977).

C 9333-GO/CGP 4540 (4-isothiocyanato-4′-nitrodiphenylamine) was originally studied for its activities against schistosomes. The toxicity is very low, the oral LD_{50} for rhesus and other animals being over 5000 mg/kg. A dose of 100 mg/kg for 5 days destroyed the macrofilariae and microfilariae of *L. carinii,* and 600 mg/kg daily for 2 days destroyed both of them in *Dipetalonema viteae* (Striebel, 1976).

It has also been used in a finely ground form to treat jirds infected with *Brugia pahangi* (Saz *et al.*, 1977). Total doses of 200–500 mg/kg given orally during 1 or 2 days were sufficient to kill all the adult worms, provided the observation period lasted 60 days. Worms removed after 30–40 days were motile and appeared normal. A 100 mg/kg dose destroyed most but not all the worms. The microfilariae diminished greatly in numbers and they became less motile, but it was not clear whether this was directly due to the drug or to the death of the parent worms. The long delay in the death of the adult worms is remarkably like that following suramin treatment. Clinical trials against human filarial infections seem to be highly desirable.

VIII. Conclusion

This survey shows that many different types of compounds manifest activity against filariae worms, but that at present the only compound for practical use in man continues to be diethylcarbamazine, with suramin for onchocerciasis.

ACKNOWLEDGMENTS

This review was initially written for the Onchocerciasis Control Project of World Health Organization. The author gratefully acknowledges the valuable assistance of the Library Staff of W. H. O., Geneva, and of Dr. B. O. L. Duke.

References

Abadie, S. H. Gonzales, R. R., Pailet, A., Bisso, R., and Samuels, M. (1969). *Mod. Vet. Pract.* **50,** 34.

Ahmed, S. A., and Gupta, B. N. (1965). *Indian Vet. J.* **42,** 140.

Allen, P. T., and Beckman, H. (1964). *Residue Rev.* **5,** 91.

Anderson, J., and Fuglsang, H. (1973). *Trans. R. Soc. Trop. Med. Hyg.* **67,** 710.

Anderson, J., Fuglsang, H., and Marshall, T. F. de C. (1976). *Tropenmed. Parasitol.* **27,** 263.

Anderson, J., Jones, B., and Fuglsang, H. (1977). WHO/ONCHO/77.137.

Aranda-Villamayor, C. (1970). *Salud Publ. Mex.* **12,** 321.

Aubrey, J. M. (1964). *Aust. Vet. J.* **40,** 161.

Baharsefat, M., Amjadi, A. R., Yamini, B., and Ahourai, P. (1973). *Cornell Vet.* **63,** 81.

Bakhle, Y. S., and Smith, T. W. (1972). *Br. J. Pharmacol.* **46,** 543P.

Bangham, D. R. (1955). *Br. J. Pharmacol. Chemother.* **10,** 397 and 406.

Baretto, M. P., and de Siqueira, A. F. de (1963). *Rev. Inst. Med. Trop. Sao Paulo* **5,** 96.

Basu, P. C., Dhar, S. K., Sundaram, R. M., Ray, S. M., and Raghavan, N. G. S. (1970). *Proc. Second Int. Congr. Parasitol. 1970,* Part 4, p. 58, abstract 962.

Benner, M., and Lowell, F. C. (1970). *J. Allergy Clin. Immunol.* **46,** 29.

Ben-Sira, I., Aviel, E., Lazar, M., Lieberman, T. W., and Leopold, I. H. (1970). *Am. J. Ophthalmol.* **70,** 741.

Benson, H. (1974). *Arch. Ophthalmol.* **91,** 313.

Berger, H., Burkhart, R. L., and Elliott, R. F. (1969). *Am. J. Vet. Res.* **30,** 611.

Bernhard, J. A., Figueroa, L. N., and Garcia Manzo, G. A. (1964). *Salud Publ. Mex.* **6,** 835.

Biagi, F. (1974). "Enfermedades Parasitarias," p. 277. La Prensa Medica, Mexicana.

Botero, D. R., Restrepo, A. M., and Velez, H. A. (1965). *Antioquia Med.* **15,** 623.

Bryceson, A. D. M., Warrell, D. A., and Pope, H. M. (1977). *Br. Med. J.* **1,** 742.

Buck, A. A., Anderson, R. I., Kawata, K., and Hitchcock, J. C., Jr. (1969). *Am. J. Trop. Med. Hyg.* **18,** 217.

Buck, A. A., Anderson, R. I., Colston, J. A. C., Jr., Wallace, C. K., Connor, D. H., Harman, L. E., Jr., Donner, M. W., and Ganley, J. P. (1971). *Bull. W. H. O.* **45,** 353.

Bueding, E. (1952). *Br. J. Pharmacol. Chemother.* **7,** 563.

Bueding, E., Saz, H. J., and Farrow, G. W. (1959). *Br. J. Pharmacol. Chemother.* **14,** 497.

Bureau, J. P., Nozais, J. P., and Botreau-Roussel, Y. (1976). *Nouv. Presse Med.* **5,** 2807.

Burka, J. F., and Eyre, P. (1974a). *Can. J. Physiol. Pharmacol.* **52,** 942.

Burka, J. F., and Eyre, P. (1974b). *Prostaglandins* **6,** 333.

Burren, C. H. (1968). *Z. Parasitenkd.* **30,** 162.

Casey, F. B., and Tokuda, S. (1973). *Int. Arch. Allergy Appl. Immunol.* **44,** 737.

Casey, H. W., Tulloch, G. S., and Anderson, R. A. (1971). *J. Am. Vet. Med. Assoc.* **159,** 1003.

Cauchie, C., Rutsaert, J., Thys, O., Bonnyns, M., and Perier, O. (1965). *Rev. Belge Pathol. Med. Exp.* **31,** 232.

Cavier, R., Leger, N., Harichaux, J.-M., and Lonne, M. C. (1971). *Ann. Parasitol. Hum. Comp.* **46,** 497.

Chapman, N. F., and Smith, A. W. (1971). *J. Am. Vet. Med. Assoc.* **138,** 605.

Chen, C. C., and Fan, P. C. (1977). *Southeast Asian J. Trop. Med. Public Health* **8,** 53.

Ch'en, T. T. (1964). *Chin. Med. J.* **83,** 625.

Connan, R., and Zurborg, J. (1966). *Southwest. Vet.* **19,** 318.

Connor, D. H., Morrison, N. E., Kerdel-Vegas, F., Berkoff, H. A., Johnson, F., Tunnicliffe, R., Failing, F. C., Hale, L. N., and Lindquist, K. (1970). *Hum. Pathol.* **1,** 553.

Cornwell, R. L., Jones, R. M., and Pott, J. M. (1972). *Vet. Rec.* **90,** 123.

Cox, J. S. G. (1967). *Nature (London)* **216,** 1328.
Dalip Singh. (1962). *Indian J. Malariol.* **16,** 27.
Danaraj, T. J. (1958). *Q. J. Med.* [N. S.] **27,** 243.
Davis, A., and Bailey, D. R. (1969). *Bull. W. H. O.* **41,** 195.
Del Castillo, J., De Mello, W. C., and Morales, T. (1964). *Br. J. Pharmacol. Chemother.* **22,** 463.
Deline, T. R., Eyre, P., and Wells, P. W. (1973). *Arch. Int. Pharmacodyn. Ther.* **205,** 192.
Denham, D. A., Ponnudurai, T., Nelson, G. S., Guy, F., and Rodgers, R. (1971). *Bull. W. H. O.* **4,** 423.
Desowitz, R. S., and Southgate, B. A. (1973). *Southeast Asian J. Trop. Med. Public Health* **4,** 179.
Downie, C. G. B. (1966). *J. R. Army Med. Corps* **112,** 46.
Duke, B. O. L. (1960). *Ann. Trop. Med. Parasitol.* **54,** 15.
Duke, B. O. L. (1961). *Ann. Trop. Med. Parasitol.* **55,** 447.
Duke, B. O. L. (1963). *Ann. Trop. Med. Parasitol.* **57,** 82.
Duke, B. O. L. (1968). *Bull. W. H. O.* **39,** 137 and 179.
Duke, B. O. L. (1974a). *Ann. Trop. Med. Parasitol.* **68,** 241.
Duke, B. O. L. (1974b). *Trans. R. Soc. Trop. Med. Hyg.* **68,** 71.
Duke, B. O. L. (1974c). *Trans. R. Soc. Trop. Med. Hyg.* **68,** 172.
Duke, B. O. L., and Anderson, J. (1972). *Trop. Doctor* **2,** 107.
Duke, B. O. L., and Moore, P. J. (1961). *Ann. Trop. Med. Parasitol.* **55,** 263.
Duke, B. O. L., Vincelette, J., and Moore, P. J. (1976a). *Tropenmed. Parasitol.* **27,** 123.
Duke, B. O. L., Moore, P. J., and Vincelette, J. (1976b). *Tropenmed. Parasitol.* **27,** 133.
Edeson, J. F. B., and Laing, A. B. G. (1959). *Ann. Trop. Med. Parasitol.* **53,** 394.
Elslager, F. E., Perricone, S. C., and Worth, D. F. (1970). *J. Heterocycl. Chem.* **7,** 543.
Ewert, A., and Emerson, G. A. (1975). *Am. J. Trop. Med. Hyg.* **24,** 71.
Eyre, P. (1971). *Br. J. Pharmacol.* **43,** 302.
Eyre, P., Lewis, A. J., and Wells, P. W. (1973). *Br. J. Pharmacol.* **47,** 504.
Fan, P. C., Wang, Y. C., Liu, J. C., and King, M. L. (1975). *Ann. Trop. Med. Parasitol.* **69,** 515.
Faulkner, J. K., and Smith, K. J. (1972). *Xenobiotica* **2,** 59.
Forbes, L. S. (1972). *Southeast Asian J. Trop. Med. Public Health* **3,** 93 and 235.
Foster, R., Pringle, G., King, D. F., and Paris, J. (1969). *Ann. Trop. Med. Parasitol.* **63,** 95.
Fowler, J. L., Warne, R. S., Furusho, Y., and Sugiyama, H. (1970). *Am. J. Vet. Res.* **31,** 903.
Fowler, J. L., Furusho, Y., and Fernaw, R. C. (1971). *Southeast Asian J. Trop. Med. Public Health* **2,** 466.
Fraser, P. J. (1972). *Indian J. Med. Res.* **60,** 1529.
Friedheim, E. A. H. (1974). *Bull. W. H. O.* **50,** 572.
Fuglsang, H., and Anderson, J. (1973). *Lancet* **2,** 321.
Fuglsang, H., and Anderson, J. (1974). *J. Helminthol.* **48,** 93.
Fuglsang, H., and Anderson, J. (1977). WHO/ONCH./77.139.
Fukamachi, H. (1960). *Endem. Dis. Bull., Nagasaki Univ.* **2,** 27.
Garcia Manzo, A., Figueroa, L. N., and Bernhard, J. A. (1965). *Salud Publ. Mex.* **7,** 209.
Gibson, D. W., Connor, D. H., Brown, H. L., Fuglsang, H., Anderson, J., Duke, B. O. L., and Buck, A. A. (1976). *Am. J. Trop. Med. Hyg.* **25,** 76.
Gonzalez Barranco, D., Arias Fernandez, T., Chévez Zamora, A., and Salazar Mallén, M. (1962). *Salud Publ. Mex.* **4,** 1079.
Gorodovich, N. M. (1971). *Tr. Dal'nevost Nauchno-Issled. Vet. Inst.* **5,** 23.
Gutman, R. A., Liu, J. C., Cheng, J. T., and Kuo, C. C. (1969). *Am. Rev. Respir. Dis.* **99,** 255.

Harada, M., Takeuchi, M., and Katagiri, K. (1971). *Dermatologica* **142,** 193.
Harned, B. K. *et al.* (1948). *Ann. N.Y. Acad. Sci.* **50,** Art. 2, 141.
Hawking, F. (1950). *Trans. R. Soc. Trop. Med. Hyg.* **44,** 153.
Hawking, F. (1952). *Br. Med. J.* **1,** 992.
Hawking, F. (1963). "Experimental Chemotherapy," Vol. I, p. 893. Academic Press, New York.
Hawking, F. (1967). *Proc. R. Soc. London, Ser. B* **169,** 59.
Hawking, F. (1973). "Chemotherapy of Helminthiasis," Vol. I, p. 437. Pergamon Press, Oxford.
Hawking, F. (1978). *Adv. Pharmacol. Chemother.* **15,** 289.
Hawking F., and Adams, W. E. (1964). *Ann. Soc. Belge. Med. Trop.* **44,** 279.
Hawking, F., and Clark, J. B. (1967). *Trans. R. Soc. Trop. Med. Hyg.* **61,** 817.
Hawking, F., and Marques, R. J. (1967). *Bull. W. H. O.* **37,** 405.
Hawking, F., Sewell, P., and Thurston, J. P. (1950). *Br. J. Pharmacol. Chemother.* **5,** 217.
Hewitt, R. I., Kushner, S., Stewart, H. W., White, E., Wallace, W. S., and SubbaRow, Y. (1947). *J. Lab. Clin. Med.* **23,** 1314.
Hujimaki, H. (1958). *Nagasaki Med. J.* **33,** Suppl., 156.
Ishimaru, T. (1972). *Res. Filariasis Schistosomiasis* **2,** 229.
Ishizaka, T., Ishizaka, K., Orange, R. P., and Austin, K. F. (1971). *J. Immunol.* **106,** 1267.
Iwamoto, I. (1971). *Trop. Med.* **13,** 1.
Jackson, R. F. (1972). *In* "Canine Heartworm Disease Second Symposium" (R. E. Bradley and G. Pacheco, eds.), p. 129. University of Florida, Gainesville.
Jaffe, J. J., and Doremus, H. M. (1970). *J. Parasitol.* **56,** 254.
Jones, B. R. (1970). *Trans. Ophthalmol. Soc. U. K.* **90,** 299.
Jones, H. L., Shrestha, B. L., Srivastava, P., and Mack, G. J. (1970). *J. Nepal Med. Assoc.* **8,** 141.
Jordan, P. (1958). *Br. J. Pharmacol. Chemother.* **13,** 318.
Kanda, T., Sasa, M., Kato, K., and Kawai, J. (1967a). *Jpn. J. Exp. Med.* **37,** 141.
Kanda, T., Tasaka, S., and Sasa, M. (1967b). *Jpn. J. Exp. Med.* **37,** 149.
Kashinskii, A. D. (1963). *Mater. Nauchn. Konf. Vses. Ova Gel'mintol, Sb.,* Part I, p. 131.
Katiyar, J. C., Govila, P., Sen, A. B., and Chandra, R. (1974). *Trans. R. Soc. Trop. Med. Hyg.* **68,** 169.
Kessel, J. F. (1957). *Bull. W. H. O.* **16,** 633.
Kessel, J. F., Siliga, N., Tompkins, H., Jr., and Jones, K. (1970). *Bull. W. H. O.* **43,** 817.
Kimura, S., and Ono, Y. (1971). *Jpn. J. Parasitol.* **20,** 34.
Kobayashi, J., Matsuda, H., Fujita, K., Sakai, T., and Shinoda, K. (1969). *Jpn. Parasitol.* **18,** 563.
Koivikko, A. (1973). *Ann. Allergy* **31,** 45.
Kono, I. (1965). *Mem. Fac. Agric., Kagoshima Univ.* **5,** 9.
Krishna Rao, C., Sundaram, R. M., Krishna Rao, P., Das, M., Koteswara Rao, N., and Rao, C. K. (1976). *J. Commun. Disord.* **8,** 193.
Kume, S. (1970). *In* "Canine Heartworm Disease First Symposium" (R. E. Bradley, ed.). University of Florida, Gainesville.
Kume, S., Ohishi, I., and Kobayashi, S. (1962). *Am. J. Vet. Res.* **23,** 1257.
Kume, S., Ohishi, I., and Kobayashi, S. (1964). *Am. J. Vet. Res.* **25,** 1521.
Kume, S., Ohishi, I., and Kobayashi, S. (1967). *Am. J. Vet. Res.* **28,** 975.
Lagraulet, J. Monjusiau, A., and Durand, B. (1964). *Bull. Soc. Pathol. Exot.* **57,** 528.
Lämmler, G. (1974). World Health Organ. Doc. WHO/FIL/74.125.
Lämmler, G. (1977). World Health Organ. Doc. WHO/FIL/77.150.

Lämmler, G., and Grüner, D. (1975). *Z. Tropenmed. Parasitol.* **26,** 359.
Lämmler, G., and Wolf, E. (1977). *Tropenmed. Parasitol.* **28,** 205.
Lämmler, G., Hertzog, H., Saupe, E., and Schütze, H. R. (1971a). *Bull. W. H. O.* **44,** 751.
Lämmler, G., Hertzog, H., and Schütze, H. R. (1971b). *Bull. W. H. O.* **44,** 757 and 765.
Lämmler, G., Hertzog, H., and Grüner, D. (1974). *World Health Organ., Tech. Rep. Ser.* **542,** 15.
Lämmler, G., Hertzog, H., and Grüner, D. (1975). *In* "Development of Chemotherapeutic Agents for Parasitic Diseases" (M. Marois, ed.), p. 157. Amsterdam.
Langham, M. E., Traub, Z. D., and Richardson, R. (1978). *Tropenmed. Parasitol.* **29,** 156.
Lapeyra, A. Z. (1970). *An. Fac. Vet. Leon, Univ. Oviedo* **16,** 171.
Lazar, M., Lieberman, T. W., Furman, M., and Leopold, I. H. (1968). *Am. J. Ophthalmol.* **66,** 215.
Lazar, M., Furman, M., and Leopold, I. H. (1969). *Isr. J. Med. Sci.* **5,** 1263.
Lazar, M., Lieberman, T. W., and Leopold, I. H. (1970). *Am. J. Trop. Med. Hyg.* **19,** 232.
Lecomte, J., and Salmon, J. (1972). *Arch. Int. Physiol. Biochim.* **80,** 161.
Leopold, I. H. (1974). *Am. J. Ophthalmol.* **78,** 759.
Lichtenstein, L. M., and De Bernardo, R. (1971). *J. Immunol.* **107,** 1131.
Lubran, M. (1950). *Br. J. Pharmacol. Chemother.* **5,** 210.
McCarthy, J. (1970). *In* "Canine Heartworm Disease First Symposium" (R. E. Bradley ed.). University of Florida, Gainesville.
McGregor, I. A., Hawking, F., and Smith, D. A. (1952). *Br. Med. J.* **2,** 908.
Manson-Bahr, P. E. C., and Wijers, D. J. (1972). *Trans. R. Soc. Trop. Med. Hyg.* **66,** 18.
Martindale, W. (1967). "Extra Pharmacopoeia," 25th ed. Pharm. Soc., London.
Martinez Baez, M. (1960). *Rev. Inst. Salubr. Enferm. Trop., Mexico City* **20,** 223.
Mazzotti, L. (1948a). *Rev. Inst. Salubr. Enferm. Trop., Mexico City* **10,** 269.
Mazzotti, L. (1948b). *Medicina (Mexico City)* **28,** 317.
Mazzotti, L. (1959). *Rev. Inst. Salubr. Enferm. Trop., Mexico City* **19,** 1.
Mazzotti, L., and Osorio, M. T. (1949). *Rev. Inst. Salubr. Enferm. Trop., Mexico City* **10,** 269.
Mellanby, H. (1955). *Parasitology* **45,** 287.
Merlin, M., Carme, B., Kauffer, H., and Laigret, J. (1977). *Bull. Soc. Pathol. Exot.* **69,** 257.
Merrit, F. R. (1970). *In* "Canine Heartworm Disease First Symposium" (R. E. Bradley, ed.). University of Florida, Gainesville.
Meyers, W. M., Connor, D. H. *et al.* (1972). *Am. J. Trop. Med. Hyg.* **21,** 528.
Miller, C. G., and Carpenter, R. (1967). *Lancet* **1,** 895.
Minning, W., and Ding, P. C. (1951). *Z. Tropenmed. Parasitol.* **2,** 535.
Mohan, R. N. (1973). *Trans. R. Soc. Trop. Med. Hyg.* **67,** 883.
Mohan, R. N. (1974). *J. Commun. Disord.* **6,** 16.
Montestruc, E., Blanche, R., and Laborde, R. (1950). *Bull. Soc. Pathol. Exot.* **43,** 275.
Mookerjee, G. C., and Das, S. K. (1977). *J. Indian Med. Assoc.* **68,** 119.
Moreau, J. P. J., and Pichon, G. C. D. (1972). *Bull. Soc. Pathol. Exot.* **65,** 98.
Natarajan, P. N., Yeoh, T. S., and Zaman, V. (1973a). *Acta Pharm. Suec.* **10,** 125.
Natarajan, P. N., Zaman, V., and Yeoh, T. S. (1973b). *Int. J. Parasitol.* **3,** 803.
Natarajan, P. N., Zaman, V., and Yeoh, T. S. (1974). *Int. J. Parasitol.* **4,** 207.
Nishimura, K. (1965). *Chemotherapia* **10,** 164.
Norton, S., and De Beer, E. J. (1957). *Am. J. Trop. Med. Hyg.* **6,** 898.
Nwokolo, C., and Imohiosen, E. A. E. (1973). *Br. Med. J.* **2,** 153.
Oomen, A. P. (1969). *Trans. R. Soc. Trop. Med. Hyg.* **63,** 548.
Orange, R. P. (1973). *Clin. Allergy* **3,** 521.

Orange, R. P., Valentine, M., and Austin, K. F. (1968). *J. Exp. Med.* **127,** 767.
Ortiz y Ortiz, L., Gonzalez-Barranco, D., and Salazar Mallén, M. (1962). *Salud Publ. Mex.* **4,** 1075.
Patra, B. B., Prabhashchandra, D., and Sikdar, S. (1969). *Bull. Univ. Coll. Med., Calcutta Univ.* **7,** 85.
Pelczarska, A. (1974). *Arch. Immunol. Ther. Exp.* **22,** 779.
Pike, E. (1960). *Exp. Parasitol.* **9,** 223.
Raether, W., and Lämmler, G. (1971). *Ann. Trop. Med. Parasitol.* **65,** 107.
Raghavan, N. G. S., Basu, P. C., and Putatunda, J. N. (1968). World Health Organ. Doc. FIL/68.82.
Rajapakse, Y. S. (1974). *J. Trop. Med. Hyg.* **77,** 182.
Ramachandran, M. (1973). *Indian J. Med. Res.* **61,** 864.
Rantanen, P. (1971). *J. Clin. Invest.* **27,** 74.
Rao, K. N., and Subrahmanyam, D. (1970). *Indian J. Med. Res.* **58,** 746.
Rée, G. H., Hall, A. P., Hutchinson, D. B. A., and Weatherley, B. C. (1978). *Trans. R. Soc. Trop. Med. Hyg.* **71,** 542.
Reinertson, J. W., and Thompson, P. E. (1955). *Antibiot. Chemother. (Basel)* **5,** 566.
Restrepo, M., Latorre, R., and Botero, D. (1962). *Antioquia Med.* **12,** 233.
Rodger, F. C. (1962). *Bull. W. H. O.* **27,** 429.
Rougemont, A., Discamps, G., Boisson, M. E., de Grandpre, E., and Colombani, H. (1974). *Med. Trop. (Marseille)* **34,** 508.
Rougemont, A., Borges da Sylva, G., Boisson, M. E., and Astier R. (1975). WHO/ONCHO/75.118.
Rougemont, A., Boisson, M. E., and Zander, N. (1976). WHO/ONCHO/76.125.
Rousett, P. (1952). *Bull. Med. AOF* **9,** 351.
Roux, J., and Picq, J. J. (1974). *Med. Armees* **2,** 877.
Ruegg, M., and Jacques, R. (1974). *Experientia* **30,** 399.
Russel, S., Sundaram, R. M., Chandrasekharan, A., and Rao, C. K. (1975). *J. Commun. Disord.* **7,** 59.
Sakuma, S., Sakuma, M., Sato, Y., Sasa, M., and Kobayashi, J. (1967). *Jpn. J. Parasitol.* **16,** 179.
Salazar Mallén, M. (1965). *Ann. Allergy* **23,** 534.
Salazar Mallén, M. (1974). *Sci. Publ. Pan Am. Hlth. Org.* No. 298, p. 112.
Salazar Mallén, M., and Chévez Zamora, A. (1965). *Rev. Inst. Salubr. Enferm. Trop., Mexico City* **25,** 163.
Salazar Mallén, M., Molina Pasquel, C., and Chavez Nuñez, M. (1962). *Salud Publ. Mex.* **4,** 1065.
Salazar Mallén, M., Gonzalez Barranco, D., and Alvares Fuertes, G. (1970). *Z. Tropenmed. Parasitol.* **21,** 212.
Sanyal, R. K. (1961). *Int. Arch. Allergy Appl. Immunol.* **18,** 193.
Sanyal, R. K., and Sinha, B. B. (1962). *Arch. Int. Pharmacodyn. Thera.* **138,** 420.
Sareen, K. N., Misra, N., Varma, D. R., Amma, M. K. P., and Gujral, M. L. (1961). *Indian J. Physiol. Pharmacol.* **5,** 125.
Sasa, M. (1974). *Prog. Drug Res.* **18,** 259.
Sasa, M. *et al.* (1963). *Jpn. J. Exp. Med.* **33,** 213.
Savage, D. C. L. (1967). *Br. Med. J.* **1,** 840.
Saxena, J. K., Bose, S. K., Sew, R., Chatterjee, R. K., Sew, A. B., and Ghatak, S. (1977). *Exp. Parasitol.* **43,** 239.
Saxena, R., Sharma, S., Iyer, R. N., and Anand, N. (1971). *J. Med. Chem.* **14,** 929.
Saz, H. J., Dunbar, G. A., and Bueding, E. (1977). *Am. J. Trop. Med. Hyg.* **26,** 574.

Schardein, J. L., Lucas, J. A., and Dickerson, C. W. (1968). *J. Parasitol.* **54,** 351.
Schofield, F. D., and Rowley, R. E. (1961). *Am. J. Trop. Med. Hyg.* **10,** 849.
Sen, A. B., Chandra, R., Katiyar, J. C., and Chandra, S. (1974). *Indian J. Med. Res.* **62,** 1181.
Sharma, L. D., Sabir, M., and Battacharya, N. K. (1976). *Ind. J. Physiol. Pharm.* **20,** 69.
Sheng, S.-k., Hsieh, C.-I., Peng, S.-H., Hsueh, Y., and Hsueh, P. (1963). *Chem. Abstr.* **60,** 13096e.
Singhal, K. C., Chandra, O. M., and Saxena, P. N. (1972a). *Jpn. J. Pharmacol.* **22,** 175 and 726.
Singhal, K. C., Saxena, P. N., and Johri, M. B. L. (1972b). *Jpn. J. Pharmacol.* **23,** 793.
Siraganian, P. A., and Siraganian, R. P. (1974). *J. Immunol.* **112,** 2117.
Sly, R. M. (1974). *J. Allergy Clin. Immunol.* **53,** 82.
Sowa, J., and Sowa, S. C. I. (1978). *Ann. Trop. Med. Parasitol.* **72,** 79–85.
Srinivas, H. V., and Antani, J. (1971). *Ann. Allergy* **29,** 418.
Streibel, H. P. (1976). *Experientia* **32,** 457.
Sturm, P. A., Henry, D. W., Thompson, P. E., Zeigler, J. B., and McCall, J. W. (1974). *J. Med. Chem.* **17,** 481.
Subbu, V. S. V., and Biswas, A. R. (1971). *Indian J. Med. Res.* **59,** 646.
Sullivan, T. J., and Hembree, S. C. (1970). *Trans. R. Soc. Trop. Med. Hyg.* **64,** 787.
Suzuki, T., and Sone, F. (1975). *Trop. Med. (Nagasaki)* **16,** 147.
Tanaka, H., Fujita, K., Kobayashi, J., Ishii, A., and Sasa, M. (1970). *Recent Adv. Res. Filariasis Schistosomiasis Jpn.* p. 217.
Tanaka, H., Eshita, Y., Takaoka, M., and Fujii, G. (1977). *Southeast Asian J. Trop. Med. Public Health* **8,** 19.
Taylor, A. E. R. (1960). *Trans. R. Soc. Trop. Med. Hyg.* **54,** 450.
Taylor, A. E. R., and Terry, R. J. (1960). *Trans. R. Soc. Trop. Med. Hyg.* **54,** 33.
Thevathasan, O. I., and Litt, M. (1971). *Clin. Exp. Immunol.* **9,** 657.
Thiruvengadam, K. V., Subramaniam, N., Devarajan, T. V., and Zachariah, M. G. M. (1974). *J. Indian Med. Assoc.* **63,** 278.
Thomas, H. (1972). *Adv. Antimicrob. Antineoplast. Chemother., Proc. Int. Congr. Chemother., 7th, 1971* p. 457.
Thompson, P. E., Boche, L., and Blair, L. S. (1968). *J. Parasitol.* **54,** 834.
Thompson, P. E., Zeigler, J. B., and McCall, J. W. (1973). *Antimicrob. Agents & Chemother.* **3,** 693.
Torroella, J. (1964). *Salud Publ. Mex.* **6,** 595.
Tulloch, G. S., and Anderson, R. A. (1972). *In* "Canine Heartworm Disease Second Symposium." (R. E. Bradley and G. Pacheco, eds.), p. 101. University of Florida, Gainesville.
Tumada, L. R., and Margono, S. S. (1973). *Southeast Asian J. Trop. Med. Public Health* **4,** 371.
Urquhart, G. M. (1960). *J. Parasitol.* **46,** 234.
Vadodaria, D. J., Vora, M. N., and Mukherji, S. P. (1968). *Indian J. Pharm.* **30,** 41.
Varqas, L., and Tovar, J. (1957). *Bull. W. H. O.* **16,** 682.
Wallace, C. F. (1970). *In* "Canine Heartworm Disease First Symposium" (R. E. Bradley, ed.). University of Florida, Gainesville.
Wallace, C. R., and Screws, R. (1972). *In* "Canine Heartworm Disease Second Symposium" (R. E. Bradley and G. Pacheco, eds.), p. 43. University of Florida, Gainesville.
Warne, R. J., Tipton, V. J., and Furusho, Y. (1969). *Am. J. Vet. Res.* **30,** 27.
Wells, P. W., and Eyre, P. (1972). *Can. J. Physiol. Pharmacol.* **50,** 255.
Wells, P. W., Eyre, P., and Lumsden, J. H. (1973). *Can. J. Comp. Med.* **37,** 119.
Wilson, T. (1950). *Trans. R. Soc. Trop. Med. Hyg.* **44,** 49.

Wiseman, R. A., Woodruff, A. W., and Pettitt, L. E. (1971). *Trans. R. Soc. Trop. Med. Hyg.* **65,** 591.

Woodruff, A. W. (1951). *Trans. R. Soc. Trop. Med. Hyg.* **44,** 479.

Wray, C., and Tomlinson, J. R. (1974). *Br. Vet. J.* **130,** 466.

Zahner, H., Weidner, E., Lämmler, G., and Soulsby, E. J. L. (1976). *Behring Inst. Mitt.* **60,** 11.

Zahner, H., Weidner, E., Lämmler, G., and Soulsby, E. J. L. (1977). *Tropenmed. Parasitol.* **28,** 273.

Zaman, V., and Natarajan, P. N: (1973). World Health Organ. Doc. WHO/FIL/73.102.

Addendum

Page 132. Sturm *et al.* (1977) prepared a large number of analogs of diethylcarbamazine and worked out a theory of structure–activity relationships in terms of the distance between the N-atoms.

Page 147. Bartholomew *et al.* (1978) have found that diethylcarbamazine has no action on microfilariae or adults of *Manzonella ozzardi* in Trinidad.

Page 147. Denham *et al.* (1978) have reported that the action of diethylcarbamazine on *Brugia pahangi* varied according to the host. In cats it rapidly brought down the microfilaria count and it killed most of the adult worms. In *Meriones unguinculatus* it had practically no effect upon either microfilariae or adults. Perhaps the absence of effect upon the microfilariae depends upon different immunological relationships in *Meriones.*

Pages 138 and 174. The possibilities of treating onchocerciasis of the eye with continuous local application of low concentrations of diethylcarbamazine have recently been investigated by Jones *et al.* (1978). It seems probable that the eyes could be cleared of microfilariae by these means without producing severe reactions; and when this had been accomplished, more complete systemic treatment by diethylcarbamazine and by suramin could be given. Improved combinations of oral diethylcarbamazine and betamethasone for the treatment of ocular onchocerciasis have also been recommended by Anderson and Fuglsang (1978).

Anderson, J., and Fuglsang, H. (1978). *Brit. J. Ophthalmol.* **62,** 450.

Bartholomew, C. F., Nathan, M. B., and Tikasingh, E. S. (1978). *Trans. R. Soc. Trop. Med. Hyg.* **72,** 423.

Denham, D. A., Suswillo, R. R., Rogers, R., and McGreevy, P. B. (1978). *J. Parasitol.* **64,** 463.

Jones, B. R., Anderson, J., and Fuglsang, H. (1978). *Brit. J. Ophthalmol.* **62,** 428.

Sturm, P. A., Cory, M., Henry, D. W., McCall, J. W., and Ziegler, J. B. (1977). *J. Med. Chem.* **20,** 1327.

ADVANCES IN PHARMACOLOGY AND CHEMOTHERAPY, VOL. 16

Pharmacology and Toxicology of Halogenated Anesthetics

THOMAS H. CORBETT*

Department of Anesthesiology
The University of Michigan Medical Center, Ann Arbor
and
Department of Anesthesiology
Wayne County General Hospital
Eloise, Michigan

I. Introduction 195
II. Halogenated Hydrocarbons 196
A. Trichloroethylene 196
B. Halothane 198
III. Halogenated Ethers 203
A. Fluroxene 203
B. Methoxyflurane 205
C. Enflurane 207
D. Isoflurane 209
IV. Summary 211
References 211

I. Introduction

In the past 10 years there have been numerous exciting advances in our knowledge of the pharmacology and toxicology of halogenated anesthetic agents.

Although inhalation anesthetics were first utilized in the 1840s, little was known about their pharmacologic and toxic effects. Chloroform was the first halogenated hydrocarbon found to have anesthetic properties, followed by trichloroethylene (1934) and halothane (1956). The first halogenated ether to be used as an inhalation anesthetic was fluroxene (1954). It was followed in relatively rapid succession by methoxyflurane (1959), enflurane (1974), and isoflurane, which is currently pending approval by the Food and Drug Administration.

The chemical and physical properties of the various halogenated anesthetics are readily available in anesthesia textbooks and will not be covered in the following discussion.

* Present address: 4271 Pratt Road, Ann Arbor, Michigan 48103; current affiliation: Flower Hospital, Toledo, Ohio.

ISBN 0-12-032916-6

II. Halogenated Hydrocarbons

A. Trichloroethylene ($CCl_2{=}CHCl$)

1. *Pharmacological Actions*

a. Uptake and Distribution. Trichloroethylene is relatively soluble in blood, and induction of anesthesia is slow, as is recovery. In clinical practice, the slow induction time if offset partially by the high anesthetic potency of the drug. The minimum alveolar concentration (MAC) necessary to maintain the first plane of surgical anesthesia is 0.17%.

b. Respiratory System. In moderate concentrations, trichloroethylene is nonirritant to the respiratory tract, and excessive secretions and salivation are not stimulated. The respiratory rate is affected by the depth of anesthesia, with increasing tachypnea occurring with increasing depth. Tidal volume decreases with increasing rate, actually resulting in a reduced minute volume with deep anesthesia.

c. Cardiovascular System. A variety of cardiac arrythmias may occur under trichloroethylene anesthesia. Bradycardia may develop under light anesthesia as a result of increased vagal tone. Nodal rhythm and partial heart block have also been reported with light anesthesia. Trichloroethylene also causes increased myocardial excitability, and ventricular arrythmias may occur especially in deeper planes of anesthesia. Because of the increased myocardial excitability, the use of epinephrine during the anesthetic period is contraindicated.

Prolonged trichloroethylene anesthesia produces decreased myocardial contractility, and rare cases of cardiac failure due to trichloroethylene anesthesia have been reported (Edwards *et al.*, 1956).

d. Liver. Although all halogenated hydrocarbons are suspect, there is no clear evidence that trichloroethylene anesthesia causes hepatic damage.

e. Skeletal Muscle. Trichloroethylene will not produce appreciable muscle relaxation when administered in safe concentrations.

f. Uterus. Anesthetic concentrations of trichloroethylene will depress uterine contractions during labor. However, analgesic concentrations have little effect on uterine muscle unless inhaled for prolonged periods.

Trichloroethylene rapidly crosses the placenta into the fetal circulation.

g. Central Nervous System. Trichloroethylene causes a rise in intracranial pressure due to cerebral vascular dilatation and increased cerebral blood flow. This effect persists even with hyperventilation and low $P_a CO_2$.

2. *Metabolism*

Trichloroethylene was the first of the inhalation anesthetics demonstrated to be biotransformed. As early as 1939, Barrett and Johnston found trichloroethylene to be metabolized to trichloroacetic acid in dogs. In 1945, Powell demonstrated that trichloroethylene was metabolized in humans to trichloroacetic acid and proposed the formation of an epoxide intermediate. In addition to trichloroacetic acid, the human urinary metabolites, trichloroethanol and monochloroacetic acid have since been identified by Soucek and Vlachova (1960). Liebman and McAllister (1967) have shown that trichloroethanol is derived from the intermediary metabolite, chloral hydrate. The biotransformation of trichloroethylene is shown in Scheme 1.

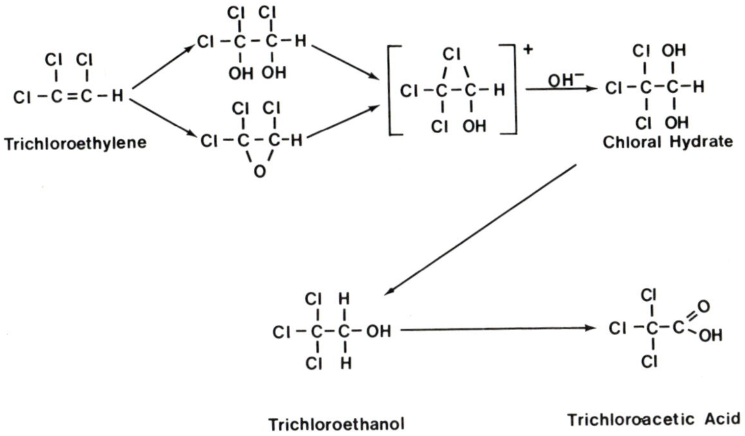

Trichloroethylene

Chloral Hydrate

Trichloroethanol

Trichloroacetic Acid

SCHEME 1

Trichloroethylene is mostly excreted by the lungs unchanged, and partly metabolized. Depending on the duration of exposure, the percentage recovery of trichloroethylene from exhalation varies from 67 to 83% of the dose (Malchy and Parkhouse, 1968). Metabolic degradation is prolonged, with metabolites present in the urine up to 18 days following a single administration.

3. *Toxicology*

Trichloroethylene has been used as an industrial solvent for many years. As a result, toxic symptoms have been observed in workers. Cranial nerve lesions are among the most common toxic manifestations seen in workers, and are caused not by trichloroethylene itself, but by its degradation products, including dichloroacetylene. The fifth cranial nerve is most commonly involved. The onset of toxic symptoms is usually characterized by numbness or coldness around the lips about 24 hours following exposure. During the next few days, the area of sensory loss spreads to involve the entire field supplied by the trigeminal nerve. There is no motor involvement. Recovery usually begins between the fifth and tenth days. Lesions of other cranial nerves have been reported (Wylie and Churchill-Davidson, 1972).

In 1971, Salvini *et al.* demonstrated that volunteers exposed to 110 ppm trichloroethylene for 4 hours had a significant decrease in performance of standard psychophysiological function tests, including parameters such as reaction time and memory recall.

In 1974, Van Duuren (1975) predicted on the basis of chemical structure and metabolism that trichloroethylene would be carcinogenic. This prediction was proven correct in tests by the National Cancer Institute in 1975. Trichloroethylene, administered in high doses orally, produced hepatocellular carcinoma in mice. Both the concentration and duration of exposure of the mice to trichloroethylene far exceeded the clinical anesthetic dose in patients and the occupationally related doses to operating room personnel. The carcinogenic risk of exposure to trichloroethylene to both patients and to operating room personnel remains unknown at this time.

B. Halothane
(2-Bromo-2-chloro-1,1,1-trifluoroethane; $CF_3CHClBr$)

1. *Pharmacological Actions*

a. Uptake and Distribution. Halothane is relatively insoluble in blood, and induction of anesthesia is relatively rapid. The minimum alveolar concentration necessary to maintain the first plane of surgical anesthesia is 0.7%. Halothane is extremely soluble in fat, allowing the body to absorb large amounts of the anesthetic. Other tissues also show a greater affinity for halothane than blood, as shown in Table I.

b. Respiratory System. Halothane is a respiratory depressant. This action is augmented by narcotic premedication. Increasing concentrations of halothane produce progressive reductions in tidal volume rather than in respiratory rate.

c. Cardiovascular System. Halothane is a myocardial depressant, and the degree of contractile depression is related to the depth of anesthesia. Halothane-induced bradycardia, reversed by atropine, suggests that the anesthetic has a parasympathetic stimulant action as well as producing myocardial depression.

TABLE I

TISSUE/BLOOD SOLUBILITY COEFFICIENTS FOR HALOTHANE

Tissue	Solubility coefficient
Kidney	1.6
Brain	2.6
Lung	2.6
Muscle	3.5
Fat	60.0

Arrythmias occurring during halothane anesthesia are related to hypercarbia from respiratory depression. Adrenaline can be used safely in the presence of halothane provided the concentration and total dose are within the acceptable limits of no more than 10 cc of a 1 : 100,000 solution during any 10 minute period.

Halothane affects the peripheral circulation by producing a persistent vasodilatation of the skin and muscle vessels with a resultant decrease in both arterial pressure and vascular resistance. Halothane does not appear to have a direct action on the vessel wall itself, but rather blocks the action of noradrenaline.

d. Liver. Halothane causes a decrease in hepatic blood flow. The association between halothane and liver damage is discussed in Section II,B,3.

e. Kidney. Halothane anesthesia produces a reduction in glomerular filtration rate, a decrease in renal blood flow, and decreased sodium excretion. Antidiuresis is observed and is probably due to both a release of antidiuretic hormone and a reduced glomerular filtration rate (Deutsch *et al.*, 1966).

f. Skeletal Muscle. Halothane has minimal neuromuscular blocking action.

Intense muscle spasms are occasionally seen in the early postanesthesia period following the use of halothane. These spasms are related to a decrease in body temperature during the anesthetic period.

g. Uterus. Halothane relaxes uterine muscle progressively with increasing depth of anesthesia. Unless carefully controlled, this uterine relaxation may fail to respond to ergot derivatives and oxytocic posterior pituitary extracts. For this reason, halothane is not recommended for obstetric anesthesia except when uterine relaxation is required.

Halothane readily crosses the placental barrier.

h. Central Nervous System. When the main arterial blood pressure and arterial pCO_2 are maintained within normal limits, halothane causes decreased cerebral vascular resistance with subsequent increased cerebral blood flow and increased intracranial pressure. This effect can be countered by decreasing the arterial pCO_2 through hyperventilation.

2. *Metabolism*

Although halothane was introduced into clinical anesthesia in 1956, the first demonstration of its metabolism was not reported until 1964 when Stier *et al.* measured urinary bromide excretion in 13 surgical patients and compared the results with nonhalothane anesthesized and with normal controls. Increased urinary bromide concentrations and elevated bromide/halide ratios were found in all patients anesthesized with halothane. Bromide concentrations peaked on the third and fifth postanesthetic days.

In 1967, Rehder *et al.* reported their findings in 2 surgical patients anesthetized for 75 minutes and followed for 23 days. Trifluoroacetic acid, bromide, and traces of inorganic fluoride were found as urinary metabolites. By measuring the total halothane absorbed and quantitating the metabolites, the amount of halothane metabolized was calculated to be between 12–20% of the total absorbed dose.

Cascorbi *et al.* (1970) studied halothane metabolism by injecting 5 anesthetists and 4 pharmacists with small doses of ^{14}C-labeled halothane and measuring radioactive nonvolatile metabolites in the urine of the subjects for a minimum of 5 days. In the anesthetists, the average recovery after 5 days was 16.9% of the injected dose. In one of the anesthetists followed for 13 days, 24.8% of the dose was eventually recovered as metabolites. For the pharmacists, the average recovery was slightly less, 14.9% of the injected dose after 5 days. These investigators also found that 2 subjects given trace doses during halothane anesthesia metabolized less of the dose than when injected during an awake period, suggesting an enzyme-inhibiting action of anesthetics at high concentrations.

Cohen *et al.* (1975) identified two additional metabolites in the urine of heart-transplant donors injected intravenously with large doses of ^{14}C-labeled halothane. In addition to trifluoroacetyl ethanolamine and *N*-acetyl-*S*-(2-bromo-2-chloro-1,1-difluoroacetyl)-L-cysteine, several additional minor metabolites were found but not identified.

The heart-transplant donor studies of Cohen *et al.* (1977) also revealed unidentified nonvolatile metabolites of halothane in a variety of tissues 6 hours following injection. Highest concentrations of these metabolites were found in liver, kidney, and gonads, with lesser concentrations in lung, muscle, blood, and fat. Approximately 1.3% of the total administered radioactivity was found to be sequestered in the liver as nonvolatile metabolites within 6 hours following administration. A large share of this radioactivity appeared to be covalently bound to lipids and proteins.

Recent studies by Van Dyke and Gandolfi (1976) indicate that halothane, in the presence of reduced oxygen tension, undergoes reductive defluorination according to the following reaction:

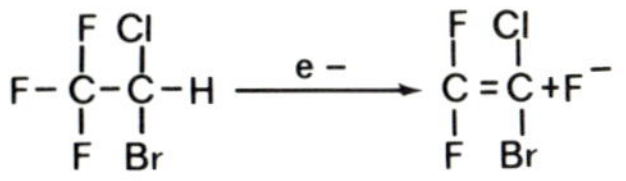

$$F-\underset{F}{\overset{F}{C}}-\underset{Br}{\overset{Cl}{C}}-H \xrightarrow{e^-} \underset{F}{\overset{F}{C}}=\underset{Br}{\overset{Cl}{C}} + F^-$$

The reaction is mediated by cytochrome P-450 and requires reduced nicotinamide adenine dinucleotide phosphate but is inhibited by oxygen. Inorganic fluoride has been identified as a metabolite of halothane, and Cohen *et al.* (1975) have identified difluorobromochloroethylene mercapturate in human urine following administration of ^{14}C-labeled halothane to heart-transplant donors.

It now appears that under conditions of low oxygen tension, the release of inorganic fluoride and covalent binding of difluorobromochloroethylene to phospholipids may occur.

Cohen and Van Dyke (1977a) have presented the overall reaction for the metabolism of halothane, as shown in Scheme 2.

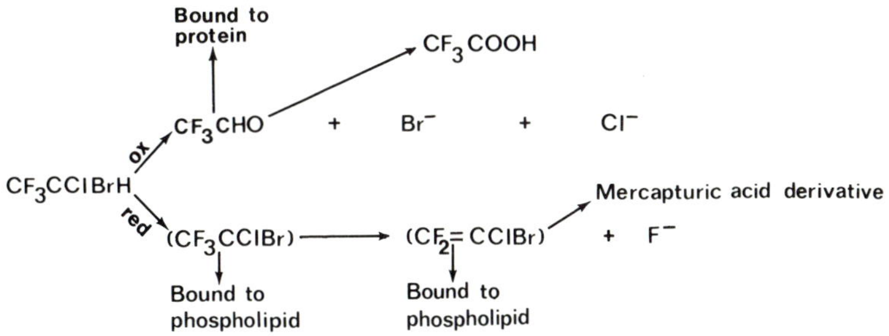

$$CF_3CClBrH \xrightarrow{ox} CF_3CHO\ (\rightarrow \text{Bound to protein};\ \rightarrow CF_3COOH) + Br^- + Cl^-$$

$$CF_3CClBrH \xrightarrow{red} (CF_3CClBr)\ (\downarrow \text{Bound to phospholipid}) \longrightarrow (CF_2{=}CClBr)\ (\downarrow \text{Bound to phospholipid};\ \rightarrow \text{Mercapturic acid derivative}) + F^-$$

SCHEME 2

3. *Toxicity*

Many halogenated hydrocarbons are known to be hepatotoxic, and at least in certain individuals, halothane is no exception. The usual clinical picture of halothane hepatitis presents with fever, leukocytosis, and with eosinophilia followed by jaundice within 5 to 21 days after anesthesia. Liver dysfunction is confirmed by finding high alkaline phosphatase, serum glutamic oxaloacetic transaminase (SGOT), and serum glutamic pyruvic transaminase (SGPT) levels.

Histologically, the outstanding feature is extensive hepatocellular necrosis, predominately central and midzonal. In most cases, the necrosis is sharply delineated, coagulative in type, and accompanied by cytoplasmic vacuolation.

The mechanism involved in the production of postanesthesia liver failure and death is still under investigation. The term "halothane hepatitis" may well be a misnomer, as the syndrome has been reported not only following the use of halothane, but following the use of methoxyflurane, enflurane, and other anesthetics as well (Bunker *et al.* (1969). Factors other than the type of anesthetic administered, such as hypoxia or hypercarbia, can increase the incidence of liver damage following ether or chloroform anesthesia. Hypotension can produce similar damage. Still, there are numerous cases in the literature reporting liver necrosis following halothane anesthesia where these other complicating factors have been nonoperative.

The production of liver damage following halothane anesthesia is thought to be related to the metabolism of the drug. Whether the necrosis is due to an abnormal metabolite or intermediate acting directly on the hepatocytes or due to a hypersensitivity reaction from a metabolite that is covalently bound to a macromolecule is the subject of considerable debate.

The usual final products of halothane biodegradation in the human (described in the preceding section) do not account for the syndrome of halothane hepatitis. The presence of an unusual final end product in patients with the syndrome has not been identified. However, the presence of highly reactive intermediate products of biodegradation appears likely in the formation of the final end products, trifluoroacetic acid, trifluoroacetyl ethanolamine, and the cysteine conjugate of 2-bromo-2-chloro-1,1-difluoroethylene. These highly reactive intermediates could, under the appropriate conditions, be responsible for the occasional hepatotoxic effects of halothane anesthesia.

Polychlorinated biphenyls (PCB's) have recently been found to enhance and alter the metabolism of halothane in rats, and pretreatment of these animals with Aroclor 1254 followed by halothane anesthesia has produced the syndrome of halothane hepatitis with widespread centrilobular necrosis and markedly elevated serum transaminase levels (Sipes and Brown, 1976). These findings suggest that perhaps PCB's and possibly other environmental pollutants may be responsible for certain cases of liver necrosis in humans following anesthesia.

The hypothesis that the liver damage is due to a hypersensitivity reaction to halothane has been suggested by the clinical findings of fever, malaise, and arthralgias, and the laboratory findings of eosinophilia and lymphocytopenia. Several *in vitro* tests dependent on the development of cell-mediated immunity, including lymphocyte transformation (Paronetto and Popper, 1970) and the appearance of mitochondrial antibodies (Rodriguez *et al.*, 1969), have been reported to have initial promise, but these findings have been inconsistent in later studies.

History of previous exposure to halothane prior to the exposure resulting in hepatitis in many of the reported cases also lends support to the sensitization hypothesis. However, the data to support this hypothesis are scant, and the toxic intermediate metabolite theory currently offers the most likely explanation.

Halothane is embryotoxic and teratogenic to rats at anesthetic concentrations (Basford and Fink, 1968). Electron-microscopic changes in brain and other tissues, with concomitant changes in behavior and intelligence have been reported in offspring of mice exposed *in utero* to concentrations of 10 ppm halothane. The effects of halothane on the human fetus are unknown.

Although the presence of highly reactive intermediate metabolites of halothane are postulated, and these metabolites may act as alkylating agents, the carcinogenic potential of halothane has not yet been determined.

Baden *et al.* (1976) were unable to demonstrate mutagenicity of halothane in two histidine mutant strains of *Salmonella typhimurium* incubated with halothane at concentrations ranging from 0.1 to 30%.

III. Halogenated Ethers

A. Fluroxene

(2,2,2-Trifluoroethyl vinyl ether; $CF_3CH_2{-}O{-}CH{=}CH_2$)

1. *Pharmacological Actions*

a. Uptake and Distribution. Fluroxene is relatively insoluble in blood. Induction and recovery are rapid, but fluroxene's anesthetic potency is low. The minimum alveolar concentration necessary to maintain the first plane of surgical anesthesia is 3.4%. The tissue solubilities of fluroxene are shown in Table II.

b. Respiratory System. With light anesthesia, the respiratory rate is increased. The tidal volume is decreased progressively with increasing depth of anesthesia. Fluroxene is not a respiratory irritant, and patients can tolerate concentrations up to 8%.

c. Cardiovascular System. Fluroxene produced decreasing blood pressure with increasing depth of anesthesia. Bradycardia may occur with

TABLE II

TISSUE/BLOOD COEFFICIENTS OF FLUROXENE

Tissue	Solubility coefficient
Brain	1.43
Liver	1.37
Muscle	2.28

deep anesthesia, as may T-wave depression. Conversion of sinus rhythm to nodal rhythm may also occur with deep anesthesia.

d. Liver. Liver function studies are normal following routine fluroxene anesthesia.

e. Kidney. Renal function is not impaired following fluroxene anesthesia.

f. Skeletal Muscle. Fluroxene produces only a moderate degree of muscle relaxation.

2. *Metabolism*

Fluroxene was the first of the fluorinated ethers to be used in human clinical anesthesia. Although introduced in the early 1950s, evidence for its metabolism was not forthcoming until 1970 when Blake and Cascorbi (1970), in a unique experiment, injected themselves with ^{14}C-labeled fluroxene intravenously and measured their own metabolites. Nonvolatile urinary metabolites accounted for 12.1 and 15.4% of the injected dose during the first 24 hours. The metabolites were not identified in this experiment.

In 1974, Gion *et al.* analyzed the urinary metabolites of patients anesthetized with fluroxene for 10 days postanesthesia and found that 10.6% of the administered dose was excreted as nonvolatile metabolites. These nonvolatile metabolites were identified as trifluoroacetic acid (7.2%), trifluoroethanol (0.27%), trifluoroethanol conjugates (0.33%), and other undetermined metabolites (2.6%). From these studies, it was determined that trifluoroacetic acid is the major urinary metabolite of fluroxene in man. This is in contrast to several animal species studied in which the toxic metabolite trifluoroethanol was formed as the predominant metabolite.

3. *Toxicity*

Fluroxene has a remarkable record of clinical safety during administration and during the postanesthesia period. However, this anesthetic has recently been found to be mutagenic in bacterial test systems (Baden *et al.*, 1977), suggesting possible long-term adverse effects including production of birth defects and carcinogenesis. No studies of exposed human populations have yet been performed.

After over one-half million fluroxene anesthetic administrations, there have been only a few reported cases of hepatotoxicity (Reynolds *et al.*, 1972; Tucker *et al.*, 1973). In the 2 fatal cases reported, both patients had been taking enzyme-inducing drugs preoperatively. It has been suggested that these patients may have metabolized a greater amount of fluroxene to trifluoroethanol than usual, thus accounting for the hepatotoxic effect. However, no data are available to prove or disprove this speculation.

B. Methoxyflurane
(2,2-Dichloro-1,1-difluoroethyl methyl ether; $CHCl_2CF_2—O—CH_3$)

1. *Pharmacological Actions*

Methoxyflurane has both anesthetic and analgesic properties, and analgesia may persist following return of consciousness. Methoxyflurane is highly soluble in blood, and induction of anesthesia is slower than with many other anesthetics. Methoxyflurane is also very fat soluble and has high anesthetic potency. The mean alveolar concentration necessary to induce the first plane of surgical anesthesia is 0.3%.

With the exception of fat, methoxyflurane is only slightly more soluble in other tissues than in blood, as shown in Table III.

a. Cardiovascular System. Methoxyflurane produces a decrease in cardiac output, systemic vascular resistance, and stroke volume, with an increase in heart rate. The resultant hypotension is mainly due to the decrease in cardiac output.

The myocardium is only minimally sensitized by methoxyflurane to epinephrine.

b. Respiratory System. Methoxyflurane depresses respiration proportional to the depth of anesthesia. The tidal volume is affected more than

TABLE III

Tissue/Blood Solubility Coefficients for Methoxyflurane

Tissue	Solubility coefficient
Brain, white matter	2.34
gray matter	1.70
Muscle	1.34
Fat	8.50

the respiratory rate. Methoxyflurane is not a respiratory irritant and does not stimulate salivation or bronchial secretions.

c. Liver. Hepatic dysfunction, jaundice, and fatal hepatic necrosis have occurred following methoxyflurane anesthesia. In most respects the clinical features seen with hepatic necrosis are similar to those seen following halothane-induced hepatitis, and the histological changes are identical.

d. Kidney. The effects of methoxyflurane on the kidney are discussed in Section III,B,3.

e. Skeletal Muscle. Methoxyflurane produces profound muscle relaxation during deep anesthesia. The muscle relaxation is thought to be due to action on the central nervous system rather than due to a peripheral effect. This anesthetic-induced muscle relaxation reduces the requirement for muscle-relaxant drugs during surgery. Because of the dose-related renal toxicity, methoxyflurane should not be administered at levels required to achieve muscle relaxation. When using nondepolarizing muscle relaxant drugs, the dosage of relaxant should be reduced by one-half.

2. *Metabolism*

Methoxyflurane is extensively metabolized in man (Holaday *et al.*, 1970; Yoshimura *et al.*, 1976): approximately 20% of the absorbed dose is exhaled unchanged; approximately 33% of the dose is biotransformed to the urinary metabolite, methoxydifluoroacetic acid; and the amounts of fluoride and oxalic acid excreted in the urine amount to approximately 10% of the dose. Other metabolites are carbon dioxide and chloride. Since not all the absorbed dose of methoxyflurane has been able to be recovered in these studies, it has been postulated that permanent binding of certain metabolites to macromolecules occurs (Yoshimura *et al.*, 1976).

3. *Toxicity*

Nephrotoxicity manifested by high-output renal failure is the major adverse effect produced by methoxyflurane anesthesia. It is caused by the release of large quantities of inorganic fluoride ion during the biotransformation of the drug. The severity of the nephrotoxicity is dose related and may occur when the serum fluoride ion concentration surpasses 40 m*M* (Cousins and Mazze, 1973). Nephrotoxicity does not occur following administration of the other fluorinated anesthetics because considerably less fluoride ion is released during biotransformation of these anesthetics.

Oxalic acid is also produced during biotransformation of methoxyflurane. However, although renal toxicity due to tubular obstruction may occur from crystalline oxalic acid deposits, the amount produced during routine methoxyflurane anesthesia is insufficient to produce toxic effects.

A number of cases of hepatitis associated with methoxyflurane have been reported. Of 24 cases reported by Joshi and Conn (1974), the clinical aspects of the hepatitis syndrome were indistinguishable from those seen in halothane-induced hepatitis, and as with the latter syndrome, the histological characteristics were identical to viral hepatitis.

The carcinogenic potential of methoxyflurane has not been determined. Mutagenicity testing in two strains of histidine-dependent *Salmonella typhimurium* has been reported to be negative (Baden *et al.*, 1977).

C. Enflurane
(2-Chloro-1,1,2-trifluoroethyldifluoromethyl ether; $CHFClCF_2—O—CF_2H$)

1. *Pharmacological Actions*

a. Uptake and Distribution. Enflurane is relatively insoluble in blood. Induction and recovery from anesthesia are rapid. The mean alveolar concentration of enflurane necessary to induce the first plane of surgical anesthesia is 1.68%.

b. Cardiovascular System. There is a decrease in blood pressure with induction of anesthesia, followed by a return to near normal with surgical stimulation. Progressive increases in depth of anesthesia produce corresponding decreases in blood pressure. The heart rate and rhythm remain stable under enflurane anesthesia. Elevation of the carbon dioxide level in arterial blood does not alter cardiac rhythm. Enflurane does not readily sensitize the human myocardial conduction system to epinephrine when moderate exogenous doses (up to 10 cc of a 1 : 100,000 solution) are used.

c. Respiratory System. Enflurane does not stimulate excess salivation or tracheobronchial secretions, nor does it affect bronchomotor tone. It reduces ventilation as depth of anesthesia increases.

d. Liver. Berman *et al.* (1976) have obtained data suggesting induction of hepatic microsomal enzymes following a single MAC dose of 9.6 hours of enflurane anesthesia. The ratio of 6β-hydroxycortisol to 17-hydrocorticosteroids (17-OHCS) in 24-hour urine specimens increased markedly in volunteers following exposure.

e. Kidney. Renal function studies are usually normal following enflurane anesthesia, although several cases of nephrotoxicity have been reported (see Section III,C,3).

f. Skeletal Muscle. At normal levels of anesthesia, enflurane produces a degree of muscle relaxation sufficient for many intra-abdominal surgical procedures. Additional muscle-relaxant drugs should be administered with caution as the nondepolarizing muscle relaxants are markedly potentiated by enflurane.

g. Central Nervous System. Increasing depth of enflurane anesthesia produces a change in the electroencephalogram characterized by high voltage, fast frequency, progressing through spike–dome complexes alternating with periods of electrical silence to frank seizure activity. The latter may or may not be associated with motor movement. When encountered, motor activity generally consists of twitching or jerking movements of various muscle groups. This is self-limiting, and can be eliminated by lowering the anesthetic concentration. The foregoing changes can be excerbated by hyperventilation-induced low arterial carbon dioxide tension. Cerebral blood flow and metabolism studies in normal volunteers during seizure patterns show no evidence of cerebral hypoxia, and recovery appears to be uncomplicated.

2. *Metabolism*

Based on the structure–activity relationships of the enflurane molecule, metabolism was predicted to occur to a lesser degree than the related haloether anesthetic, methoxyflurane.

Chase *et al.* (1971) studied the biotransformation of enflurane in 7 healthy patients. Urinary fluoride excretion was studied for 10 days postanesthesia. Inorganic fluoride excretion peaked after 7 hours, with a half-life of 1.55 days. Organic fluoride excretion peaked on the second day with a half-life of 3.69 days. The total nonvolatile fluorinated metabolites in urine represented 2.4% of the enflurane absorbed during anesthesia. The majority of the metabolites were recovered as organic fluoride (1.91% organic fluoride, 0.51% inorganic fluoride).

Serum inorganic fluoride levels in patients anesthetized with 1.4% enflurane were studied by Cousins *et al.* (1976). Peak serum inorganic fluoride levels of 22.2 m*M* were attained 4 hours postanesthesia, and dropped significantly by 48 hours postanesthesia.

3. *Toxicity*

Although fluoride ion is released during metabolism of enflurane, the concentrations seen in serum are considerably lower than following anesthesia with methoxyflurane. Nevertheless, several cases of nephrotoxicity following enflurane anesthesia have been reported. One patient had severe preexisting renal disease with only modest increase in serum fluoride (Loehning and Mazze, 1974), whereas another developed renal failure following 6 hours of enflurane anesthesia. In the latter case, serum fluoride levels peaked at 93 m*M* and returned to normal by the thirteenth postanesthesia day. The patient had received enflurane anesthesia 6 weeks previously, and enzyme induction may have caused the increased rate of enflurane metabolism in this patient (Eichorn *et al.*, 1976). The possible role of enzyme induction in enflurane toxicity is further suggested in a study by Cousins *et al.* (1976) showing that increased fluoride production occurred following enflurane anesthesia in a patient receiving enzyme-inducing drugs.

Carcinogenicity testing of enflurane has not been reported. Mutagenicity testing has been reported as negative (Baden *et al.*, 1977).

D. Isoflurane
(2,2,2-Trifluoro-1-chloroethyl difluoromethyl ether; $CF_3CHCl—O—CF_2H$)

1. *Pharmacological Actions*

a. Uptake and Distribution. Anesthetic induction and recovery are more rapid than with halothane. The mean alveolar concentration necessary to induce surgical anesthesia is 1.3%.

b. Respiratory System. Fourcade *et al.* (1971) compared the ventilatory effects of isoflurane with those of halothane in human volunteers and found that when equivalent anesthetic doses were considered, less isoflurane than halothane was needed to increase P_a CO_2 and depress the slope of the CO_2 curve. In contrast to halothane, isoflurane in increasing concentrations, did not cause progressive increases in respiratory frequency. For this reason, isoflurane produces a more profound respiratory depression than halothane.

c. Cardiovascular System. Stevens *et al.* (1971) demonstrated that isoflurane, in human volunteers, under conditions of constant arterial carbon dioxide tension and body temperature, maintained normal myocardial function but produced progressive vasodilatation as anesthesia deepened. The cardiac output was maintained by an increased heart rate that compensated for a decreased stroke volume.

Cromwell *et al.* (1971) found that isoflurane, under conditions of spontaneous ventilation with the concomitant increase in arterial carbon dioxide tension, produced an increase in heart rate and cardiac output over and above that seen under conditions of normal arterial carbon dioxide tension.

d. Liver. Bromsulfophthalein (BSP) retention is increased in normal subjects receiving isoflurane in oxygen (Stevens *et al.*, 1973). Induced hypercapnea during isoflurane anesthesia did not increase the BSP retention. No significant changes were observed in SGPT or lactic dehydrogenase (LDH) values; however, decreases were found in serum cholesterol and alkaline phosphatase values in subjects receiving isoflurane in 70% nitrous oxide.

e. Kidney. Stevens *et al.* (1973) found that normal subjects receiving isoflurane anesthesia had significantly decreased blood urea nitrogen levels postanesthesia. Creatinine levels did not change significantly, however. Uric acid levels were significantly higher the seventh day following anesthesia compared to the first day postanesthesia in subjects receiving isoflurane in oxygen. There were no significant changes in serum and urine lysozyme levels. Urine pH tended to increase slightly, and the specific gravity decreased on the first day following exposure to isoflurane. These parameters returned to normal by the seventh postexposure day. Mazze *et al.* (1974) found that renal function, including the response to vasopressin, was normal in subjects anesthesized with isoflurane. In their studies, intra-anesthesia depressions of renal blood flow (51% of control) and urinary flow rate (63% of control) occurred during isoflurane anesthesia.

f. Central Nervous System. Results of studies in volunteers by Miller *et al.* (1971) suggest that isoflurane has neuromuscular effects qualitatively similar to those of other halogenated inhalation anesthetics. Twitch height was not altered. However, the average neuromuscular refractory period increased and the ability to sustain tetanus decreased with increasing isoflurane concentrations. These investigators found that isoflurane has greater neuromuscular depressant effects both alone and in combination with *d*-tubocurarine than equivalent doses of halothane. In fact, isoflurane appears to potentiate *d*-tubocurarine more than any other inhalation agent, including diethyl ether.

2. *Metabolism*

Less than 1% of the administered dose of isoflurane is metabolized in normal subjects. Stevens *et al.* (1971) showed a small increase in serum fluoride ion concentration in 3 out of 4 volunteers up to 7 days following exposure. In 9 surgical patients receiving isoflurane anesthesia, Mazze *et al.* (1974) found a mean peak serum inorganic fluoride concentration of 4.4 m*M*/liter 6 hours after anesthesia. In a series of 189 patients, Dobkin *et al.* (1971) found a mean serum inorganic fluoride level at the end of anesthesia of 3.6 m*M*/liter, with 12 m*M*/liter the highest value reported. The mean duration of anesthesia was 178 minutes.

3. *Toxicity*

To date, no significant toxic effects from isoflurane anesthesia have been reported. The small amount of fluoride produced appears insufficient to produce the nephrotoxicity seen with methoxyflurane anesthesia.

A preliminary report suggesting carcinogenic activity from isoflurane or a metabolite in mice has been published (Corbett, 1976). However, it was later learned that the mice used in the experiment were contaminated with polybrominated biphenyls, which may have themselves produced the hyperplastic nodules seen in livers of exposed animals. The possibility of interaction between polybrominated biphenyls and isoflurane to produce the nodules must also be entertained. Mutagenicity testing of isoflurane to date has been negative (Baden *et al.*, 1977).

IV. Summary

The recent advances in the pharmacology and toxicology of halogenated, inhalation anesthetic agents have resulted in changes in both administration of these anesthetics to patients and in operating room personnel exposure. Considerable care is now taken in choosing a particular anesthetic for a particular patient. Of particular importance is the patient's medication history and any history of disease of the various organ systems that may be exacerbated by a particular anesthetic.

The potential threat to the health of operating room personnel from acute (impaired mental abilities) or chronic (possible carcinogenicity/teratogenicity) exposure to low concentrations of the halogenated anesthetic agents in the operating room environment has been countered with the installation of gas-scavenging devices on anesthesia machines. These devices capture escaping anesthetic gases and vapors and shunt them from the operating room rather than allowing them to be dispersed throughout the operating room.

References

Baden, J. M., Brinkenhoff, M., Wharton, R. S., Hitt, B. A., Simmon, V. F., and Mazze, R. I. (1976). *Anesthesiology* **45,** 311.

Baden, J. M., Kelley, M., and Hitt, B. A. (1977). *Anesthesiology* **46,** 346.

Barrett, H. M., and Johnston, J. (1939). *J. Biol. Chem.* **127,** 765.

Basford, A., and Fink, R. A. (1968). *Anesthesiology* **29,** 1167.

Berman, M. L., Green, O. C., Calverley, R. K., Smith, N. T., and Eger, E. I. (1976). *Anesthesiology* **44,** 496.

Blake, D. A., and Cascorbi, H. F. (1970). *Anesthesiology* **32,** 560.

Bunker, J. P., Forrest, W. H., Mosteller, F., *et al.* (1969). "The National Halothane Study: A Study of the Possible Association Between Halothane Anesthesia and Postoperative Hepatic Necrosis." US Govt. Printing Office, Bethesda, Maryland.

Cascorbi, H. F., Blake, D. A., and Helrich, M. (1970). *Anesthesiology* **32,** 119.

Chase, R. E., Holaday, D. A., Fiserova-Bergerova, V., Saidman, L. J., and Mack, F. E. (1971). *Anesthesiology* **35,** 262.

Cohen, E. N., and Van Dyke, R. A. (1977a). *Addison-Wesley Publ.* No. 72.

Cohen, E. N., and Van Dyke, R. A. (1977b). *Addison-Wesley Publ.* No. 142.

Cohen, E. N., Trudell, J. R., Edmunds, H. N., Watson, E. (1975). *Anesthesiology* **43,** 392.
Corbett, T. H. (1976). *Ann. N. Y. Acad. Sci.* **271,** 58–66.
Cousins, M. J., and Mazze, R. I. (1973). *J. Am. Med. Assoc.* **225,** 1161.
Cousins, M. J., Greenstein, L. R., Hitt, B. A., and Mazze, R. I. (1976). *Anesthesiology* **44,** 44.
Cromwell, T. H., Stevens, W. C., Eger, E. I., Shakespeare, T. F., *et al.* (1971). *Anesthesiology* **35,** 17.
Deutsch, S., Goldbery, M., Stephen, G. W., and Wu, W. H. (1966). *Anesthesiology* **27,** 793.
Dobkin, A. B., Byles, P. H., Ghanooni, S., *et al.* (1971). *Can. Anaesth. Soc. J.* **18,** 264.
Edwards, G., Morton, H. J. V., Pask, E. A., and Wylie, W. D. (1956). *Anaesthesia* **11,** 194.
Eichorn, J. H., Hedley-Whyte, J., Steinman, T. I., *et al.* (1976). *Anesthesiology* **45,** 557.
Fourcade, H. E., Stevens, W. C., Larson, P., Cromwell, T. H., *et al.* (1971). *Anesthesiology* **35,** 26.
Gion, H., Yoshimura, N., Holaday, D. A., *et al.* (1974). *Anesthesiology* **40,** 553.
Holaday, D. A., Rudofsky, S., and Treuhaft, P. S. (1970). *Anesthesiology* **33,** 579.
Joshi, P. H., and Conn, H. V. (1974). *Ann. Intern. Med.* **80,** 395.
Liebman, K. C., and McAllister, W. J. (1967). *J. Pharmacol. Exp. Ther.* **157,** 574.
Loehning, R. W., and Mazze, R. I. (1974). *Anesthesiology* **40,** 203.
Malchy, H., and Parkhouse, J. (1968). *Can. Anaesth. Soc. J.* **16,** 119.
Mazze, R. I., Cousins, M. B., and Barr, G. A. (1974). *Anesthesiology* **40,** 536.
Miller, R. D., Eger, E. I., Way, W. L., Stevens, W. C., *et al.* (1971). *Anesthesiology* **35,** 38.
Paronetto, F., and Popper, H. (1970). *N. Engl. J. Med.* **283,** 277.
Powell, J. F. (1945). *Br. J. Ind. Med.* **2,** 142.
Rehder, K., Forbes, J., Alter, H., *et al.* (1967). *Anesthesiology* **28,** 711.
Reynolds, E. S., Brown, B. R., and Vandam, L. D. (1972). *N. Engl. J. Med.* **286,** 530.
Rodriguez, M., Paronetto, F., Schaffner, F., *et al.* (1969). *J. Am. Med. Assoc.* **208,** 148.
Salvini, M., Binaschi, S., and Riva, M. (1971). *Br. J. Ind. Med.* **28,** 293.
Sipes, I. G., and Brown, B. R. (1976). *Anesthesiology* **45,** 622.
Soucek, B., and Vlachova, D. (1960). *Br. J. Ind. Med.* **17,** 60.
Stevens, W. C., Cromwell, T. H., Halsey, M. J., Eger, E. I., *et al.* (1971). *Anesthesiology* **35,** 8.
Stevens, W. C., Eger, E. I., Joas, T. A., Cromwell, T. H., White, A., and Dolan, W. M. (1973). *Can. Anaesth. Soc. J.* **20,** 357.
Stier, A., Alter, H., Hessler, O., *et al.* (1964). *Anesth. Analg.* (*Cleveland*) **43,** 723.
Tucker, W. K., Munson, E. S., Holaday, D. A., *et al.* (1973). *Anesthesiology* **39,** 104.
Van Duuren, B. L. (1975). *Ann. N. Y. Acad. Sci.* **246,** 258.
Van Dyke, R. A., and Gandolfi, A. J. (1976). *Drug Metab. Dispos.* **4,** 40.
Wylie, W. D., and Churchill-Davidson, H. C. (1972). *3rd Ed. Yearb. Med. Publ.* **314.**
Yoshimura, N., Holaday, D. A., and Fiserova-Bergerova, V. (1976). *Anesthesiology* **44,** 372.

Magnetically Responsive Microspheres and Other Carriers for the Biophysical Targeting of Antitumor Agents

KENNETH J. WIDDER, ANDREW E. SENYEI, AND DAVID F. RANNEY*

Departments of Pathology, Microbiology-Immunology and Surgery and the Northwestern University Cancer Center Northwestern University Medical and Dental Schools Chicago, Illinois

I. Introduction 213
II. Goals and Problems of Targeted Cancer Chemotherapy 215
III. Biodegradable Encapsulation Carriers 218
A. Erythrocyte Ghosts 219
B. Other Cells 222
C. Liposomes 223
D. Albumin Microspheres 233
E. Magnetically Responsive Albumin Microspheres 239
F. Discussion 259
IV. Exposed Carriers and Targeted Natural Products 261
V. Summary 264
References 265

I. Introduction

One of the major challenges in cancer chemotherapy is the targeting of antineoplastic agents to restricted anatomic sites and specific target cells. The need for targeting stems from two general conditions that apply to most tumor-bearing patients at the time of clinical diagnosis. First, various biological activities and surface properties of malignant cells interfere with their recognition and elimination. This leads to a progressive biological imbalance between successful tumors and their hosts. For a brief description of the major contributory factors, see Byers and Levin (1976). Second, biochemical differences between tumor and host cells are almost always minimal and frequently quantitative rather than qualitative (Broome, 1961; Papanastassiou *et al.*, 1966; Tsou *et al.*, 1967; Hurwitz *et al.*, 1975; Rowland *et al.*, 1975). This makes it difficult to overcome the tumor–host imbalance using nontargeted agents. These problems have re-

* Present address: Department of Pathology, University of Texas Health Science Center, 5323 Harry Hines Blvd., Dallas, Texas 75235.

ISBN 0-12-032916-6

sulted in efforts to focus the effects of existing agents and treatments on tumor cells and spare their effects on normal cells. The major clinical and experimental approaches are outlined in Table I.

This review emphasizes and compares the properties of biodegradable, encapsulation carriers that have the potential to target a wide spectrum of antineoplastic agents. It concentrates on their demonstrated capabilities as targeting vehicles in model systems and compares their chemical, biological, and distribution characteristics with those of other pertinent carriers listed in Table I. In addition to providing a general review of drug carriers, this article summarizes our recent studies on the area-specific localization of adriamycin using a newly developed carrier consisting of magnetically responsive, albumin microspheres. Included are brief re-

TABLE I

PARTITIONING OF DRUG AND THERAPEUTIC EFFECTS IN MEDICINE[a]

Method	Agent or procedure
I. Biophysical	
A. Treatments	Local irradiation Hyperthermia
B. Encapsulation drug carriers	
1. Nonbiodegradable	Glass beads, plastic beads, polyacrylamide gel, ferrosilicone gel, surfactant membranes
2. Biodegradable	
a. Vesicular carriers	
(1) Cells	Erythrocyte ghosts, leukocytes, hepatocytes
(2) Synthetic systems	Lactic acid polymers, liposomes and macrovesicles, ufasomes (unsaturated fatty acid spheres)
b. Particulate carriers	Oil emulsions, albumin microspheres, magnetically responsive albumin microspheres
II. Chemical	
A. Treatments	Hyperoxia
B. Drugs	Solubility partitioning
III. Biochemical	
A. Drugs	Prodrugs, lectins, toxins, and bacteriocins
B. Exposed drug carriers	Drug–metal complexes; drug–macromolecular complexes with albumin, fibrinogen, dextran, DNA, glycoproteins, immunoglobulins
IV. Surgical	Regional perfusion of drugs; local installation and implantation of drugs; release of agents from magnetically responsive paraoperational devices (M-PODS); vascular occlusion with magnetically responsive carbonyl iron

[a] Adapted in part from Gregoriadis (1977).

views on the development of albumin microspheres, the magnetic guidance of intravascular particles, and the potential side effects of magnetically responsive iron oxides.

II. Goals and Problems of Targeted Cancer Chemotherapy

The comprehensive goal of targeted chemotherapy is to reduce tumor–host imbalance by altering the distribution, uptake, or effects of drug(s) such that tumor cells are damaged substantially more than normal cells. The targeting of intravascularly administered agents involves three distinct stages that are classified as first-order, second-order, and third-order targeting. *First-order targeting* refers to the restricted distribution of carrier and drug to the capillary bed of a predetermined target site, organ, or tissue. For solid tumors, this includes transendothelial migration of either the drug–carrier complex or the drug alone. For leukemias and tumors of the reticuloendothelial system, the endothelial barrier may be reduced or absent (Studer and Potchen, 1971). *Second-order targeting* refers to the selective direction of carrier or drug to tumor cells versus normal cells. For solid tumors, this can occur only after the drug–carrier complex or drug itself has gained access to the tissue parenchyma. *Third-order targeting* refers to the carrier-directed release of drug at selected intracellular sites. This is based on the ability of some drug carriers to enter target cells by either endocytosis or cell fusion (see Section III,C).

An ideal carrier for the targeting of intravascularly administered, antitumor agents has the following characteristics: (*1*) it restricts the distribution of drug to the desired target area, organ, or tissue; (*2*) it undergoes uniform, capillary-level distribution throughout the target circulation; (*3*) it maintains prolonged control over the localization of drug; (*4*) it affords the drug ready access to tissue parenchyma; (*5*) it delivers drug preferentially to tumor cells or enhances its effects on those cells; (*6*) it provides a controllable and predictable rate of drug release; (*7*) it has the capacity to carry a wide spectrum of agents (including high molecular weight, drug–macromolecular complexes); (*8*) it incorporates and releases these agents without significantly reducing their biological activities; (*9*) it contains a sufficient quantity of drug per unit carrier to release therapeutic concentrations at the target site without excessively loading the host with carrier products; (*10*) it minimizes the leakage of free drug during intravascular transit; (*11*) it protects the agent from inactivation by plasma enzymes; (*12*) it protects the host from immediate allergic responses to encapsulated agents or surface products; (*13*) it avoids carrier-induced modulation of tumor cell growth; (*14*) it exhibits biocompatible surface properties and negligible antigenicity; and (*15*) it undergoes biodegradation, with prompt elimination and minimal toxicity of the breakdown products. For optimal utility in adjuvant chemotherapy, the drug–carrier complex must be easily prepared and available for use either intraoperatively or during the immediate postoperative period. These criteria should be considered as the various carrier systems are evaluated.

Although a number of the carriers listed in Table I are quite innovative and several have been therapeutically efficacious, most have not solved the problem of first-order targeting. There are two major reasons. First, as a class, encapsulation carriers that are small enough (<1.4 μm) to avoid extensive embolization of the target organs and lungs (Ring *et al.*, 1961; Wagner *et al.*, 1969b; Zolle *et al.*, 1970), are rapidly sequestered by mononuclear phagocytes of the reticuloendothelial system (Saba, 1970; McDougall *et al.*, 1974; Segal *et al.*, 1974). For most tumors, this localizes drug at a site distant from its desired target and produces a weak local drug gradient. Second, all carriers that are designed to afford second-order targeting to tumor cells within an organ must first traverse the capillary endothelium.

The endothelial barrier has severely frustrated attempts at *in vivo* targeting that are based on surface differences between normal and malignant cells. With the possible exception of angiomas, there is no necessary relationship between the surface antigens of tumor neovascular endothelium and the tumor-associated antigens of malignant cells in the adjacent tissue parenchyma. This markedly impairs the efficiency of drug targeting using carriers directed against tumor-associated antigens. Consequently, targeted carriers must either take advantage of naturally occurring differences in the permeability of tumor neovascular endothelium or selectively induce changes in that permeability.

In normal tissues, low molecular weight drugs partition between the intravascular and extravascular spaces based on gradients in the hydrostatic and osmotic pressures and the concentration of agent (Landis, 1927; Zweifach and Intaglietta, 1968). The extravascular movement of larger molecules, small vesicles, and particles appears to be regulated by the size of "tight" junctions between capillary endothelial cells (Landis and Pappenheimer, 1963; Karnovsky, 1967) and the rate of active transport through these cells via pinocytic vesicles (Palade, 1953; Karnovsky, 1967). Major ultrastructural differences in capillary endothelial cells and tight junctions occur among the organ systems of the normal human body. These have been reviewed and classified by Majno (1965). The three general categories are as follows: (Class I) capillaries that exhibit a continuous endothelium and low molecular permeability (including the central nervous system, striated and cardiac muscle, lung, small intestinal muscle, and skin); (Class II) fenestrated capillaries that exhibit intracellular openings and intermediate molecular permeability (including the adrenals, kidney, and lamina propria of the intestine); and (Class III) discontinuous capillaries that exhibit large intercellular gaps or sinusoidal structure and very high permeability, including permeability to colloids (represented by the liver and spleen). The blood–brain barrier is unique in that it has both tight, nonpenetrable endothelial junctions and a paucity of endocytic transport vesicles (Reese and Karnovsky, 1967). The choroid plexus differs to the extent that it exhibits fenestrations and allows significant intercellular and transcellular passage of large (40,000-dalton) molecules, such as horseradish peroxidase (Brightman, 1968). Functional studies, using labeled serum albumin, have also been performed to investigate these organ-dependent differences in capillary permeability (Studer and Potchen, 1971). The results are generally consistent with the ultrastructural findings just summarized. Based on these two types of studies, it can be predicted that intravascularly administered macromolecular carriers, vesicles, and microspheres will be preferentially cleared by the liver and spleen, and to a lesser extent by the kidneys. Indeed, this organ pattern is commonly observed and difficult to alter. The most promising attempts involve blockading the reticuloendothelial system prior to administering the carrier (see Section III,C).

Preliminary indications suggest that tumor tissues exhibit variable increases in capillary permeability (Potchen *et al.*, 1971; Gregoriadis *et al.*, 1974c; Dapergolas *et al.*, 1976). When this is observed, it appears to result from alterations in the microvascular circulation within tumor tissue, and additional changes related to tumor-induced inflammation. The neovasculature of many tumors is characterized by increased distances between capillary endothelial cells (Potchen, *et al.*, 1971). This increases the passage of larger molecules and small vesicles from the intravascular to the extravascular space. In addition, tumors often exhibit a deficiency of small lymphatic vessels (Potchen *et al.*, 1971). The resulting decrease in lymphatic drainage may prolong the extravascular residence of substances that have entered from the bloodstream. Tumor-induced inflammation contributes to the enhanced extravascular transport of large materials in at least two ways. It promotes the physical separation of endothelial cell junctions (Buchner, 1956; Anderson and McCutcheon, 1966) and induces the directed movement (chemotaxis) of leukocytes out of the bloodstream into the extravascular space (Snyderman and Mergenhagen, 1976). These leukocytes can actively phagocytize macromolecules, vesicles, and particles, and transport them into the tumor parenchyma (see Sections III and IV). One agent whose extravascular filtration is facilitated by this process is the "tumor-seeking" radionuclide, ^{67}Ga (Hayes *et al.*, 1970; Ito *et al.*,

1971; Higasi *et al.,* 1972). Gallium-67 binds to serum proteins and extravasates as a protein-bound complex (Ito *et al.,* 1971). Its preferential uptake by neoplastic lesions is based, in part, on the enhanced endocytic and phagocytic activities of both inward-migrating inflammatory cells and resident tumor cells (Hayes *et al.,* 1970; Ito *et al.,* 1971; Higasi *et al.,* 1972; Gregoriadis and Neerunjun, 1975b).

Tumor cells also can exhibit a moderate-to-marked enhancement of endocytic activity (Gregoriadis and Neerunjun, 1975b; Nicolson *et al.,* 1976). This characteristic feature has suggested a potential approach to second-order targeting based on endocytosis of appropriately designed drug carriers. Unfortunately, this property has been difficult to exploit for three reasons. First, despite changes in tumor neovascular permeability, most endocytizable carriers are rapidly cleared by the reticuloendothelial system (see Sections III and IV) and are not locally available for uptake by the tumor. Moreover, the presence of clinically detectable neoplasms increases rather than decreases the systemic reticuloendothelial clearance of such carrier materials (Salky *et al.,* 1967; Sheagren *et al.,* 1967). Second, only the smaller encapsulation carriers undergo preferential uptake by tumor tissue compared to the surrounding normal tissue (see Section III,C). Third, since they are actively endocytic, intralesional macrophages also take up significant quantities of cytotoxic agents that are delivered by endocytizable carriers. This damages or destroys one of the important local host defenses that retards tumor growth and metastasis (Lohmann-Matthes, 1976; Tevethia *et al.,* 1976). Thus, second-order targeting has been largely unsuccessful because it requires prior solutions to the problems of first-order targeting and more sophisticated approaches to second-order targeting than those depending on differences between the endocytic activities of malignant cells and host macrophages.

Third-order targeting will be discussed in Section III,C.

III. Biodegradable Encapsulation Carriers

This classification includes all three-dimensional carriers that physically separate the incorporated agent from the surrounding environment. The group can be divided into vesicular and particulate carriers. Vesicular carriers commonly consist of water-insoluble envelopes that encapsulate the respective drug. These can be subdivided into biologically derived preparations, such as erythrocyte ghosts, leukocytes, and hepatocytes; and biosynthetic preparations, such as liposomes, macrovesicles, and lactic acid polymers. Particulate carriers are characterized by homogeneous, oil or solid-phase matrices that entrap the respective drug. They can be subdivided into oil emulsions and microspheres.

As a class, encapsulation carriers prevent or retard the release of drug during intravascular transit of the drug–carrier complex. By minimizing the interaction of encapsulated drugs with blood enzymes, antibodies, and white cells, these carriers diminish intravascular catabolism of the drugs and prevent them from initiating allergic reactions. They also alter the clearance, organ distribution, and excretion of drugs. Clearance and first-order targeting are determined by the route of carrier administration, the rate of drug release from the carrier, and various properties of the carrier. These include size, chemical composition, the presence of surface groups that confer either charge or receptor specificity, and the responsiveness of carrier constituents to external magnetic fields. For intravascularly administered preparations, the distribution of carrier and drug will be similar if the spontaneous release of drug is slow. Conversely, if this release is rapid, significant quantities of drug will circulate and distribute in a pattern identical to the free agent.

A. Erythrocyte Ghosts

Drug-bearing erythrocyte ghosts were originally devised to provide an approach to the treatment of Gaucher's disease (Ihler *et al.,* 1973), characterized by the accumulation of β-glucocerebroside in cells of the reticuloendothelial system and kidneys. To date, their use as carriers for antitumor agents has been limited to experimental animal systems.

1. *Preparation and in Vitro Characteristics*

Loading of erythrocytes with enzymes, drugs, and drug–macromolecular complexes has been achieved by hypotonic lysis of human, murine, and rat erythrocytes at 4°C, in the presence of the desired pharmacological agent (Ihler *et al.,* 1973; Fiddler *et al.,* 1974; Tyrrell and Ryman, 1976). The entry of drugs is rapid. Under optimal conditions, maximal entrapment occurs about 60 seconds after the initiation of lysis. The erythrocyte membranes are resealed by exposure to iso-osmotic sodium chloride. This produces osmotically intact ghosts that have lost their characteristic erythroid shape and are increased in average volume from 102 to 139 μm^3.

Depending on the experimental conditions, the efficiency of entrapment can vary from 3.2 to 16.6% for drugs such as methotrexate and adriamycin (Tyrrell and Ryman, 1976), and from 24 to 60% for enzymes such as β-galactosidase and β-glucosidase (Ihler *et al.,* 1973). The major factors influencing entrapment of a given agent are its extracellular concentration and molecular weight. Increasing the extracellular concentration enhances the absolute quantity of drug entrapped (Tyrrell and Ryman, 1976). Low molecular weight products and smaller proteins are incorporated to a greater extent than high molecular weight substances such as DNA. In studies using ^{35}S-labeled proteins from *Escherichia coli,* optimal entrapment was observed for proteins of approximately 90,000 daltons (Ihler *et al.,* 1973). Similar results were reported for dextrans of various molecular sizes (Marsden and Ostling, 1959). Although the incorporation of *E. coli* β-galactosidase (MW 540,000) has been accomplished, the efficiency of entrapment is lower than for smaller molecules (Ihler *et al.,* 1973). During attempts to entrap adriamycin–DNA complexes, the apparent entrapment of DNA (60.0%) was greater than that of adriamycin (16.6%) (Tyrrell and Ryman, 1976). A significant quantity of adriamycin separated from its DNA complex. Moreover, much of the DNA was associated with, rather than entrapped in the resealed ghosts. This selectivity toward the size of entrapped molecules appears to depend on the functional diameter of membrane pores formed during reversible osmotic lysis of the erythrocyte. Such a carrier system would be expected to accommodate best water-soluble agents of less than 100,000–200,000 daltons. This property may place an upper limit on the molecular size of agents that can be targeted by erythrocyte ghosts that are prepared by hypotonic lysis.

More recently, bovine and human erythrocyte ghosts have been prepared by dielectric breakdown of the cell membranes (Zimmermann *et al.,* 1975, 1976). These ghosts have been shown to spontaneously reseal at 37°C. Their ultimate sizes have been varied by altering the concentration of inorganic phosphates during preparation and resealing (Zimmermann *et al.,* 1975, 1976). Respresentative entrapment of exogenous agents has ranged from 20% for the enzyme, urease (Zimmermann *et al.,* 1976), to greater than 50% for methotrexate (Zimmermann *et al.,* 1978).

In vitro studies indicate that the spontaneous leakage of even low molecular weight agents from erythrocyte ghosts occurs quite slowly. Methotrexate is lost at a rate of 10% per hour on incubation in serum at 37°C (Tyrrell and Ryman, 1976; Zimmermann *et al.,* 1978). This property and those described in the foregoing suggest that the release of entrapped agents during intravascular transit should be minimal. The complete release of agents requires destruction of the erythrocyte ghosts, resulting in a rate of release which is almost instantaneous.

2. *Distribution and Targeting*

The major target organs for intravascularly administered ghosts are the liver and spleen. As evaluated by distribution studies using ^{99m}Tc-labeled ghosts in rats (Tyrrell and Ryman, 1976) and mice (Fiddler *et al.,* 1974;

Zimmermann *et al.*, 1978), the liver receives 65–70% of the injected carrier and the spleen approximately 18%. It has been suggested that this pattern could be altered by modifying the carrier's surface charge (Tyrrell and Ryman, 1976; Gregoriadis, 1975) or oxidizing its surface sulfhydryl groups (Rifkind, 1966). However, at best, such changes appear to result in preferential uptake by the spleen versus the liver. Therefore, the principal target remains one or more organs of the reticuloendothelial system. A potential approach to this problem has been suggested by Zimmermann *et al.* (1978). This would involve the entrapment of small (4–20 nm) para-, ferro-, or ferrimagnetic particles that could permit the subsequent, intravascular targeting of resealed ghosts using extracorporeal magnets.

After first-order targeting has occurred, the natural fate of erythrocyte ghosts is similar to that of endogenously damaged erythrocytes. These cells undergo erythrophagocytosis and degradation by mononuclear cells of the liver and spleen (Rifkind, 1966). Entrapped enzymes and drugs are released intracellularly. On crude subfractionation of the liver, these agents are found primarily in the lysosomal and mitochondrial fractions (Tyrrell and Ryman, 1976; Fiddler *et al.*, 1974). Therefore, erythrocyte-borne drugs might be expected to enter preferentially tumor cells that exhibit enhanced phagocytic activity. However, given the current limitations on modification of first-order targeting, this second-order mechanism could be used to advantage only for tumors of the reticuloendothelial system. Erythrocyte ghosts do not easily penetrate the tight junctions between normal capillary endothelial cells (Gregoriadis, 1977). They would be expected to penetrate tumor neovascular endothelium rather poorly.

3. *Metabolism, Antigenicity, and Toxicity*

Erythrocyte ghosts are catabolized by lysosomal glycosidases and lipases within the mononuclear phagocytes of the reticuloendothelial system (Rifkind, 1966). Their toxicity is negligible in hosts whose liver and spleen cells have a normal complement of lysosomal enzymes. Theoretically, toxicity could become a problem if the recipient were deficient in one or more enzymes required to catabolize the glycoprotein and β-glucocerebroside constituents contributed by the erythrocyte membranes themselves. Erythrocyte ghosts should exhibit negligible antigenicity in donor–recipient pairs that bear identical major blood group antigens. However, this carrier has been shown to act as an immunological adjuvant and thereby enhance the antigenicity of entrapped, heterologous proteins (Tyrrell and Ryman, 1976). A similar enhancement would also be predicted to occur for heterologous DNA or other foreign macromolecules that are entrapped in the form of drug–macromolecular complexes.

4. *Current and Projected Utility in Cancer Chemotherapy*

The incorporation of methotrexate, adriamycin, and adriamycin–DNA complexes into erythrocyte ghosts (Tyrrell and Ryman, 1976; Zimmermann *et al.*, 1978) has introduced the possibility of using this carrier as a targeting vehicle for antitumor agents. However, current limitations on modifying the usual pattern of organ distribution appear to restrict these applications to relatively uncommon malignancies of the reticuloendothelial system, such as histiocytic medullary reticulosis in man (Tyrrell and Ryman, 1976). This restriction may be overcome by the successful introduction of magnetically responsive materials, as suggested above. The major remaining disadvantage of such drug-carrier preparations would be their relatively short shelf lives.

B. Other Cells

Model systems exist for the use of viable cells as vehicles for targeting drugs to homologous organs. To date, these experimental systems have been limited to the reconstitution of enzyme deficiencies using human peripheral blood leukocytes (Knudson *et al.*, 1971) and rat hepatocytes (Matas *et al.*, 1976). In the human system, intravenously administered, normal peripheral blood leukocytes (consisting of 70–90% lymphocytes) have been used to contribute an as yet unidentified "corrective factor" to a patient with Type II mucopolysaccharidosis. This treatment briefly normalized his urinary secretion of glycosaminoglycans. In the rat system, suspensions of normal hepatocytes have been infused into the portal vein of animals lacking the enzyme uridine diphosphate glucuronyltransferase. This produced a transient decrease in the concentration of serum bilirubin.

In both of the above cases, the corrective factor or enzyme was synthesized by the cells themselves. However, it is also possible to introduce exogenous chemotherapeutic agents into such cells by *in vitro* incubation with drug-bearing liposomes (see Section III,C). The loaded cells could then be injected as targeted drug carriers. For example, peripheral blood leukocytes may be removed from a patient in moderate numbers, loaded with liposome-encapsulated drug, and reinjected. The lymphocytes present in this cell preparation will circulate throughout the blood and lymphatic systems. A significant fraction of these cells home to target areas within lymphoid and reticuloendothelial organs (Woodruff, 1974). Such homing appears to be based on interactions between lymphoid cell-surface glycoproteins and tissue determinants. Peripheral blood leukocytes have the additional property of readily migrating across vascular endothelium in areas of inflammation (Snyderman and Mergenhagen, 1976), such as those frequently surrounding malignant tumors. Despite these potential advantages, three major problems have prevented the widespread use of leukocytes as targeted drug carriers: (*1*) viable cells represent inefficient drug carriers because only a small fraction of the cell volume represents usable drug space; (*2*) an extremely large number of cells are required to physically saturate the system-wide target organs; and (*3*) intracellular enzymes potentially can inactivate a substantial portion of encapsulated drug before cellular lysis and drug release could occur. Consequently, only a low percentage of the drug would be made available to act on adjacent target cells.

The targeting of hepatocytes to liver is dependent on their administration via the portal vein. Theoretically, an adequate saturation of the liver with carrier cells could be achieved by this route. Practically, such transplantation would require the use of large numbers of hepatocytes from unrelated donors. Although the liver does represent an immunologically protected site with respect to allograft rejection (Matas *et al.,* 1976), such protection is relative. A large number of foreign donor cells would be expected to overcome this protection and elicit a vigorous immune response. This would lead to substantial intrahepatic inflammation and tissue destruction. Moreover, hepatocytes are even more active than leukocytes with respect to the intracellular degradation of chemotherapeutic agents. Therefore, at present, it appears that the use of viable cells as vehicles for targeting antitumor agents will remain theoretical. Their clinical applications probably will be limited to cases where the therapeutic goal involves intracellular synthesis and release of a deficient natural product, rather than uptake and targeting of exogenous drugs.

C. Liposomes

Liposomes have received considerable attention as experimental carriers of antitumor agents in animals and patients. This interest is based on studies showing that they can alter the systemic distribution of entrapped agents (Gregoriadis and Ryman, 1971), decrease the required dosage of drugs (Gregoriadis and Allison, 1974), minimize allergic reactions to encapsulated foreign proteins (Neerunjun and Gregoriadis, 1976), increase the cellular uptake of poorly transported agents (Papahadjopoulos *et al.,* 1974a), and delay the clearance and excretion of water-soluble drugs (Juliano and Stamp, 1975).

1. *Preparation and in Vitro Characteristics*

The term, liposome, was first proposed by Bangham *et al.* (1965). According to current usage, *liposomes* are vesicles consisting of one or more concentrically ordered assemblies of polar phospholipid bilayers. The most commonly used phospholipids are egg phosphatidylcholine, synthetic dipalmitoyl-DL-α-phosphatidylcholine, brain-derived and synthetic phosphatidylserine, sphingomyelin, phosphatidylinositol, and ovolecithin (Fendler and Romero, 1977). Liposomes can be subdivided into three major structural classes: monolamellar (single compartment) vesicles, multilamellar vesicles, and macrovesicles (Fendler and Romero, 1977). Multilamellar liposomes are commonly prepared by evaporating a volatile organic solution containing the phospholipids, cholesterol, and other hydrophobic adducts. The resulting organic film is shaken with an aqueous solution, forming large multilamellar liposomes with concentric aqueous compartments. Sonication of these vesicles produces smaller monolamellar liposomes that can be separated from the parent structures by gel filtration or ultracentrifugation. Liposomes range in size from 8.5 nm for monolamellar structures to several microns for multilamellar ones (Gregoriadis, 1976a, 1977). Macrovesicles are formed by the slow injection of a lipid–ether solution into warm aqueous buffer (Deamer and Bangham, 1976). This produces single-compartment structures that are 0.13 ± 0.06 μm in diameter.

Liposomes can be made to entrap both hydrophobic and water-soluble drugs. Hydrophobic drugs are added to the original organic solution and become entrapped in the lipid film. Water-soluble drugs are dissolved in the aqueous solution that is later mixed with the organic film. The efficiency of drug entrapment depends on the drug's solubility in either aqueous or nonpolar solvents and on the sizes of the liposome's aqueous and lipid compartments (Fendler and Romero, 1977). Agents that are highly soluble in either aqueous or nonpolar solvents will undergo extensive entrapment. Representative entrapment of enzymes and synthetic polynucleotides ranges from 2.5-5% for horseradish peroxidase (Magee *et al.*, 1974), 4–6.5% for amyloglucosidase (Gregoriadis *et al.*, 1974a), 12% for L-asparaginase (Fishman and Citri, 1975), and 14–26% for polyuridilic acid (Kulpa and Tinghitella, 1976). For relatively soluble, low molecular weight agents, entrapment ranges from 0.7–5.4% for 8-azaguanine (Fendler and Romero, 1976), 20% for cyclic AMP (Papahadjopoulos, *et al.*, 1974a), and up to 60% for bleomycin (Gregoriadis *et al.*, 1976; Dapergolas *et al.*, 1976). Agents that are poorly soluble in both aqueous and nonpolar solvents undergo meager entrapment. For example, only 0.1–0.5% of 6-mercaptopurine is incorporated under standard conditions (Tsujii *et al.*, 1976). However, both the solubility and entrapment of such drugs can be enhanced by either adjusting the pH to produce ionized functional groups or forming charge-transfer complexes between the parent drug and acceptors such as chloranil (Tsujii *et al.*, 1976). Molecular size does not appear to limit entrapment. For example, macrovesicles can be made to encapsulate sucrose, polynucleotides (poly I: poly C), large proteins (ferritin) and viruses (poliovirus) (Papahadjopoulos and Vail, 1978), and DNA of up to 5000 base pairs (Hoffman *et al.,* 1978). However, these large vesicles experience differences in clearance, organ distribution, and access to tumors when compared to smaller vesicles (see the following). The efficiency of drug entrapment is also influenced by physical properties of the liposome. For example, multilamellar liposomes contain larger aqueous spaces than their smaller monolamellar counterparts. Consequently, the former entrap higher percentages of polar drugs (Gregoriadis, 1973; Fendler and Romero, 1976).

Entrapped drugs are liberated by either leakage through the lipid bilayer or destruction of the vesicle. Spontaneous leakage is influenced by the lipid composition, charge interactions between the drug and liposomal membrane, and the molecular size of the entrapped agent. Such leakage is maximal when the bilayer is near its characteristic phase-transition temperature (Haest *et al.,* 1972; Papahadjopoulos *et al.,* 1973; Inoue, 1974; Nicholls and Miller, 1974; Blok *et al.,* 1975, 1976; Lawaczek *et al.,* 1976; Breisblatt and Ohki, 1976a). Cholesterol is generally added to the mixture of phospholipids to produce an intermediate membrane fluidity (Ladbrooke *et al.,* 1968; Breisblatt and Ohki, 1976a,b) and to decrease membrane permeability at biologically relevant temperatures (Papahadjopoulos *et al.,* 1971; de Gier *et al.,* 1968). The leakage of selected agents also can be reduced by the addition of sterols (Gregoriadis, 1977) and by the alteration of surface charge. A positive charge is conferred by the incorporation of long-chain amines (usually stearylamine), and a negative charge by phosphatidylserine or dicetyl phosphate (Fendler and Romero, 1977). Liposomes composed of only cholesterol and phospholipid are electrostatically neutral. Charge interactions between the drug and lipid bilayer are exemplified by the enhanced uptake and slower release of methotrexate by positively charged liposomes (Kimelberg, 1976). In general, large molecules such as invertase (Gregoriadis and Ryman, 1972a) and neuraminidase (Gregoriadis *et al.,* 1974b), are released more slowly than smaller molecules. Low molecular weight, chemotherapeutic agents complexed to macromolecules behave as large molecules. For example, daunomycin and melphalan are retained longer when complexed to DNA or polyglutamic acid (Gregoriadis, 1977). The spontaneous leakage of smaller molecules is variable. Drugs such as 5-fluorouracil (Gregoriadis, 1974) and penicillin (Gregoriadis, 1973) undergo rapid diffusion. By contrast, actinomycin (Gregoriadis, 1973), bleomycin (Dapergolas *et al.,* 1976; Gregoriadis and Neerunjun, 1975a), and colchicine (Juliano and Stamp, 1975) are released quite slowly. Actinomycin, which is soluble in both polar and nonpolar solvents, is released from liposomes more rapidly when entrapped in the aqueous phase compared to the lipid phase (Rahman *et al.*, 1975). These differences in leakage lead to differences in drug distribution (see Section III,C,2).

As illustrated by the preceding discussion, maximal encapsulation and minimal leakage depend on optimizing the liposome's size and lipid composition for each chemotherapeutic agent. The resulting properties do not always afford maximal distribution of the carrier to tumor tissues. For example, small liposomes gain the best access to neoplastic tissues (see Section III,C,2). However, compared to larger vesicles, they often allow a faster leakage of low molecular weight drugs and place constraints on the entrapment of high molecular weight drug complexes.

2. *Distribution and Targeting*

The targeting of liposomes is determined by their size, lipid composition, charge, and specific surface receptors. It is also influenced by external factors, including the route of injection, binding of serum proteins, and the state of the reticuloendothelial system. These variables have been extensively reviewed by Gregoriadis (1977, 1976a) and Fendler and Romero (1977).

Initial considerations of targeting must address the problems of blood clearance and organ distribution. The rate of clearance is based predominantly on carrier size and charge. Small vesicles are cleared more slowly than larger ones (Juliano and Stamp, 1975; Gregoriadis and Neerunjun, 1974). Postively charged liposomes are cleared more slowly than those that are neutral or negatively charged (Juliano and Stamp, 1975; Gregoriadis and Neerunjun, 1974). Regardless of size and charge, circulating liposomes and their contents are taken up predominantly by the liver and spleen, and to a lesser extent by the lungs, bone marrow, and kidneys (Segal *et al.*, 1974, 1976; Gregoriadis and Ryman, 1972b; Wisse and Gregoriadis, 1975; Rahman and Wright, 1975; Gregoriadis, 1973). In humans, approximately 81% of liposome-encapsulated albumin is cleared by the liver within 6 hours of injection (Gregoriadis *et al.*, 1974c). In monkeys, the 4-hour accumulation of radiolabeled liposomes by the spleen, liver, bone marrow, and lungs is 2.2, 0.35, 0.09, and 0.05% per gram of tissue, respectively, (Kimelberg *et al.*, 1975, 1976). The corresponding values for other organs are less than 0.02% per gram of tissue. Thus, reticuloendothelial organs commonly achieve concentrations 5–100 times those attained by other organs. Such a predilection for reticuloendothelial clearance may be mediated by the spontaneous adsorption of α_2-macroglobulins present in serum (Black and Gregoriadis, 1976; Tyrrell *et al.*, 1977).

This has been shown to promote the phagocytosis of lipoid particles by fixed macrophages of the liver and spleen (Gregoriadis, 1976a).

In vivo studies in the murine system indicate that bleomycin gains better access to solid tumors ($6C_3HED$ and Meth "A") when encapsulated in small versus large liposomes (Dapergolas *et al.*, 1976). This may result from an improved passage of small liposomes through tumor neovascular endothelium, a slower hepatic clearance of small liposomes, or both. Although small liposomes facilitate the absolute uptake of bleomycin by tumors, they have an adverse effect on the ratio of drug that localizes in the liver compared to the tumor. For example, the administration of free bleomycin to mice with $6C_3HED$ tumors results in concentrations of 1.18 and 1.81% bleomycin per gram of liver and tumor tissue, respectively. This represents a liver-to-tumor ratio of 0.65 : 1. By contrast, bleomycin encapsulated in small liposomes produces liver and tumor concentrations of 25.6 and 6.82% per gram of tissue, respectively. This represents a liver-to-tumor ratio of 3.75:1. Therefore, the liposome-mediated improvement of drug concentrations within the tumor is achieved at the expense of a sixfold increase in the fraction of drug that partitions to the liver. Moreover, recent work by Ryman *et al.* (1978) has indicated that small liposomes may not be preferentially concentrated by human tumors as they are by animal tumors. Hence, the access of small liposomes to tumors appears to vary with the system under study and to require further investigation.

Liposomes have been shown to enhance the transport of cytosine arabinoside across the blood–brain barrier (Mayhew *et al.*, 1978), suggesting that they may be of particular value for the delivery of chemotherapeutic agents to tumors of the central nervous system.

A final important factor that influences the distribution of liposome-borne agents is their rate of leakage from the carrier. Agents that undergo moderately rapid leakage (actinomycin D entrapped in the aqueous phase) distribute according to an organ pattern approaching that of the free drug (Rahman *et al.*, 1975). By contrast, agents that undergo slower leakage (actinomycin D entrapped in the lipid phase) distribute with the carrier to the liver and spleen.

The problem of carrier uptake by the reticuloendothelial system has been recognized as a serious impediment to selective organ and tissue targeting of encapsulated agents (Gregoriadis, 1976a, 1977). Two approaches have been pursued in attempt to reduce this uptake. The first consists of blockading the reticuloendothelial system prior to administering liposome-borne agents. In initial attempts, intravenously administered carbon particles were used (Gregoriadis and Neerunjun, 1974). Paradoxically, this actually increased rather than decreased the hepatic localization of liposomal agents. More recent attempts have employed concomitant treatment with either a large number of empty (non-drug-bearing) liposomes (Gregoriadis and Neerunjun, 1974; Gregoriadis *et al.*, 1977) or a high dose of free methyl palmitate (Tanaka *et al.*, 1975). Both treatments substantially delayed the hepatic uptake of a smaller number of concomitantly administered active (drug-bearing) liposomes. In preliminary studies, treatment with empty liposomes has been reported not to interfere with the accumulation of active liposomes by tumors (Gregoriadis *et al.*, 1977; Haynes and Kang, 1978). This important initial finding remains to be further documented and explored.

A second approach to the problem of selective organ targeting involves the incorporation of specific receptors into the external surface of the lipid bilayer. Such components include desialylated fetuin, erythrocyte membrane glycoprotein, heat-aggregated immunoglobulins, and native immunoglobulins. The first of these, desialylated fetuin, has been shown to alter the organ distribution of liposomes by associating with relevant receptors on hepatocytes (Gregoriadis and Neerunjun, 1975a). Although this does modulate the standard pattern of organ distribution, it accentuates rather than solves the problem of reticuloendothelial drug localization. The other components listed above modify second-order targeting in preference to organ distribution. They will be discussed in further detail below.

In order for second-order targeting to occur, there must be an absence of anatomic barriers between the intended target cells and the derivatized liposomes. These conditions are ideally met by experimental systems in which liposomes are delivered to tumor cells *in vitro,* within the peritoneal cavity or by vascular distribution to the reticuloendothelial system (Wisse, 1970). If one adheres to these favorable systems, effective second-order targeting can be demonstrated. It is generally accomplished by incorporating either purified receptor molecules or antireceptor molecules into the external surface of the liposome. As one example, the major sialoglycoprotein receptor of the red cell membrane has been purified (Marchesi *et al.*, 1972) and incorporated into the lipid bilayer of liposomes (Juliano and Stamp, 1976). This preparation selectively binds to erythrocytes in the presence of multivalent plant lectins that cross-link the common sialoglycoprotein. The result is a mixed agglutination reaction between liposomes and erythrocytes (Juliano and Stamp, 1976). This exact system is not practical for *in vivo* use because intravascular agglutination would rapidly ensue. Nevertheless, it introduces the possibility of liposomal homing based on complementary interactions between liposome-bound glycoproteins and tissue glycoproteins. For example, in the presence of an adequate reticuloendothelial blockade, vesicles bearing purified lymphoid cell-surface determinant(s) might be useful for concentrating drugs in the lymphoid organs (Woodruff, 1974) of patients with disseminated lymphomas. This represents a potential future application and is, at present, highly theoretical.

A second approach to receptor–receptor interaction takes advantage of the property that a high proportion of mononuclear phagocytes displays surface receptors for denatured immunoglobulins. The incorporation of heat-aggregated IgM into liposomes results in their preferential uptake by these cells (Weissmann *et al.*, 1975). Although this manipulation provides another intriguing model for cell-specific homing, it also accentuates rather than decreases reticuloendothelial clearance.

Experimental approaches to the use of antireceptor molecules have employed undenatured immunoglobulins directed against target cell surface determinants. This has involved the incorporation of hyperimmune IgG into the liposome such that the Fc ("tail") portion of the molecule is entrapped in the lipid phase, and the $F(ab)'_2$ (antigen-binding) portion is oriented externally (Gregoriadis and Neerunjun, 1975a; Gregoriadis, 1977). Liposome-bound antibody then can interact with specific antigens on the target cell surface. This molecular orientation of antibody theoretically minimizes its own antigenicity by burying the most antigenic Fc portion in the lipid bilayer. The latter consideration is important because immune IgG is usually raised in an unrelated animal. The administration of this foreign protein to a sensitized recipient can result in severe allergic reactions. *In vitro* tests using liposomes bearing anti-HeLa cell IgG have demonstrated a twenty-five-fold increase in the uptake of encapsulated bleomycin by HeLa cells compared to non-cross-reactive fibroblasts (Gregoriadis and Neerunjun, 1975a). In a reciprocal fashion, liposomes bearing antifibroblast IgG afforded a fivefold differential uptake of the drug by fibroblasts versus HeLa cells. Similar results have been obtained using liposomes with antibody directed against AKR-A murine leukemia cells (Gregoriadis and Neerunjun, 1975a). Although these *in vitro* results appear encouraging, the usefulness of such techniques for *in vivo* targeting continues to be limited by the problems of first-order distribution. If these problems can be overcome, antibody-mediated, second-order targeting could provide a valuable approach to the cellular focusing of chemotherapeutic agents.

Liposomes have the capacity to enter target cells and release their contents intracellularly. Their potential for localizing agents at preselected intracellular sites introduces the possibility of achieving third-order (intracellular) targeting. Although it is still somewhat controversial, liposomes appear to enter cells by two distinct processes—endocytosis and fusion (Grant and McConnell, 1973; Gregoriadis and Buckland, 1973; Inbar and Shinitzky, 1974; Gregoriadis *et al.*, 1974c; Papahadjopoulos *et al.*, 1974b;

Pagano and Huang, 1975; Rahman and Wright, 1975; Wisse and Gregoriadis, 1975; Gregoriadis, 1976a,b; Martin and MacDonald, 1976; Poste and Papahadjopoulos, 1976; Roerdink *et al.*, 1976). The ratio of one process to the other depends in part on the liposome's composition. Endocytosis usually constitutes the major pathway.

The enhanced endocytic activity exhibited by some, but not all, animal tumors (Gregoriadis and Neerunjun, 1975b) is partially responsible for their ability to concentrate liposome-encapsulated agents (Gregoriadis *et al.*, 1974c; Dapergolas *et al.*, 1976). Liposomes that enter predominantly by endocytosis are transported into the cell as membrane vesicles. These fuse with primary lysosomal granules to form secondary lysosomes. Destruction of the vesicles takes place within secondary lysosomes. This liberates the encapsulated agent. Depending on its molecular size and susceptibility to enzymatic degradation, the agent will diffuse through the lysosomal membrane into the cytoplasm and affect intracellular processes (Black and Gregoriadis, 1974; Colley and Ryman, 1974; Gregoriadis and Buckland, 1973; Roerdink *et al.*, 1976). Small molecules, such as actinomycin D, are able to do this (Black and Gregoriadis, 1974). Liposomal delivery of actinomycin D prolongs its intracellular retention compared to that of free drug (Black and Gregoriadis, 1974). However, the resulting sequestration of drug in secondary lysosomes decreases its peak concentration in the nuclear fraction. The net antitumor effect depends on multiple metabolic variables.

If the composition of lipids and fluidity of the lipid bilayer are appropriate, liposomes also may enter the target cell by fusion with the plasma membrane (Papahadjopoulos *et al.*, 1974b; Inbar and Shinitzky, 1974). This allows the release of water-soluble agents directly into the cytoplasmic compartment and also leads to the incorporation of lipid-soluble agents into the cell membrane. Cyclic AMP has been introduced into cells using liposomes that enter at least in part by fusion (Papahadjopoulos *et al.*, 1974b). The result is a rapid decrease in the rate of cell growth due to intracytoplasmic effects of the drug. These considerations of third-order targeting will gradually shift from the realm of the theoretical to the practical as better techniques for achieving first-order and second-order targeting are developed.

3. *Metabolism, Antigenicity, and Toxicity*

Liposomes are catabolized by lysosomal lipases within reticuloendothelial phagocytes and other target cells (Roerdink *et al.*, 1976; Black and Gregoriadis, 1974; Gregoriadis and Buckland, 1973; Colley and Ryman, 1974). Studies on liposomal toxicity are scarce (Gregoriadis, 1976a). Preliminary work indicates that intravenously administered liposomes consisting of egg lecithin, cholesterol, phosphatidic acid, and similar lipids produce no overt toxicity or histochemical changes in rats (Gregoriadis, 1976a) and no detectable side effects in tumor-bearing patients (Gregoriadis *et al.*, 1974c). However, the intravenous injection of small liposomes composed of phospholipids from bovine brain has been reported to increase catecholamine metabolism in the brains of mice, to cause the release of acetylcholine from the cortical areas of rat brains, and to modify tissue glucose distributions (Bruni *et al.*, 1976). The active component has been identified as phosphatidyl serine. Also, the incorporation of certain charged lipids into the liposomal bilayer (stearylamine and dicetyl phosphate), but not others (phosphatidic acid), leads to seizures and cerebral necrosis when these liposomes are injected intracerebrally (Gregoriadis, 1976a). The same liposomes should be less toxic when administered by the intravascular route because charged materials do not readily cross the blood–brain barrier. This remains to be determined.

The antigenicity of liposomal lipids has not been extensively investigated. Generally, lipids of this molecular size produce negligible immune responses. One characteristic that liposomes do display is the ability to act as immunological adjuvants (Allison and Gregoriadis, 1974; Gregoriadis and Allison, 1974; Heath *et al.*, 1976) and thereby augment the immune responses to entrapped foreign proteins, toxins, and enzymes. This property is undesirable if the patient requires subsequent treatment with the free agent. However, it does not interfere with recurrent treatments if the agent is again given in the encapsulated form. Although this seems paradoxical, it occurs because the lipid bilayer physically separates the agent from blood constituents. Hence, the agent cannot initiate allergic reactions because it cannot interact with circulating sensitized lymphocytes and serum antibodies (Gregoriadis and Allison, 1974). Adjuvant activity, on the other hand, occurs later during local processing of the liposomes and their contents by phagocytic cells of the immunologically competent, reticuloendothelial system.

Currently, there are no reports indicating that empty liposomes alter the rate of tumor cell growth. However, antitumor IgG has been shown to accelerate the growth of certain tumors (see Section IV). This has important implications with respect to the derivatization of liposomes with immune IgG as a means to enhance the specificity of second-order targeting.

4. *Current and Projected Uses in Cancer Chemotherapy*

Liposomes have now been used as carriers for a large number of experimental and applied, antitumor and immunopotentiating agents (Table II).

TABLE II

LIPOSOMES AS EXPERIMENTAL AND APPLIED DRUG CARRIERS FOR ANTITUMOR AND IMMUNOPOTENTIATING AGENTS[a]

Agent	Reference
Chemotherapeutic agents, growth inhibitors, and toxins	
Actinomycin D	Gregoriadis, 1973; Neerunjun and Gregoriadis, 1974; Rahman *et al.*, 1974; Black and Gregoriadis, 1974; Gregoriadis and Neerunjun, 1975b; Segal *et al.*, 1975; Papahadjopoulos *et al.*, 1976; Juliano and Stamp, 1978
Asparaginase	Neerunjun and Gregoriadis, 1976
8-Azaguanine	Fendler and Romero, 1976
Bichloroethyl nitrosourea	Rutman *et al.*, 1976
Bleomycin	Gregoriadis and Neerunjun, 1975a; Gregoriadis *et al.*, 1976; Dapergolas *et al.*, 1976; Segal *et al.*, 1976
Colchicine	Juliano and Stamp, 1975
Daunomycin	Juliano and Stamp, 1978
Cyclic 3′:5′-adenosine monophosphate	Papahadjopoulos *et al.*, 1974a,b
Cytosine arabinoside and derivatives	Kobayashi *et al.*, 1975; Mayhew *et al.*, 1976; Juliano and Stamp, 1978; Ryman *et al.*, 1978
Diphtheria toxoid	Gregoriadis and Allison, 1974
5-Fluorouracil	Gregoriadis, 1974; Segal *et al.*, 1975
Mechlorethamine	Rutman *et al.*, 1976
Methotrexate	Gregoriadis *et al.*, 1974c; Kimelberg *et al.*, 1975; Colley and Ryman, 1975; Kimelberg *et al.*, 1976
Neuraminidase	Rahman *et al.*, 1974; Gregoriadis *et al.*, 1974b; Almeida *et al.*, 1975
Vinblastine	Juliano and Stamp, 1978
Immunopotentiating/antiviral agents	
Poly I: poly C	Straub *et al.*, 1974; Magee *et al.*, 1976

[a] Adapted and updated from Gregoriadis (1977) and Fendler and Romero (1977).

Generally, these encapsulated agents have retained their characteristic antitumor activities in most of the experimental systems tested (Gregoriadis, 1976a, 1977; Fendler and Romero, 1977). There are conflicting reports concerning their ability to enhance the concentration of antitumor agents selectively in human tumor tissue compared to adjacent normal tissue (Gregoriadis *et al.*, 1974c; Ryman *et al.*, 1978). The therapeutic efficacy of liposome-encapsulated drugs has usually been demonstrated in animals bearing ascites tumors (Rahman *et al.*, 1974) or other neoplasms where there is no endothelial barrier between the tumor cells and liposomes (Martius *et al.*, 1975). Liposome-mediated delivery of antitumor agents may be particularly useful for tumors of the central nervous system (see

Section III,C,2) and tumor cells that have developed drug resistance due to a decrease in the rate of drug transport. For example, the dose of actinomycin D required for maximal inhibition of RNA synthesis in drug-resistant, DC-3F/ADX, Chinese hamster tumor cells can be reduced by a factor of 200 if the drug is encapsulated in liposomes (Bangham, 1972; Papahadjopoulos *et al.,* 1976).

Despite the potential applications described above, the major problems relating to first-order targeting of intravascularly administered liposomes have not been overcome. Solutions to these problems will require more effective measures to block reticuloendothelial clearance selectively and overcome the endothelial barrier that separates potentially targetable liposomes from tumor cells. If these major obstacles can be surmounted, the full potential of liposomes to serve as targeted drug carriers *in vivo* can be realized.

D. Albumin Microspheres

Microspheres of various size and composition have been used extensively for lung scans and circulatory studies in animals and human subjects (Taplin *et al.,* 1964; Rhodes and Wagner, 1969; Buchanan *et al.,* 1969; Rhodes *et al.,* 1969; Warren and Ledingham, 1974, 1975; Arruda *et al.,* 1974; Utley *et al.,* 1974; Kaplan *et al.,* 1975; McDevitt and Nies, 1976). For a complete review of this area, see Wagner *et al.* (1969b). Earlier microspheres were composed of silica (Prinzmetal *et al.,* 1947), wax (Sirsi and Bucher, 1953), plastic (Parker *et al.,* 1958), and ceramics (Grotenhuis, 1966). These materials were not ideal for human use because of their nonbiodegradability and potential toxicity. Microspheres consisting of aggregated human serum albumin (Halpern *et al.,* 1956; Rhodes *et al.,* 1969) were developed to circumvent these problems. Their use as experimental carriers of antitumor agents is relatively new.

1. *Preparation and in Vitro Characteristics*

Albumin microspheres are prepared by emulsifying water solutions of human serum albumin in cottonseed oil (Rhodes *et al.,* 1969). The resulting microspheres are stabilized by heat denaturation at temperatures above 100°C (Rhodes *et al.,* 1969) or by chemical cross-linking (Senyei *et al.,* 1978; Widder *et al.,* 1978a, 1979). The cottonseed oil is removed by extraction with ether. Microspheres prepared without homogenization or sonication range from 7 to 250 μm in diameter. By mechanical sieving, it is possible to obtain fractions that are fairly uniform in size (Buchanan *et al.,* 1969). Smaller microspheres (0.2–1.2 μm in diameter) can be produced by homogenizing or sonicating the original emulsion at controlled temperatures (Scheffel *et al.*, 1972; Kramer, 1974). It is common for albumin microspheres to swell from 20 to 50% on prolonged reexposure to aqueous solutions (Zolle *et al.*, 1970). Since a 50% enlargement of 1.2-μm particles leads to a significant increase in their capillary retention (Taplin *et al.*, 1964), it is important that the time interval between rehydration and injection of the carrier be kept to a minimum.

The addition of water-soluble drugs and particulate materials to the water–oil emulsion leads to their entrapment in the albumin matrix (Kramer, 1974; Kramer and Burnstein, 1976; Widder *et al.*, 1978a, 1979). Drugs of even meager water solubility are entrapped with a high degree of efficiency. For example, 87% of the poorly soluble drug, mercaptopurine hydrate, becomes entrapped (Kramer, 1974). On the other hand, the absolute quantity of drug entrapped per milligram of carrier is directly limited by its solubility. For example, the entrapment of agents that exhibit high solubility (adriamycin), intermediate solubility (daunomycin), and low solubility (mercaptopurine hydrate) is, respectively, 90, 8, and 3.5 μg of drug per milligram of albumin (Kramer, 1974; Widder *et al.*, 1978a, 1979). These considerations should not restrict the general applicability of this carrier because both drug solubility and the extent of entrapment can be enhanced by chemical procedures (see Section III,C). Although it has not been extensively investigated, the entrapment of even lipid-soluble agents should be possible. This can be accomplished by the addition of appropriate organic solvents to the reaction mixture. At this writing, the largest chemotherapeutic agent that has been tested for entrapment and subsequent *in vitro* biological activity is the enzyme, urokinase (K. Widder and A. E. Senyei, unpublished observations). However, it is quite probable that drug–macromolecular complexes also will be well entrapped.

Various classes of drugs exhibit differences in temperature and chemical sensitivity. If these properties are anticipated, the biological activity of entrapped agents can be preserved by selecting a nondestructive method for stabilization of the albumin matrix. For example, adriamycin (Widder *et al.*, 1978b) and mercaptopurine hydrate (Kramer, 1974) are heat-stable at 135° and 175°C, respectively. Thus, carrier stabilization can be achieved by brief heating of the entrapment complex. However, for heat-sensitive drugs, the carrier must be stabilized by chemical cross-linking. This has been successfully accomplished for adriamycin-bearing microspheres. These have been stabilized using both formaldehyde and 2,3-butanedione without chemically altering the released drug (Widder *et al.*, 1979) (see Section III,E).

Entrapped drug exists in two forms. A portion of the agent, usually 40%, appears to be associated with the carrier surface and is rapidly released by brief sonication (Widder *et al.*, 1979). The majority of drug is associated with the interior portion of the albumin matrix and is released at a slower rate that parallels the rate of matrix hydration (Widder *et al.*, 1979). This, in turn, is related to the extent of matrix stabilization. By varying the latter property, drug can be made to release at a controllable and predictable rate that ranges from less than 2% to greater than 20% per hour (Scheu *et al.*, 1977; Widder *et al.*, 1978b, 1979). Because the sequestration of intravascular microspheres occurs quite rapidly, this entire range of kinetics is consistent with delivering 95% or more of the slowly releasable drug to a predetermined target. Once the target has been reached, the rate of drug release continues to be governed by carrier stability. Release times have been projected to vary from minutes to days (Widder *et al.*, 1978b, 1979).

The ability of albumin microspheres to afford a continuous release of drugs has several implications with respect to their *in vivo* capabilities. They do not have to be phagocytized or otherwise destroyed in order to release the entrapped drug. Consequently, substantial quantities of drug can be made available at extracellular sites. This potentially allows the drug-carrier complex to modulate its own entry into tissues. For example, the spontaneous release of entrapped histamine or other inflammatory substances can be used to modify capillary permeability and thereby enhance the penetration of carrier into the tissue parenchyma. This property also enhances the effects of agents for which the initial site of release must be extracellular in order for them to act. Examples include chemotactic factors and selected antibiotics. In addition to providing these advantages of extracellular release, albumin microspheres can also deliver a variable fraction of drug to intracellular sites. This is based on their propensity to be phagocytized (see Section III,D,2).

2. *Distribution and Targeting*

The first-order distribution of underivatized microspheres is determined almost entirely by their size. Following intravenous injection, more than 90% of microspheres smaller than 1–1.4 μm in diameter are removed by the liver and spleen (Ring *et al.*, 1961; Taplin *et al.*, 1964). Conversely, microspheres larger than 10 μm in diameter are almost entirely trapped in the lungs by arteriolar and capillary blockade (Taplin *et al.*, 1964). Following intra-arterial injection, small microspheres are again cleared by the reticuloendothelial system, but large microspheres are sequestered in the first capillary bed encountered (Taplin *et al.*, 1964; Wagner *et al.*, 1969b; Blanchard *et al.*, 1975). The immediate spillover of large microspheres into secondary capillary systems is negligible. However, as they begin to degrade, matrix products are released from the target circulation and gradually accumulate in the retriculoendothelial system (Taplin *et al.*, 1964; Zolle *et al.*, 1970; Petriev *et al.*, 1976). The rate at which this occurs is determined by the extent of matrix stabilization. Since albumin microspheres swell following hydration, their functional classification as small or large particles depends on three factors: the dehydrated particle size, the degree of matrix stabilization, and the time of hydration prior to injection. If one adheres to the usual brief interval of hydration, most carrier preparations will distribute *in vivo* as predicted by their dehydrated particle size. Regardless of size, albumin microspheres are rapidly cleared from the general circulation. Following intravenous injection, they are completely removed in 2–10 minutes, depending on the dose (Wagner *et al.*, 1963).

The partitioning of albumin microspheres within a target circulation is proportional to the regional blood flow (Wagner *et al.*, 1965). Hence, these particles undergo homogeneous arteriolar-capillary distribution. The first-order targeting of small microspheres can be modified to a minimal degree by incorporating various surface derivatives or altering the surface charge, as described for liposomes. However, unlike the situation for liposomes, an additional method exists for producing major alterations in their organ distribution. This involves the incorporation of magnetically responsive material into the albumin matrix. The resulting preparation is injected into a predetermined arterial supply and held at the desired capillary bed using an extracorporeal magnetic field (see Section III,E).

The initial distribution of microsphere-entrapped drugs depends on their rate of release during vascular transit. Their delayed distribution depends on the rate at which carrier particles migrate into the extravascular space where released drug is no longer subject to direct circulatory clearance.

There is an isolated report that intravascularly administered microspheres will distribute to tumor tissue in preference to the surrounding normal tissue. This has been demonstrated in rabbits bearing intrahepatic V2 carcinomas (Blanchard *et al.*, 1965). The concentration of microspheres in tumor tissue is reported to reach levels 4 times higher than those found in adjacent normal tissue. This effect is observed only when microspheres are administered via the hepatic artery and not when they are given by the portal vein. Moreover, it has not been possible to demonstrate this effect for solid tumors located outside the liver.

By virtue of their particulate nature, albumin microspheres are actively internalized by tumor cell lines that exhibit enhanced endocytic and phagocytic activity. This has been demonstrated for HeLa cells, KB tumor cells, and human glioblastoma cells (Kramer, 1974; Kramer and Burnstein, 1976). The fraction of entrapped drug that is delivered to intracellular versus extracellular sites depends on two factors: the rate of drug release from the carrier and the rate of phagocytic uptake of the carrier. The former can be modulated as previously described. The latter can be varied by entrapping pharmacological agents that enhance or depress phagocytosis. As described for liposomes, the indiscriminate second-order "targeting" of microspheres based on endocytosis and phagocytosis may lead to undesirable cytotoxic effects on intralesional macrophages. This potential problem can be surmounted by employing a carrier of intermediate stability that affords a rapid release at predominantly extracellular sites.

Because albumin microspheres can enter target cells by only a single mechanism, namely phagocytosis (Kramer, 1974; Kramer and Burnstein, 1976), their range of third-order targeting is restricted to intracellular lysosomes. This contrasts with the situation for liposomes, where agents can be selectively targeted to either of two intracellular sites.

3. *Metabolism, Antigenicity, and Toxicity*

Albumin microspheres are biodegradable (Wagner *et al.*, 1969a; Zolle *et al.*, 1970). Hence they are efficiently removed from target capillary beds and subsequently catabolized by mononuclear phagocytes (Taplin *et al.*, 1964; Wagner *et al.*, 1968; Petriev *et al.*, 1976). The time required for 50% clearance of the localized carrier material can vary from 2 hours to 8 days (Rhodes *et al.*, 1969; Zolle *et al.*, 1970; Petriev *et al.*, 1976). This is directly related to the extent of matrix stabilization.

At this writing, toxicity studies have been reported mainly for large, nonmagnetic albumin microspheres (greater than 7 μm in diameter). Particles of this size produce embolic infarction within the first capillary bed encountered. Consequently, their clinical usage has been limited to diagnostic situations in which only tracer doses are required. This minimizes the ischemic disruption of cellular function in the target organs (Arfors *et al.*, 1976). Experimental toxicity studies, on the other hand, have employed doses of microspheres large enough to produce massive embolism within the lungs and other target organs. As a result, the toxic effects to be discussed represent primarily the sequelae of embolic ischemia rather than direct chemical toxicity induced by metabolites of the albumin matrix. These sequelae are expected to be minimal for small microspheres because the latter do not appear to disrupt capillary blood flow substantially (see Section III,E).

Large albumin microspheres have now been used for lung scans in more than 1000 patients without reports of significant toxicity (Rhodes and Wagner, 1969; Rhodes *et al.*, 1969). These studies employed doses of up to 50 mg per patient. In a subgroup study, no significant changes were reported in the electrocardiogram, pulmonary artery pressure, systemic blood pressure, pulse, or respiratory rate. Moreover, no allergic reactions were observed in 50 patients who received serial injections of microspheres over a course of 3 weeks to 12 months (Rhodes *et al.*, 1969). Microspheres composed of human serum albumin have been shown to induce skin sensitivity in guinea pigs (Rhodes *et al.*, 1969). However, serial injections of the microspheres did not elicit anaphylactic responses. Therefore, even in genetically unrelated species, these microspheres appear to be nontoxic from the standpoint of generating serious allergic responses directed against surface antigens. There are some indications that macroaggregates of albumin and large albumin microspheres promote intravascular coagulation (Wagner *et al.*, 1969b). However, this has not resulted in significant clinical problems. Therefore, as currently employed, albumin microspheres appear to be clinically safe.

In mice, the LD_{50} for large albumin microspheres is greater than 200 mg/kg (Rhodes *et al.*, 1969). Deaths in all cases are due to pulmonary embolization. Lower doses (9.6 mg/kg) produce foci of hemorrhagic infarction that subsequently resolve (Szymendera *et al.*, 1977). Using a sensitive system such as the choriocapillary circulation of rhesus monkeys, even small doses of these microspheres can be shown to produce isolated microvascular infarction (Stern and Ernest, 1974). A syndrome consisting of delayed, irreversible shock has been described for rats receiving injections of large albumin microspheres (Stahl *et al.*, 1977). However, this required direct introduction of the particles into both renal arteries in quantities sufficient to produce total cessation of renal blood flow. These toxic side effects can be reduced or eliminated by the use of small microspheres (see Section III,E).

4. *Current and Projected Utility in Cancer Chemotherapy*

The use of albumin microspheres as carriers for antitumor agents was first suggested by Kramer (1974). To date, they have been employed as experimental carriers for several of these drugs (Table III). Based on their

TABLE III

ALBUMIN MICROSPHERES AS EXPERIMENTAL CARRIERS FOR ANTITUMOR AGENTS

Agent	Reference
Adriamycin	Widder *et al.*, 1978a; Widder *et al.*, 1978b; Widder *et al.*, 1979
Daunomycin HCl	Kramer, 1974
6-Mercaptopurine and derivatives	Kramer, 1974; Kramer and Burnstein, 1976

compatibility with a broad range of water-soluble drugs and their minimal chemical toxicity, albumin microspheres should represent ideal carriers for the targeted delivery of antitumor agents. However, to date their use has been limited to experimental animal systems. There are several reasons for this. Microspheres larger than 7 μm in diameter cannot achieve a homogeneous saturation of target tissues without producing massive infarction of the microvascular circulation. Because of their large size, these microspheres cannot deliver drugs to the arteriolar-capillary level where diffusional distances and vascular barriers are minimal. Consequently, only small microspheres are feasible for the delivery of drugs. Although small microspheres avoid the problems of extensive tissue infarction, they largely pass through the intended target circulation and localize in the reticuloendothelial system (Ring *et al.*, 1961; Taplin *et al.*, 1964; Kramer, 1974). Without further modification, their use as carriers for antitumor agents would be limited to tumors of the reticuloendothelial system. However, if a means were found to localize these microspheres within a predetermined capillary bed, they potentially could enjoy widespread use as targeted carriers for the treatment of severe localized disease. The authors have taken a biophysical approach to the solution of this problem, as described in the following section.

E. Magnetically Responsive Albumin Microspheres

Magnetically responsive, small albumin microspheres were recently developed and tested by the authors (Senyei *et al.*, 1978; Widder *et al.*, 1978a,b, 1979). To date, their use has been restricted to *in vitro* culture systems and small animals. Discussion of this work will be prefaced by a short history of the magnetic guidance of intravascular materials.

1. *Magnetic Guidance of Intravascular Materials*

The feasibility of localizing intravascular materials using magnetic fields was first demonstrated by Meyers *et al.* (1963). In this study, particles of micronized iron, 1–3 μm in diameter, were held at specific sites within a large artery using external permanent magnets. By ^{59}Fe labeling, it was demonstrated that some of the particles remained at the target area for up to 7 days after magnetic localization. It was suggested but not proved that they had migrated into the arterial wall under the initial influence of the magnetic field. Magnetic localization was first employed clinically for the selective thrombosis of intracerebral arterial aneurysms (Alksne *et al.*, 1966). Together, these studies demonstrated that 1–3 μm particles of carbonyl iron could be retained at a specified intravascular site, even at arterial flow rates, in the presence of a sufficiently intense magnetic field. Based on this initial work, Meyers *et al.* (1963), suggested that carbonyl iron might be used as a vehicle for the targeted delivery of chemotherapeutic agents. However, the problem of coating sufficient drug onto the surface of these particles without significantly increasing their diameter represented a formidable obstacle to their successful application as drug carriers. Moreover, this and other magnetically responsive materials were found to aggregate irreversibly upon exposure to magnetic fields (Nakamura *et al.*, 1971). Aggregation of drug delivery vehicles was undesirable because it prevented them from achieving a homogeneous distribution at the capillary level and caused them to embolize and infarct portions of the target circulation. Because of these problems, the early applications of magnetic fields to the delivery of clinical agents were restricted to selective angiography using catheters tipped with large (2-cm) magnetically responsive paraoperational devices (M-PODS) (Tillander, 1951, 1956, 1970; Frei *et al.*, 1966), and selective arterial thrombosis with carbonyl iron (Alksne *et al.*, 1966). The problem of irreversible particle aggregation was eventually overcome by Nakamura *et al.* (1971), who demonstrated that it could be reduced or eliminated by coating the magnetizable material with charged polymers and proteins such as albumin. These findings provided the basis for the authors' current approach. This involved polymerizing human serum albumin into small microspheres, each forming a matrix, or drug space, that surrounded and functionally coated the magnetically responsive material (see Section III,E,2).

The development of clinically applicable delivery vehicles was paralleled by the development of electromagnets suitable for these biomedical applications. In early studies, fixed permanent magnets that generated relatively low field intensities were used. These magnets were positioned either extracorporeally in a bipolar configuration across various body extremities (Meyers *et al.*, 1963) or internally as unipolar probes next to diseased intracerebral arteries (Alksne *et al.*, 1966). In more recent studies, permanent magnets have been replaced by helium-cooled superconducting magnets. The latter generate field intensities of up to 7000 Oe at distances of 10 cm (Rand and Mosso, 1972; Mosso and Rand, 1973; Hilal *et al.*, 1974). Superconducting magnets have been used clinically to localize magnetically responsive ferrosilicone for selective thrombosis of the vascular supply to hypernephromas (Turner *et al.*, 1975). These studies have demonstrated that currently available electromagnets can generate field intensities sufficient for intravascular retention of small microspheres in deep organs within the major body cavities. Such magnets are positioned extracorporeally and used to generate strong fields and field gradients of unipolar configuration.

The putative biological effects, both toxic and beneficial, of high-intensity magnetic fields (4000 to 100,000 Oe) represent a still controversial area. Physiological and cellular effects have been discussed at length in separate reviews (M. F. Barnothy, 1964, 1969, 1974). There are isolated reports of cocarcinogenic effects during the experimental induction of rat sarcomas (Kogan and Kulitskaya, 1977) and transforming effects on frozen cell lines (Malinin *et al.*, 1976). Also, the chronic exposure of C3H mice to magnetic fields of 4200 G has been reported to produce reversible changes in their rate of growth and their differential white blood cell counts (Barnothy *et al.*, 1956). On the other hand, significant toxicity has not been reported in patients undergoing magnetically guided catheterization for selective angiography (Hilal *et al.*, 1974) or selective vascular occlusion of intracerebral aneurysms and hypernephromas (Mosso and Rand, 1973; Hilal *et al.*, 1974; Turner *et al.*, 1975). Further studies of potential toxicity are justified by the increasing importance of magnetic guidance in the therapy of human disease. Nevertheless, initial and continuing clinical experience suggests that these effects will be minimal and tolerable in patients whose diseases are severe enough to warrant targeted chemotherapy.

2. *Preparation and in Vitro Characteristics*

During development of the current drug delivery vehicle, a number of magnetizable materials and three-dimensional carrier systems were tested. The rationale for selecting albumin for the matrix and magnetite (Fe_3O_4) as the magnetically responsive material can be briefly summarized as follows. It was technically possible to produce small albumin spheres (<1.4 μm) that would avoid microvascular embolization. These had been shown to be biodegradable, minimally reactive with blood components, and clinically nontoxic from the standpoints of chemical and immunological reactivity. The carrier system could accommodate a wide spectrum of water-soluble agents. In contrast to liposomes, the albumin matrix could be stabilized by heating or chemical cross-linking to afford a broad spectrum of release kinetics. The albumin coating already had been shown to minimize intravascular conglutination of magnetically responsive materials. In pilot studies, the albumin matrix was demonstrated to stabilize the spatial distribution of Fe_3O_4 within each microsphere such that it could not be altered by subsequent exposure to a magnetic field. In turn, maintenance of this initial distribution was found to be an important determinant of the magnetic responsiveness of the preparation (see the following). Magnetite was found to have the desired degree of magnetic responsivity, and it was commercially available as a ferrofluid. Furthermore, the individual magnetite particles were much smaller (10–20 nm) than the microsphere matrix and, consequently, occupied a tiny fraction of the potential drug space. In reported studies, Fe_3O_4 was found to have minimal inflammatory and toxic properties (see Section III,E,4).

Adriamycin was chosen as a prototype drug for several reasons. It had demonstrated activity against a broad range of solid tumors (Blum, 1975). Also, the drug was directly active at the target site and did not require hepatic microsomal activation. Its characteristic photofluorescence afforded rapid determinations of drug concentrations in test solutions and body tissues. The presence of well-defined fluorescent degradation products allowed a straightforward determination of the effects of entrapment and release on the chemical integrity of the drug. The high water solubility of adriamycin assured extensive entrapment.

The carrier–adriamycin complex has been produced by the method of emulsion polymerization (Widder *et al.*, 1978a). Briefly, an aqueous solution of human serum albumin, bulk-purified adriamycin (Adria Laboratories) and 10–20 nm particles of Fe_3O_4 (Ferrofluidics Corporation) is emulsified with cottonseed oil. For experimental purposes, trace amounts of bovine serum albumin-^{125}I are added to radiolabel the microsphere matrix. The resulting emulsion is homogenized by brief sonication at 4°C. This produces small, noncrosslinked microspheres, 0.25–1.35 μm in diameter, that contain adriamycin. Matrix cross-linking is then carried out by one of two procedures: heat denaturation at temperatures between 100° and 165°C or treatment with ether-soluble cross-linking reagents, such as 0.1 *M* formaldehyde or 0.2 *M* 2,3-butanedione. The extent of matrix hardening is varied by changing either the temperature used for denaturation or the duration of chemical treatment. The reagents used for chemical cross-linking are removed by ether extraction. The resulting preparation of microspheres is lyophilized and stored at 4°C for later use. The latter two procedures are designed to leave the preparations free of viable microorganisms and to give them a prolonged shelf life.

The adriamycin content of standard microsphere preparations is approximately 9% (w/w), including parent drug and fluorescent drug products. Of this, more than half, 4.0–5.4% (w/w), represents slowly releasable drug. This constitutes 40–54 μg of adriamycin per milligram of albumin carrier. The content of Fe_3O_4 has been varied experimentally from 20 to 50% (w/w). By scanning electron microscopy, these preparations consist of small spheres that range from 0.25 to 1.35 μm in diameter and have a mean size of 1.0 μm (Fig. 1). By transmission electron microscopy, each albumin matrix is seen to contain clumps of Fe_3O_4 distributed largely around the periphery of the particle (Fig. 2, main panel and inset A). Occasional spheres also contain electron-lucent spaces that are

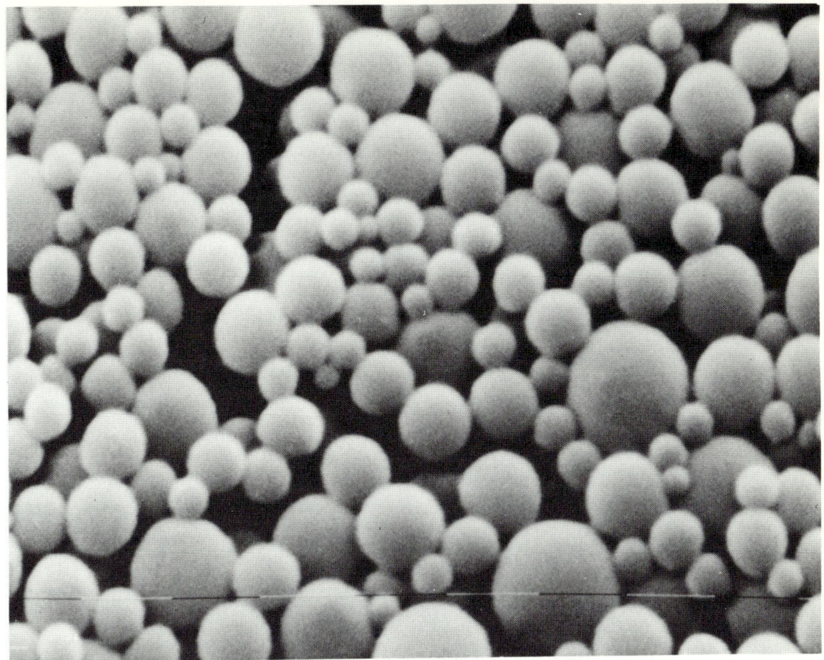

FIG. 1. Scanning electron micrograph of magnetically responsive small albumin microspheres following evaporation from an ether suspension. Magnification = ×8500. Calibration line = 1 μm. (Reproduced from Widder *et al.*, 1978a, by permission of Academic Press.)

thought to represent vacuoles of air. The addition of a cationic surfactant during polymerization results in a homogeneous rather than peripheral distribution of magnetite within the microspheres (Fig. 2, inset B). This alters their responsivity to magnetic fields (see the following).

Optimal delivery of drug *in vivo* requires that the carrier be retained predominantly within the arteriolar-capillary vasculature. Therefore, it was necessary to determine which combination of carrier properties and ambient magnetic field conditions would produce an optimal retardation of microspheres at arteriolar-capillary flow rates. In normal human subjects, the linear rates of blood flow range from mean values of 31 cm/sec in major arteries to 0.05 cm/sec in capillary vessels. Therefore, it was desirable to design the present system such that it would afford maximal particle retention at flow rates of 0.05 to 0.10 cm/sec. For this purpose, an *in vitro* apparatus was used to reproduce physiological flow rates. This apparatus employed a syringe pump that delivered solution through a 1.7-mm polyethylene tubing at constant flow rates of 0.05 to 10.0 cm/sec. The car-

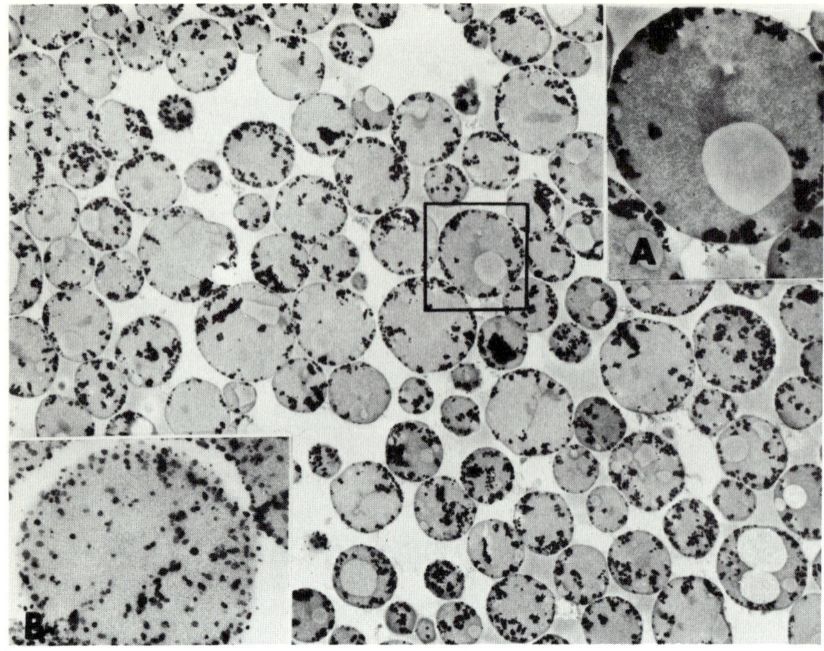

FIG. 2. Transmission electron micrograph of microspheres prepared as in Fig. 1. Main panel, standard preparation of microspheres (magnification = ×8500). Inset A, enlargement of a standard microsphere containing peripherally oriented electron-dense clumps of Fe_3O_4, a medium dense albumin matrix, and an eccentric electron-lucent vacuole (magnification = ×38,250). Inset B, enlargement of a microsphere prepared with cationic surfactant, exhibiting a homogeneous distribution of Fe_3O_4 (magnification = ×19,040). (Adapted from Widder *et al.*, 1978a.)

rier fluids consisted of either 0.15 *M* NaCl or heparinized whole human blood. Boluses of ^{125}I-microspheres (0.1 mg in 0.1 ml) were introduced through a proximal injection port at various flow rates and their retention by a distal, bipolar magnetic field was evaluated. The fraction of microspheres retained in the section of tubing circumscribed by the magnetic field was determined by allowing adequate dilutional flow past the retained particles. This piece of tubing, together with its contents, was clamped, removed, and counted for ^{125}I-gamma radiation. Appropriate controls revealed negligible nonspecific adherence of microspheres to the tubing. Three preparations of microspheres were tested: ones containing 20% Fe_3O_4 (w/w) and 50% Fe_3O_4 (w/w) distributed in the peripheral configuration and ones containing 50% Fe_3O_4 (w/w) distributed homogeneously throughout the particles. The latter were prepared by the addition of a cationic surfactant.

More than 90% of the microspheres from all preparations were retained at arteriolar-capillary flow rates of 0.05 to 0.10 cm/sec (Fig. 3). Whereas spheres composed of 20% Fe_3O_4 were allowed to pass at faster (arterial-arteriolar) flow rates of 1 to 5 cm/sec (Fig. 3, A), spheres containing 50% Fe_3O_4 were substantially retained (Fig. 3, B). Microspheres with a homogeneous distribution of magnetite were less responsive (Fig. 3, C) than standard microspheres with a peripheral configuration (Fig. 3, B). Because surfactant-treated microspheres had a lower magnetic responsivity and an increased potential for *in vivo* toxicity, they were excluded from further studies.

In order to predict whether or not the standard preparations of microspheres could be effectively retained in deep body cavities by currently available unipolar electromagnets, *in vitro* flow-retention studies were repeated using a unipolar field. The resulting curves were similar to those obtained with bipolar fields (Senyei *et al.*, 1978). Moreover, similar fractional retentions were achieved at a significantly lower field strength of 600 Oe and field gradient of 300 Oe/cm. A detailed analysis indicated that the retention of microspheres under flow conditions depended not only on the field strength but also on the field gradient. This is described in a separate publication (Senyei *et al.*, 1978).

In order to evaluate the effects of erythrocytes and other blood ele-

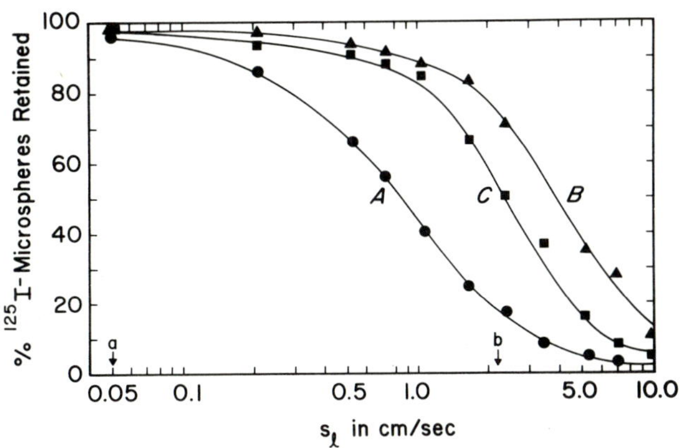

FIG. 3. Magnetic retention of heat-stabilized ^{125}I-microspheres suspended in 0.15 *M* NaCl at various rates of laminar flow. S_l = linear flow speed. Ambient field = 0 ± 1,120 Oe (2% error) and field gradient = 13,300 ± 300 Oe/cm (2% error). (Curve *A*), Standard microspheres containing 20% Fe_3O_4 (w/w); (curve *B*) standard microspheres containing 50% Fe_3O_4 (w/w); (curve *C*) microspheres prepared in the presence of cationic surfactant, containing 50% Fe_3O_4 (w/w). Physiological rates of blood flow in humans are indicated for capillaries (a) and arteries (b). (Reproduced from Senyei *et al.*, 1978, by permission of the American Institute of Physics.)

ments on the retention of microspheres, similar studies were performed using whole blood (Senyei *et al.*, 1978). Identical retention curves were obtained. Thus, the introduction of blood elements did not require any significant modification of the particle properties or magnetic fields. Hence, microspheres containing 20% Fe_3O_4, prepared without surfactant, were projected to have the ideal magnetic properties for arteriolar-capillary localization.

Having produced microspheres that exhibited the desired properties, it was important to determine if the processes of entrapment and carrier stabilization affected the chemical integrity of released adriamycin. Microspheres were prepared, as just described, and stabilized by either brief heating at 115° or 135°C, or cross-linking with 0.1 *M* formaldehyde or 0.2 *M* 2,3-butanedione (Widder *et al.*, 1978b, 1979). These preparations were suspended in media and allowed to release 20% of the initially incorporated drug. The released products were chromatographed on thin-layer silica gel developed in chloroform:methanol:acetic acid:water (60:20:14:6) (Widder *et al.*, 1979). The migration of processed drug and its major fluorescent breakdown products (aglycones) was determined by comparing the positions of fluorescent spots on experimental chromatograms to the corresponding R_f values for native adriamycin and its known aglycones. The ratio of degradation products to parent drug was determined by extracting appropriate areas of the chromatogram with acid alcohol and determining their quantitative fluorescence by a modification of the technique described by Bachur *et al.* (1970). In the absence of carrier stabilization, there was no chemical degradation of the drug (Widder *et al.*, 1978b, 1979). Heat stabilization at 115°C and chemical cross-linking also produced no detectable alteration. Stabilization at 135°C for 10 minutes produced 26% degradation of the parent drug to aglycones. These results showed that adriamycin could be entrapped and released from variously stabilized microspheres with negligible to minimal chemical degradation.

The effect of stabilization on the kinetics of drug release was determined as follows. Microsphere preparations were suspended in release medium, sonicated, and washed to remove the rapidly releasable fraction of adriamycin. The particles were resuspended and the kinetic release of the slowly diffusible fraction was determined by sampling the supernatant at various time intervals for adriamycin fluorescence. The release of drug was slowed substantially by increasing the temperature of matrix stabilization (Fig. 4). However, for both preparations, a very high proportion of the slowly releasable adriamycin traveled with and subsequently diffused from magnetically responsive microspheres compared to unresponsive microspheres (see Fig. 4 caption). Similar results (not shown in Fig. 4)

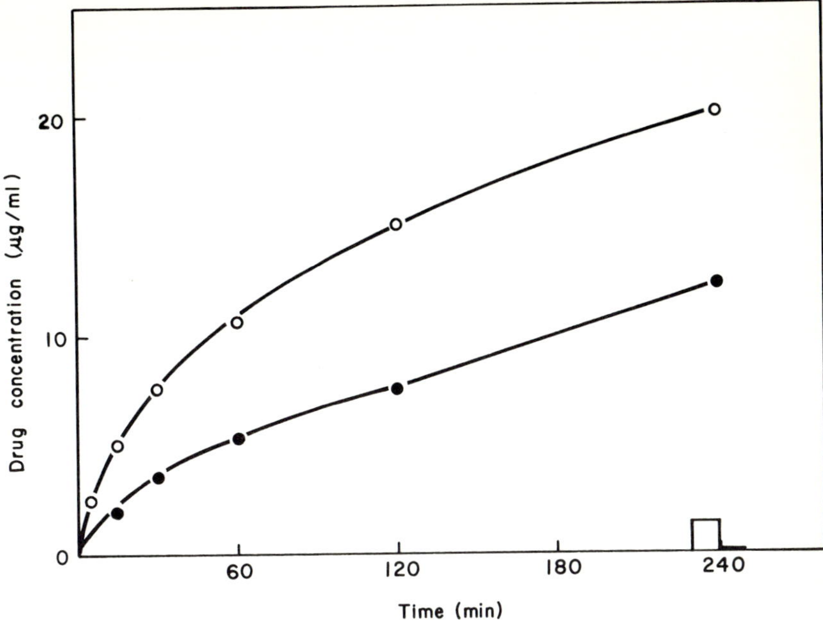

FIG. 4. Kinetic release of chemically determined adriamycin from albumin microspheres stabilized at 115°C (○) and 135°C (●). Both preparations contained 40 μg of slowly diffusible adriamycin per milligram of carrier prior to the onset of release. Drug concentrations represent micrograms of adriamycin per milliliter of RPMI 1640 release medium. Actual values at 240 minutes = 20.0 and 12.2 μg/ml, respectively, for the 115° and 135°C preparations. The proportions of slowly releasable drug that traveled with and subsequently diffused from magnetically responsive microspheres (circles at 240 minutes) versus unresponsive microspheres (bars at 240 minutes) = 15:1 and 147:1, respectively, for the 115° and 135°C preparations (Widder *et al.*, 1978b).

were obtained with microspheres stabilized by chemical cross-linking. These kinetics were highly reproducible. Hence, it was relatively simple to make preparations that afforded a slow, intermediate, or rapid release of chemically unaltered drug.

The final *in vitro* test of this carrier system was to determine if the released drug retained biological activity. This was done using an assay system employing a Fisher 344 rat fibrosarcoma that had been induced with methyl nitrosourea and adapted by the authors for growth as an *in vitro* cell line (Widder *et al.*, 1978b). This line retained its malignant characteristics as evaluated by electron microscopy and recurrent growth in syngeneic rats. The quantity of biologically active adriamycin released by a given preparation of microspheres was determined by allowing known concentrations of the spheres to release drug for standard time intervals. The resulting supernatants were added to newly plated microtiter cultures of the fibrosarcoma. Initially, this assay was performed according to the method of Levy *et al.* (1975). Cells were exposed to supernatant for 2 hours, pulse-labeled with uridine-5-^{3}H for an additional 4 hours, harvested by precipitation with cold 5% trichloroacetic acid, and solubilized for scintillation counting. The effect on gross cellular RNA synthesis was estimated from the decrement of radiolabel incorporation. This assay was later modified by the authors to allow rapid processing of large sample numbers. The modification involved trypsinizing and harvesting whole tumor cells on a multiple, automated sample harvester (Widder *et al.*, 1978b). Standard dose–response curves were generated for each harvesting procedure by incubating cells with known concentrations of free adriamycin (Fig. 5). Since the two procedures generated identical dose–response curves, the newer technique was used for all subsequent bioassays.

The kinetic release of biologically active drug was determined by assay-

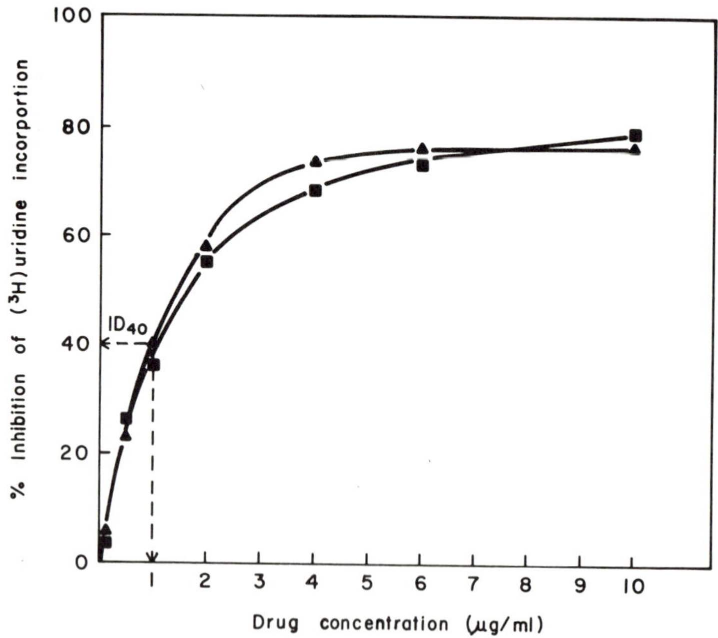

FIG. 5. Dose–response inhibition of uridine-^{3}H incorporation by free adriamycin. Target cells: malignant Fisher 344 rat fibrosarcoma line. Harvesting techniques: (▲) precipitation of uridine-^{3}H-labeled macromolecules with 5% trichloroacetic acid; (■) harvesting of whole-cell radiolabel using a multiple automated sample harvester (see text). The correspondence of 1.00 μg/ml adriamycin to 40% inhibition is later used for the quantitation of drug activities in unknown supernatants (see Fig. 7) (Widder *et al.*, 1978b).

ing the supernatants of prewashed microspheres (1 mg/ml) (Fig. 6). A controlled continuous release was observed for microspheres stabilized at both 115° and 135°C. The rate of release was substantially slower for the more highly stabilized (135°C) preparation. These curves corresponded well to the chemical release curves (see Fig. 4). Again, for both preparations, a very high proportion of the biologically active drug traveled with and later diffused from the magnetically responsive fraction of microspheres (Fig. 6 caption). This result corroborated the previous chemical data (see Fig. 4). Importantly, non-drug-bearing microspheres were biologically inert in this assay system (Fig. 6).

The effect of carrier stabilization on the biological activity of released drug was quantitated by a dose–response analysis. This analysis was performed using the ID_{40} correspondence from the standard free drug curve (Fig. 5). The 115° and 135°C preparations released, respectively, 20.0 and 9.5 μg/ml equivalents of biologically active drug after 240 minutes of incu-

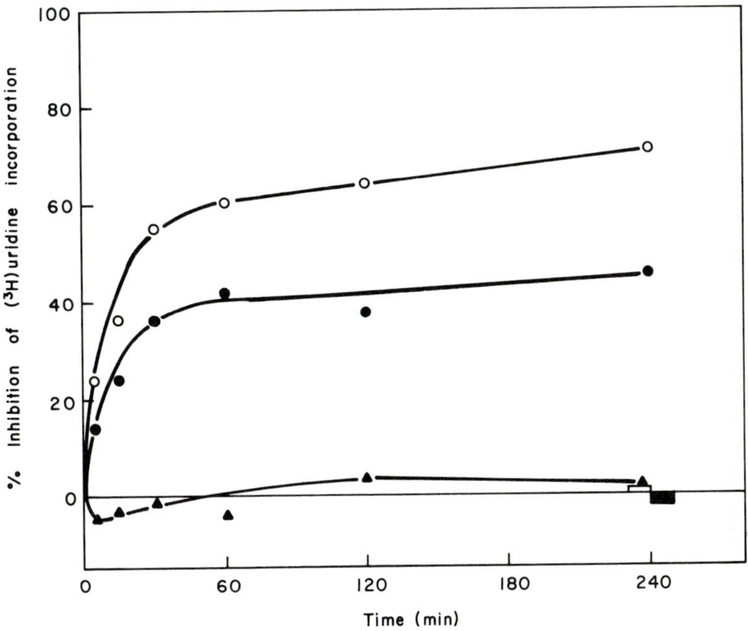

FIG. 6. Kinetic release of biologically active adriamycin by microspheres stabilized at 115° (○) and 135°C (●), and biological effects of products released by empty (non-drug-bearing) microspheres (▲). Assay system as in Fig. 5. Bioassays performed by adding 1:6 final dilutions of the supernatants shown in Fig. 4. The quantities of slowly releasable drug that traveled with and subsequently diffused from magnetically responsive microspheres versus unresponsive microspheres are indicated, respectively, by the circles and bars at 240 minutes (Widder *et al.*, 1978b).

bation (Fig. 7). The resulting ratios of biological activity to chemically determined activity were 1.00 (20.0 μg/ml/20.0 μg/ml) for the 115°C preparation and 0.78 (9.5 μg/ml/12.2 μg/ml) for the 135°C preparation. Thus, heat stabilization at 115°C produced no biological degradation of released adriamycin, and stabilization at 135°C produced a moderate but tolerable 22% decrease. These results correlated well with the chromatographic analysis of adriamycin degradation to aglycones and corroborated the accuracy of this method as a quantitative assay for biologically active drug.

Further analysis of the 135°C preparation indicated that 20% of the active drug was released during the first hour and 80% remained for subsequent release (Widder *et al.*, 1978b). Although relatively slow, this rate was considerably faster than the rate of matrix degradation (<3% in 48 hours) (Widder *et al.*, 1979). Hence, the kinetics of drug release appeared to approximate more closely the rate of matrix hydration than matrix degradation.

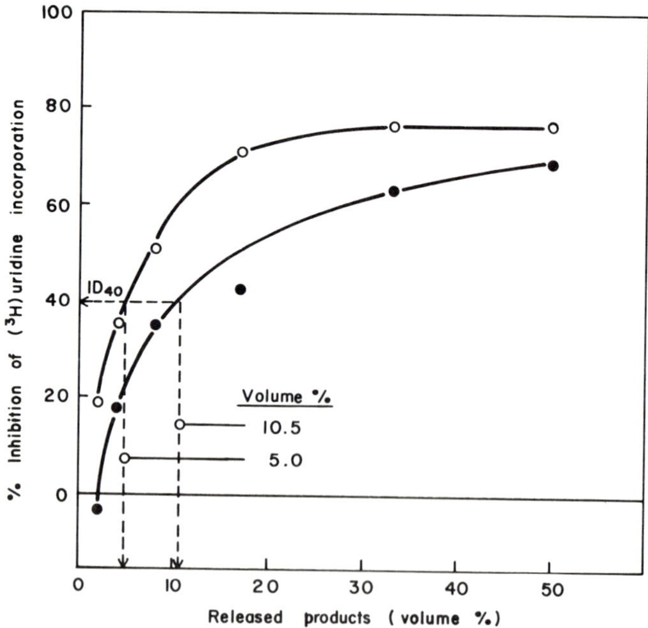

FIG. 7. Dose–response quantitation of biologically active drug products released from 0 to 240 minutes of incubation by microspheres stabilized at 115° (○) and 135°C (●). Concentrations of biologically active drug are calculated as (100/ID_{40} volume % of unknown supernatant) × (ID_{40} equivalent of 1.00 μg/ml for the free drug [from Fig. 5]). The actual values = 20.0 and 9.5 μg/ml, respectively, for the 115° and 135°C preparations. Both preparations were identical to those used in Fig. 4, and contained 40 μg of slowly diffusible adriamycin per milligram of carrier (Widder *et al.*, 1978b).

3. *Distribution and Targeting*

The tail vasculature of large Sprague-Dawley rats was chosen as the initial model system for *in vivo* localization of microspheres. In these studies, the tail was demarcated into four sections, each measuring 3.5–4.0 cm in length. The carrier preparation was introduced into the ventral caudal artery through a small polyethylene catheter inserted proximally, at tail segment 1. The microspheres were localized in tail segment 3, 6.5 cm distal to the point of injection, using bipolar magnetic fields of selected intensities. Iodine-125-labeled microspheres (0.5 mg in 0.5 ml) were infused at a rate of 0.6 ml/minute. This corresponded to the normal rate of blood flow in the ventral caudal artery. Following infusion, the catheter was removed and resumption of arterial flow was verified using a transcutaneous Doppler apparatus. The magnet was left in position for an additional 30 minutes before sacrificing the animals. The tail segments and major organs were removed and counted for gamma radioactivity.

The localization of microspheres in tail segment 3 increased with the intensity of the ambient field (Fig. 8). At field strengths of 8000 Oe, more than 50% of the carrier was retained in the target segment. The other segments (1, 2, and 4) that were not circumscribed by the field exhibited negligible retention. The discrepancy between *in vitro* retention (>90%) (see the foregoing) and *in vivo* retention (±50%) appeared to result from two factors: the small configuration of the magnetic field and the vascular anatomy of the rat tail. The ventral caudal arterial system typically has perforating arteries that communicate between its superficial and deep branches. This and associated venous return allow proximal shunting of a portion of blood and injected microspheres away from the magnetic field. Recently, such shunting has been minimized by advancing the injection catheter in a caudal direction to the leading edge of the target segment. Alternatively, it could be reduced by applying a more uniform field over the entire capillary bed supplied by the ventral caudal artery.

Further evaluation of the tissue for carrier radioactivity indicated that approximately 60% was present in the skin and subcutaneous tissues of the target segment and 40% in bone, muscle, and tendons. Transmission electron micrographs of the tail skin at 30 minutes revealed that the majority of microspheres had become attached to small arteriolar and capillary endothelial cells (Widder *et al.*, 1978a). Some of the spheres had already begun to migrate from the vascular space into and between adjacent endothelial cells. No microvascular obstruction, embolization, or infarction was observed.

Recent experiments using ^{125}I-microspheres have shown that nearly 100% of the initially localized spheres remained at the target site for ≥24 hours in the absence of a continued magnetic field (K. Widder and A. E.

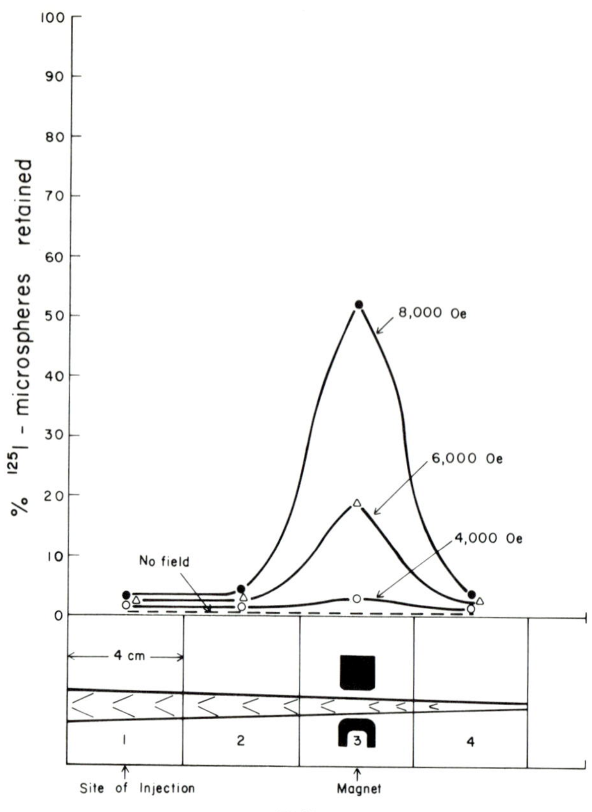

FIG. 8. Magnetic retention and distribution of small albumin microspheres in the tail skin of Sprague-Dawley rats. Iodine-125-labeled magnetically responsive microspheres, 0.5 mg in 0.5 ml of 0.15 *M* NaCl containing 0.1% Tween 80, infused into the proximal, ventral caudal artery of 400-gm rats, 10 per experimental group. (Adapted from Widder *et al.*, 1978a,b.)

Senyei, unpublished observations). Hence, an initial 30-minute exposure to the field appears to be sufficient for protracted localization of the microspheres. This is highly desirable because the particles can then provide a local depot of drug for subsequent controlled release.

Magnetic targeting produced a dramatic effect on the first-order distribution of microspheres (Table IV). The ratios of carrier that localized at the target site compared to the liver and heart were, respectively, 8.6:1 and 215:1. This was associated with an actual decrease in the concentration of microspheres in the liver and spleen (Table IV). These differentials are substantially higher than those afforded by any other type of encapsulation carrier.

TABLE IV

In Vivo DISTRIBUTION OF ^{125}I-LABELED MAGNETICALLY RESPONSIVE MICROSPHERES[a]

	Target								
	Tail segment (μg/gm)			Organs (μg/gm)					
Category	No. 2	No. 3	No. 4	Heart	Kidney	Lung	Liver	Spleen	Remainder of carcass (μg/gm)
Control	<1	<1	<1	<1	<1	31 ± 2	40 ± 2	50 ± 2	<1
Magnet[b]	<1	215 ± 18	<1	<1	<1	27 ± 2	25 ± 2	40 ± 2	<1

[a] Protocol as described in Fig. 8 caption. Limits of detection ≤1.0 μg of microspheres per gram of tissue (wet weight). Adapted from Widder *et al.* (1978a,b).

[b] Ambient magnetic field of 8000 Oe for 30 minutes over tail segment 3.

Initial experiments also have been performed to see if the carrier preparations could be localized in deep organs within the major body cavities (A. E. Senyei and K. Widder, unpublished observations). In these studies, 0.2-mg boluses of ^{125}I-microspheres were injected into the tail veins of BDF_1 mice and targeted to the lungs using an extracorporeal unipolar magnet producing an ambient field of 800 Oe. Approximately 50% of the injected carrier was localized in the experimental group compared to 6–18% in the controls. These results indicated that deep organ targeting of microspheres is indeed feasible. Again, it is anticipated that an even greater retention could be achieved by slowing the rate of infusion and appropriately adjusting the magnetic field vector, intensity, and gradient.

After it had been established that the carrier preparations could be efficiently targeted, investigations to determine whether or not the prototype drug, adriamycin, would distribute stoichiometrically with the carrier were performed (Widder *et al.*, 1978a,b). For this purpose, the above infusions and 30-minute magnetic localizations were repeated. The drug–carrier preparation in this study consisted of microspheres that were stabilized at 135°C and contained approximately 36 μg of slowly releasable adriamycin per milligram of carrier. Tissue concentrations of adriamycin were determined using a modification of the method of Bachur *et al.* (1970). Adriamycin was solubilized from tail skin and other organs by overnight extraction with cold 0.5 *N* acetic acid. This was shown not to interfere with the measurement of drug. Drug concentrations were quantitated by specific fluorescence, as described in Section III,E,2.

In the presence of an 8000-Oe bipolar magnetic field and a field gradient of ±4000 Oe/cm, 3.9 μg of carrier-delivered adriamycin was localized per gram of target tail skin (Table V). More than 85% of the carrier-delivered drug remained at the target site after 30 minutes of magnetic localization. No drug was detectable in the nontarget tail segments or in the liver. By contrast, a 100-fold higher dose of free adriamycin was required to obtain comparable local tissue concentrations (Table V). Unlike the carrier-delivered drug, this resulted in liver concentrations of 15 μg/gm and a liver-to-target ratio of 4.5:1. Carrier localization was followed by the appearance of diffuse adriamycin fluorescence in the tissues surrounding the drug-bearing microspheres (A. E. Senyei and K. Widder, unpublished observations). This indicated that a portion of the released drug had diffused into the target tissues. Further studies are currently in progress to determine, for different carrier preparations, the fractions of drug that remain at the target site and the fractions that undergo systemic clearance. Regardless of clearance, all preparations should afford high, local drug gradients when compared to other types of carriers that partition mainly to the reticuloendothelial system.

TABLE V

In Vivo LOCALIZATION OF CARRIER-DELIVERED AND FREE ADRIAMYCIN[a]

Form of drug	Dose (mg/kg)	Magnetic field[b]	Tissue concentrations (μg/gm) Target tail skin	Liver
Carrier-delivered	0.05	0	<1	<1
	0.05	+	3.9	<1
Free	0.05	0	<1	<1
	5.00	0	3.3	15.0

[a] Protocol as described in Fig. 8 caption. Limits of detection ≤1.0 μg of drug per gram of tissue (wet weight).

[b] Ambient magnetic field of 8000 Oe for 30 minutes over target tail segment (No. 3).

4. *Metabolism, Antigenicity, and Toxicity*

The metabolism, antigenicity, and toxicity of the albumin matrix have been described in Section III,D,3. However, the present carrier has potential differences in toxicity due to its smaller size and the inclusion of Fe_3O_4 as a matrix component. In order to evaluate these differences, acute (7-day) and chronic (90-day) toxicity studies were performed on BDF_1 mice (Widder *et al.*, 1978a). The protocol consisted of injecting intravenously 0.04–400 mg/kg of the drug-free carrier containing 20% Fe_3O_4 (w/w). The mice were then followed for signs of acute respiratory distress, maintenance of weight, histopathological changes in representative organs, and death. At the highest dose (400 mg/kg), 2 acute deaths occurred in a group of 10 animals. On histopathological examination, these deaths were caused by pulmonary embolization. This appeared to result from clumping of the microspheres, which occurs when they are suspended at extremely high concentrations. No other major toxic signs or findings were observed in the entire study. Consequently, the LD_{20} for small microspheres was reached only at tremendous overdoses of 400 mg/kg. By contrast, the LD_{50} for large albumin microspheres was reported to occur at a significantly lower dose of 200 mg/kg (Rhodes *et al.*, 1969). These results indicated that small albumin microspheres, even those containing magnetically responsive material, are less toxic than their larger counterparts. This difference appears to be based on a difference in their propensity to cause microvascular obstruction.

At this writing, there are no other published studies describing the toxicity of intravenously administered Fe_3O_4. However, extensive human studies have been performed to evaluate the effects of the inhaled material. These studies revealed that the respiratory intake of moderately large quantities of Fe_3O_4, in the absence of other irritants such as asbestos, does not cause significant inflammation, fibrosis, or alteration of pulmonary function (Bates *et al.*, 1971; Jones and Warner, 1972; Cohen, 1973). Based on these results, it is reasonable to predict that intravascularly administered microspheres will also induce minimal inflammatory responses. Although accumulation and removal of systemically administered Fe_3O_4 are not well understood, the clearance, catabolism, and excretion of another nonionic form of iron, carbonyl iron, have been investigated (Meyers *et al.*, 1963). In the absence of magnetic targeting, a substantial fraction of carbonyl-^{59}Fe is cleared by the reticuloendothelial system shortly after injection. Two weeks later, this pool has become markedly depleted. A portion of the iron is excreted in the urine. This rate of excretion is accelerated by the administration of desferrioxamine B, a chelator of ionic iron. These results suggest that cells of the reticuloendothelial system can convert a portion of the nonionic iron to the ionic form, in preparation for its subsequent renal excretion. Studies using $^{59}Fe_3O_4$ are currently in progress to determine if this form of nonionic iron is similarly metabolized and excreted.

The quantity of carrier-borne Fe_3O_4 required to localize therapeutic concentrations of adriamycin is actually quite small. According to Harris *et al.* (1975), concentrations of adriamycin in the tumors of animals and humans undergoing therapeutic responses range from 0.2 to 1.0 μg/gm of wet tumor weight. Using microspheres composed of 20% Fe_3O_4 (w/w) and assuming that the site-specific localization is 50% efficient, the total iron required to deliver high therapeutic concentrations of adriamycin (1 μg/gm) to a 1000-gm tumor would be less than 7 mg. This represents only 3–4 times the daily absorption of iron in a normal adult. Moreover, it constitutes a relatively insignificant load when compared to the iron pools of 150, 1000, and 2500 mg that are contained, respectively, in the bone marrow, reticuloendothelial system, and circulating red blood cells. Therefore, it should be possible to administer multiple courses of carrier-delivered adriamycin to patients with relatively large tumors without exceeding the maximal tolerable dose of Fe_3O_4.

Both the initial localization and serial accumulation of Fe_3O_4 can be determined by taking advantage of its magnetic properties. The material itself will become magnetized during initial localization and/or subsequent exposure to an external magnetic field (Cohen, 1975). It then will emit a remanent magnetic field that can be used to locate and quantitate the amount of Fe_3O_4 present. Two types of instruments have been used for this purpose: the highly sensitive, superconducting quantum interference device (SQUID) magnetometer and the less sensitive fluxgate gradiometer. Both devices are currently available for the noninvasive localization and quantitation of this carrier material. Radiological techniques can also be used to provide an initial assessment of carrier delivery (see Section III,E,5).

5. *Current and Projected Utility in Cancer Chemotherapy*

Adriamycin microsphere preparations are currently undergoing tests for antitumor activity *in vivo*. If efficacious, this carrier system could enjoy wide utility in the treatment of patients with severe residual disease where the majority of tumor is located in anatomic regions with well-defined blood supplies. The two major advantages of this carrier over other delivery systems are its high efficiency of targeting under *in vivo* conditions and its controlled release of drug at the microvascular level. In addition, the carrier exhibits minimal toxicity at doses required for the therapy of even large tumors. Targeting could be determined easily and precisely under clinical conditions by either magnetic means (see the preceding) or radiological visualization. The latter can be accomplished by injecting tracer microspheres that carry water-soluble radiocontrast agents, such as Hypaque. Furthermore, this carrier represents a universal vehicle that potentially is compatible with both low and high molecular weight chemotherapeutic agents, synthetic and natural products. It affords a means to achieve uniform organ distributions of water-soluble immunopotentiating agents, such as muramyl dipeptide (MDP), levamisole, and glucan. Hence, the system may offer the first practical approach to the immunotherapy of solid tumors. In the cases of weakly antigenic tumors or tumor-induced immunosuppression, these microspheres also may permit the localized delivery of inflammatory agents, such as histamine. This could initiate the directed chemotaxis and inflammatory activities of blood monocytes, segmented neutrophils, and recirculating thymus-derived lymphocytes (T cells).

The versatility of this carrier matrix allows the simultaneous delivery of multiple agents. Moreover, the ease and rapidity of drug-carrier preparation potentially allow the tailoring of combination chemotherapy, or chemoimmunotherapy, to individual malignancies whose drug sensitivities are determined by histopathological and biological analysis of the resected primary tumor mass. Near-term postoperative availability of the drug-carrier complex also enhances its practicality for targeted adjuvant chemotherapy. Such targeting should preserve a higher level of specific antitumor immunity by directing the cytotoxic agents toward the tumor mass and away from systemic lymphoid organs. This might be expected to decrease the biological imbalance between tumor and host rather than to produce a parallel suppression of both entities.

By delivering agents that themselves undergo second-order targeting, these microspheres could be used as the first stage of a two-stage delivery system. For example, toxic lectins and drug–antibody complexes might be encapsulated, efficiently localized, and released within the desired tissue, where they could subsequently home to tumor cells in preference to normal cells.

Finally, the albumin matrix is capable of incorporating a variety of radionuclides for use in antitumor therapy. This can potentially afford an optimal homogeneous distribution of radioactivity within the desired target and avoid radiation damage to adjacent critical organs and tissues.

6. *Other Uses*

The availability of this targeted carrier system suggests potential uses in a number of other localized disease states. It may be of particular value for the delivery of antibiotics in patients with bacterial or fungal abscesses and other resistant or sequestered infections such as prostatitis and osteomyelitis. The foregoing studies indicated that 40% of the carrier that was delivered to a body extremity became localized in bone and associated connective tissues. Hence, the carrier should achieve and maintain high therapeutic concentrations of drug within bone.

Another area of potential utility involves the delivery of fibrinolytic agents in the treatment of thrombophlebitis and pulmonary embolism. Current systemic therapy is associated with the problems of inadequate local enzyme concentrations and systemic bleeding. Both of these problems can be overcome by targeted chemotherapy using agents such as urokinase in conjunction with the present delivery system.

Other potential uses include the delivery of anti-inflammatory and immunosuppressive agents to sites of severe, localized inflammatory processes and immunopathological disorders, such as acute glomerulonephritis, autoimmune and immune-complex nephritis, recurrent hepatitis, and severe localized arthritis. Also, this carrier should be of considerable value for the localized suppression of acute allograft rejection in patients with systemic infection that would otherwise mandate surgical removal of the transplanted organ.

By employing a combination of Hypaque-loaded microspheres and pulsed magnetic fields, the system may be of use for transient tissue scanning in situations where it is undesirable for the particles to remain for long periods in the target tissue.

In addition to its potential clinical utility, this carrier should prove extremely valuable as a research tool. For example, there is currently no good method for restricting to specific organs the distribution of systemically administered carcinogens and promoter substances. The present carrier provides an ideal method for isolating and accentuating the effects of these agents on nonhepatic organ systems. It also provides a method to evaluate the requirement for hepatic microsomal activation of procarcinogens to metabolites that may be carcinogenic in other organ systems. Additional applications include its use as an appropriately derivatized solid-phase support for radioimmunoassay and rapid cell sorting. The current fluorescent methods of cell sorting are slow and tedious. Hence, it is difficult to separate, by serological means, the large number of viable cells required for subsequent functional studies in *in vivo* systems. Derivatization of the microsphere surface with antibodies of appropriate specificity will allow the almost instantaneous magnetic separation of large numbers of cells that bear complementary surface determinants. The relatively low nonspecific reactivity of the albumin matrix with cellular elements should make this an ideal preparation for use in these separations.

F. Discussion

Of the various biodegradable encapsulation drug carriers discussed in this section, liposomes and small albumin microspheres exhibit the physical and biological characteristics most appropriate for broad clinical applications. The major problem experienced by both of these carriers, in the underivatized form, is their rapid particulate clearance by the reticuloendothelial system. This problem has not been overcome by any type of nonmagnetic encapsulation carrier. For example, compared to the first-order distribution of free drugs, liposome-mediated delivery actually decreases rather than increases the average tumor-to-liver drug concentration ratios by approximately 0.5 log. By contrast, magnetically responsive, small albumin microspheres enhance the target-to-liver ratio by nearly 1 log and the target-to-cardiac ratio by more than 2 logs. This pattern of first-order distribution has the potential to enhance local therapeutic effects and to reduce systemic toxicity for a wide variety of antitumor agents. It also should lead to a major decrease in cardiotoxicity for the prototype drug, adriamycin.

Additional studies by the authors have indicated that it is much more feasible to achieve magnetic targeting using microspheres than liposomes. It has been exceedingly difficult to prepare liposomes containing Fe_3O_4 that exhibit either adequate or reproducible magnetic responsivity. This is probably due to their lack of a matrix equivalent that, once polymerized, stabilizes and maintains the optimal peripheral distribution of Fe_3O_4. Albumin microspheres have an additional advantage compared to liposomes. With microspheres, it should be possible to alter the matrix properties and the attendant rate of drug release to fit the clinical situation.

Two larger, three-dimensional systems have been used in attempts to obtain high local concentrations of drugs. The first consists of intravascular, magnetically guided catheters and magnetically responsive macrocapsules positioned by such catheters (see Section III,E,1). There are several problems associated with these paraoperational devices. Drug is released at the arterial level rather than the microvascular level. Consequently, the barriers to extravascular diffusion are great. As a result, the majority of drug flows through the target organ and experiences systemic distribution and clearance. Also, either the catheter or the capsular device must be left in place during the entire period of infusion. In the latter instance, this may necessitate subsequent recovery of the indwelling capsule.

The second system consists of extravascular, general-purpose capsules composed of silicone rubber (Schmidt *et al.,* 1972; Dziengiel, 1973), synthetic polypeptides (Mason *et al.,* 1976; Schwope *et al.,* 1976; Sidman *et al.,* 1976), glycerides (Sullivan and Kalkwarf, 1976), and other polymers (Capozza *et al.,* 1976) that range in size from 100 μm to several centimeters in diameter. These capsules are designed for injection directly into tissues, insertion into body cavities, or application to the surface of skin and internal organs. Although they do afford a localized, depot-type release, the agent is again subjected to substantial diffusional barriers. As a result, these capsules are generally incapable of achieving uniform distributions of drugs within larger tissue masses and organs. Such capsules are not designed primarily for drug targeting, but rather, for the treatment of disorders requiring long-term systemic therapy, such as narcotic addiction.

The use of magnetically responsive albumin microspheres or any other targeted carrier system constrains the classes of applicable drugs to ones that are directly active at the target site and do not require prior activation by hepatic microsomal enzymes. Fortunately, this includes not only adriamycin but also a wide variety of clinically useful antitumor agents. A second general constraint that applies to area-specific antitumor therapy involves the precision with which the location of tumor masses can be determined. With the advent of computerized axial tomography and other sophisticated diagnostic techniques, this should no longer represent a major limiting factor. Hence, it would appear that both the diagnostic and therapeutic capabilities exist to proceed with targeted chemotherapy on an experimental clinical basis. Based on the targeting capabilities and release characteristics of the available encapsulation carriers, it appears that magnetically responsive, small albumin microspheres currently represent an optimal prototype system for the area-specific delivery of antitumor agents.

IV. Exposed Carriers and Targeted Natural Products

This classification includes all complexed or covalently conjugated carriers that potentially expose the cytotoxic agent to the surrounding environment. It can be subdivided into two groups. The first consists of lectins, toxins, and bacteriocins. Here, either the carrier itself or one of its naturally occurring subunits constitutes the toxic moiety and another molecular region or subunit constitutes the specific binding moiety. The second group consists of carriers that are artifically bound to the cytotoxic agent. These include macromolecular carriers, such as serum proteins, glycoproteins, nonspecific and specific immunoglobulins, hormones, DNA, dextran, and synthetic polymers; and low molecular weight chelators, such as divalent cations.

As a class, exposed drug carriers and natural products are larger than free drugs and smaller than encapsulation carriers. Compared to the latter, they theoretically should experience decreased rates of blood clearance and gain better access to extravascular sites. Although this is sometimes observed, there are a number of offsetting properties that dimish their utility as targeting vehicles. For example, most of these carriers represent foreign macromolecules. Consequently, many become sequestered in the reticuloendothelial organs by both nonimmunological and immunological clearance. This counteracts the apparent advantage of tissue access and diminishes the therapeutic index of bound cytotoxic agents. Foreign macromolecules have the potential to induce specific immunity and elicit anaphylactic responses on repeated administration. Moreover, drug–carrier conjugates often induce immunity against the drug as well as the carrier. This can accelerate the development of severe drug sensitivity and preclude subsequent administration of the free drug. Because at least a portion of the drug is exposed to serum enzymes, it is susceptible to degradation during intravascular transit. Finally, depending on the carrier system, its capacity for drug delivery, on a weight basis, is often substantially lower than that of encapsulation carriers.

A detailed comparison of exposed drug carriers is beyond the scope of this article. A brief discussion of antitumor antibody is presented later in this section. For discussions of the targeting capabilities and antitumor effects of other systems, the reader is referred to the following papers and reviews: abrin and ricin (Lin *et al.*, 1970; Hsu *et al.*, 1974; Nicolson *et al.*,

1976; Robbins *et al.*, 1977), diphtheria toxin (Buzzi and Maistrello, 1973; Iglewski and Rittenberg, 1974; Pappenheimer, 1977), bacteriocins (Farkas-Himsley, 1976), drug–protein complexes (Szekerke *et al.*, 1972a,b; de Duve *et al.*, 1974; Shier *et al.*, 1976; Szekerke and Driscoll, 1977), drug–DNA complexes (Trouet *et al.*, 1972, 1974; Atassi *et al.*, 1974, 1975; Marks and Venditti, 1976), synthetic polymeric antitumor agents (Levy *et al.*, 1969; Regelson and Munson, 1970; Breslow *et al.*, 1973; Noronha-Blob *et al.*, 1977; Chu and Whiteley, 1977), drug–hormone complexes (Kaplan, 1976), and drug–metal chelates (Yesair *et al.*, 1974).

Specific antibodies represent a special class of exposed drug carrier. First, they are uniquely able to recognize the subtle surface differences that are frequently, but not always demonstrable between normal and malignant cells. Second, they afford a potential approach to the targeted therapy of disseminated malignancies.

Satisfactory covalent coupling of antibodies to daunomycin and adriamycin (Hurwitz *et al.*, 1975), chlorambucil (Ghose *et al.*, 1972a,b), and other alkylating agents (Rowland *et al.*, 1975) has been achieved with good retention of both drug and antibody activities at low ratios of substitution (Guclu *et al.*, 1976). By radionuclide labeling, these preparations have been shown to undergo tumor-specific targeting in cell culture (Ghose *et al.*, 1975a). Initial studies in murine and human systems indicate that intravenously administered antitumor antibodies also target to tumors under *in vivo* conditions (Davies and O'Neill, 1973; Ghose *et al.*, 1975a). This targeting is antigen-specific. In an isolated report, the tumor-to-liver ratio of radiolabeled antibody reached levels as high as 37:1 (Ghose *et al.*, 1975a).

Preliminary studies of *in vivo* efficacy have shown that chlorambucil–antibody complexes will inhibit the growth of Ehrlich ascites tumors more effectively than chlorambucil alone, antibody alone, or chlorambucil bound to nonspecific immunoglobulins (Ghose *et al.*, 1972a). Further reports indicate that human malignant melanoma responds more favorably to drug–antibody complexes than to drug alone (Ghose *et al.*, 1972b). The interpretation of these effects as the direct result of antibody-mediated drug targeting has been called into question by studies showing that equivalent effects are obtained when drug and antibody are administered separately (Davies and O'Neill, 1973; Ghose *et al.*, 1977). These findings have suggested that specific antibody acts synergistically to enhance the antitumor effects of concomitantly administered nontargeted drugs. The exact basis for this effect is not known. However, studies by Shearer and Parker (1975) and Shearer *et al.* (1973, 1974, 1975) have provided a possible explanation. These revealed that, under appropriate conditions, cytotoxic antitumor antibodies actually stimulate rather than suppress the growth of tumors. Stimulation usually occurs at low-antibody concentrations in either the presence or absence of complement. This effect depends on divalent antibody of the IgG class. Studies of possible mechanisms have revealed that growth stimulation is preceded by an increase in the turnover of tumor membrane phospholipids (Shearer, 1977). This and the requirement for divalent antibody strongly suggest that antibody acts by cross-linking tumor cell-surface receptors, perturbing the cell membrane, and thereby initiating cell division.

Progressive growth of clinical tumors is commonly associated with a decrease in the fraction of cycling cells (Byers and Levin, 1976). Noncycling cells have a lower sensitivity to the "cycle-specific" agents that have been used in most of the reported studies. Therefore, it is quite possible that drug–antibody synergism results from antibody-initiated cycling and attendant sensitization of quiescent tumor cells. Although such immunostimulation has produced beneficial effects in a small number of reported cases, extensive studies will be required to determine if it is advisable to employ this form of adjuvant immunotherapy on a broader scale. Until these studies have been completed, it is prudent to proceed with caution in the use of antibody as a targeted carrier for antitumor therapy.

In addition to its direct modulatory effect on tumor growth, specific antibody has a number of other drawbacks as a carrier system. Since antitumor globulins are almost always raised in heterologous animal systems, they represent foreign proteins in human recipients. Consequently, they can induce specific immunity and elicit anaphylactic reactions (Ghose *et al.*, 1977). The foreign character of the molecules together with the low ratio of specific antitumor antibody to total immunoglobulin (usually 1:100) result in a substantial first-order clearance by the reticuloendothelial system (Ghose *et al.*, 1976, 1977). This diminishes the efficiency of targeting and decreases the therapeutic index of the complexed drug. Due to the lack of extensive cross-reactivity among tumor-associated antigens, even for tumors within a given organ system (Ghose *et al.*, 1975b), it may be necessary to prepare specific carrier antibody on an individual basis, using the patient's own primary tumor. The time required for immunization, purification of the immunoglobulin fraction, and coupling of drug would preclude the use of antibody as a carrier for adjuvant chemotherapy during the immediate postoperative period. Furthermore, although the immunoglobulin fraction of immune serum is relatively easy to prepare, additional purification required to increase the ratio of immune to nonimmune globulin is considerably more involved. Hence, it may be impractical, on an individual basis, to produce immunoglobulin whose specific activity is high enough to eliminate clearance by the reticuloendothelial system. Nevertheless, specific antibodies currently represent the best available approach to the treatment of widely disseminated malignancies. If practical solutions to these problems are forthcoming, the full potential of antibody to serve as a targeted drug carrier can be realized.

V. Summary

This chapter has compared the major encapsulation carriers that have been tested for targeting of antitumor agents. A new, nontoxic carrier system was introduced for the *in vivo* localization of these agents. This consisted of magnetically responsive small albumin microspheres that are injected intra-arterially and localized at specific target sites by the application of appropriately directed magnetic fields. The new drug delivery vehicle could be targeted much more efficiently than any other type of nonmagnetic encapsulation carrier. It appears to have overcome the major problem characteristic of encapsulation carriers, namely, their rapid clearance by organs of the reticuloendothelial system. This preparation has the additional advantage of affording various rates of drug release that can be tailored to *in vivo* requirements. A prototype drug, adriamycin, was encapsulated and was found to distribute with the carrier. Thc released drug retained its biological activity.

The relative advantages and disadvantages of encapsulation carriers and exposed drug carriers were compared. Based on a high efficiency of targeting, magnetically responsive albumin microspheres appear to represent the optimal currently available vehicle for delivery of antitumor agents to regionally localized tumors with well-defined blood supplies. Although there are still significant problems attending their uses as carrier systems, specific antitumor antibodies appear to represent the best currently available approach to the treatment of widely disseminated tumors. A hybrid approach, involving two-stage delivery, was discussed as a potential method for further augmenting the efficiency of drug targeting. This would involve the first-order (site-specific) targeting of an encapsulation carrier containing drug–macromolecular complexes that could diffuse and undergo second-order (cellular) targeting. Although still theoretical, this type of stacked system could potentially achieve the dual goals of localizing a reservoir of drug at the desired target and focusing the released drug onto specific tumor cells. Hopefully, the emergence of magnetically targetable albumin microspheres, specific antibodies, and additional new carrier systems will pave the way for highly efficient, experimental and clinical focusing of antitumor therapy.

Acknowledgments

The authors' research summarized in this chapter was supported in part by the Department of Pathology of Northwestern University Medical and Dental Schools, the Northwestern University Cancer Center, and a grant from the National Cancer Institute (NIH CA26031).

The authors would like to thank the following individuals for their excellent technical support: Miss Sandra Garretson for editorial and library assistance, Miss Mary Paylo and Ms. Rikki Horne for information retrieval, coordination of data and preparation of the manuscript, Miss Twee Moy for library assistance and preparation of art work, and Mr. Odell Minick for preparation of the electron micrographs. Dr. Alfred Quattrone, Ms. Elizabeth Gilchrist, and Mrs. Betsy Jones were also of invaluable help in the initial and final stages of this work.

References

Alksne, J. F., Fingerhut, A., and Rand, R. (1966). *Surgery* **60,** 212.

Allison, A. C., and Gregoriadis, G. (1974). *Nature (London)* **252,** 252.

Almeida, J. D., Brand, C. M., Edwards, D. C., and Heath, T. D. (1975). *Lancet* **2,** 899.

Anderson, W. A. D., and McCutcheon, M. (1966). *In* "Pathology" (W. A. D. Anderson, ed.), p. 13. Mosby, St. Louis, Missouri.

Arfors, K. E., Forsberg, J. O., Larsson, B., Lewis, D. H., Rosengren, B:, and Odmon, S. (1976). *Nature (London)* **262,** 500.

Arruda, J. A. L., Boonjarern, S., Westenfelder, C., and Kurtzman, N. A. (1974). *Proc. Soc. Exp. Biol. Med.* **146,** 263.

Atassi, G., Tagnon, H. J., and Trouet, A. (1974). *Eur. J. Cancer* **10,** 399.

Atassi, G., Duarte-Karim, M., and Tagnon, H. J. (1975). *Eur. J. Cancer* **11,** 309.

Bachur, N. R., Moore, A. L., Bernstein, J. G., and Liu, A. (1970). *Cancer Chemother. Rep.* **54,** 89.

Bangham, A. D. (1972). *Chem. Phys. Lipids* **8,** 386.

Bangham, A. D., Standish, M. M., and Watkins, G. C. (1965). *J. Mol. Biol.* **13,** 238.

Barnothy, M. F., ed. (1964). "Biological Effects of Magnetic Fields," Vol. 1. Plenum, New York.

Barnothy, M. F., ed. (1969). "Biological Effects of Magnetic Fields," Vol. 2. Plenum, New York.

Barnothy, M. F. (1974). *Prog. Biometerol.* **1,** No. 1A, 392.

Barnothy, J. M., Barnothy, M. F., and Boszormenyi-Nagy, I. (1956). *Nature (London)* **177,** 576.

Bates, D. V., Macklem, P. T., and Christie, R. V. (1971). *In* "Respiratory Function and Disease," pp. 367 and 371. W. B. Saunders Co., Philadelphia.

Black, C. D. V., and Gregoriadis, G. (1974). *Biochem. Soc. Trans.* **2,** 869.

Black, C. D. V., and Gregoriadis, G. (1976). *Biochem. Soc. Trans.* **4,** 253.

Blanchard, R. J. W., Grotenhuis, I., LaFave, J. W., and Perry, J. F., Jr. (1965). *Proc. Soc. Exp. Biol. Med.* **118,** 465.

Blok, M. C., van der Nuet-Kok, E. O. M., van Deenen, L. L. M., and de Gier, J. (1975). *Biochim. Biophys. Acta* **406,** 187.

Blok, M. C., van Deenen, L. L. M., and de Gier, J. (1976). *Biochim. Biophys. Acta* **433,** 1.

Blum, R. H. (1975). *Cancer Chemother. Rep.* **6,** 247.

Breisblatt, W., and Ohki, S. (1976a). *J. Membr. Biol.* **23,** 385.

Breisblatt, W., and Ohki, S. (1976b). *J. Membr. Biol.* **29,** 127.

Breslow, D. S., Edwards, E. I., and Newburg, N. R. (1973). *Nature (London)* **246,** 160.

Brightman, M. W. (1968). *Prog. Brain Res.* **29,** 19.
Broome, J. D. (1961). *Nature* (*London*) **191,** 1114.
Bruni, A., Toffano, G., Leon, A., and Boarato, E. (1976). *Nature* (*London*) **260,** 331.
Buchanan, J. W., Rhodes, B. A., and Wagner, H. N., Jr. (1969). *J. Nucl. Med.* **10,** 487.
Buchner, F., ed. (1956). "Handbuch der Allgemeine Pathologie," p. 313. Urban & Schwarzenberg, Munich.
Buzzi, S., and Maistrello, I. (1973). *Cancer Res.* **33,** 2349.
Byers, V. S., and Levin, A. S. (1976). *In* "Basic and Clinical Immunology" (H. Fudenberg *et al.,* eds.), p. 242. Lange Med. Publ., Los Altos, California.
Capozza, R. C., Schmitt, E. E., and Sendelbeck, L. R. (1976). *In* "Narcotic Antagonists: The Search for Long-Acting preparations" (R. Willette, ed.), p. 39. Natl. Inst. Drug Abuse, Rockville, Maryland.
Chu, B. C. F., and Whiteley, J. M. (1977). *Mol. Pharmacol.* **13,** 80.
Cohen, D. (1973). *Science* **180,** 745.
Cohen, D. (1975). *IEEE Trans. Magn.* **mag-2,** 694.
Colley, C. M., and Ryman, B. E. (1974). *Biochem. Soc. Trans.* **2,** 871.
Colley, C. M., and Ryman, B. E. (1975). *Biochem. Soc. Trans.* **3,** 157.
Dapergolas, G., Neerunjun, E. D., and Gregoriadis, G. (1976). *FEBS Lett.* **63,** 235.
Davies, D. A. L., and O'Neill, G. J. (1973). *Br. J. Cancer* **28,** Suppl. I, 285.
Deamer, D., and Bangham, A. D. (1976). *Biochim. Biophys. Acta* **443,** 629.
de Duve, C., de Barsy, T., Poole, B., Trouet, A., Tulkens, P., and van Hoof, F. (1974). *Biochem. Pharmacol.* **23,** 2495.
de Gier, J., Mandersloot, J. G., and van Deenen, L. L. M. (1968). *Biochim. Biophys. Acta* **150,** 666.
Dziengiel, S. L. (1973). *Am. J. Med. Technol.* **39,** 175.
Farkas-Himsley, H. (1976). *IRCS Libr. Compend.* **4,** 291.
Fendler, J. H., and Romero, A. (1976). *Life Sci.* **18,** 1453.
Fendler, J. H., and Romero, A. (1977). *Life Sci.* **20,** 1109.
Fiddler, M. B., Thorpe, S. J., Krivit, W., and Desnick, R. J. (1974). *In* "Enzyme Therapy in Lysosomal Storage Diseases" (J. M. Tager *et al.,* eds.), p. 182. North-Holland Publ., Amsterdam.
Fishman, Y., and Citri, N. (1975). *FEBS Lett.* **60,** 17.
Frei, E. H., Driller, J., Neufeld, H. N., Barr, I., Bleiden, L., and Askenazy, H. M. (1966). *Med. Res. Eng.* **5,** 11.
Ghose, T., Path, M. R. C., and Nigam, S. P. (1972a). *Cancer* **29,** 1398.
Ghose, T., Norvell, S. T., Guclu, A., Cameron, D., Bodurtha, A., and MacDonald, A. S. (1972b). *Br. Med. J.* **3,** 495.
Ghose, T., Guclu, A., Tai, J., MacDonald, A. S., Norvell, S. T., and Aquino, J. (1975a). *Cancer* **36,** 1646.
Ghose, T., Tai, J. Aquino, J., Guclu, A., Norvell, S. T., and MacDonald, A. S. (1975b). *Radiology* **116,** 445.
Ghose, T., Tai, J., Guclu, A., Norvell, S. T., Bodurtha, A., Aquino, J., and MacDonald, A. S. (1976). *Ann. N.Y. Acad. Sci.* **277,** 671.
Ghose, T., Norvell, S. T., Guclu, A., Bodurtha, A., Tai, J., and MacDonald, A. S. (1977). *J. Natl. Cancer Inst.* **58,** 845.
Grant, C. W. M., and McConnell, H. M. (1973). *Proc. Natl. Acad. Sci. U.S.A.* **70,** 1238.
Gregoriadis, G. (1973). *FEBS Lett.* **36,** 292.
Gregoriadis, G. (1974). *Biochem. Soc. Trans.* **2,** 117.
Gregoriadis, G. (1975). *Biochem. Soc. Trans.* **3,** 613.
Gregoriadis, G. (1976a). *N. Engl. J. Med.* **295,** 704.

Gregoriadis, G. (1976b). *N. Engl. J. Med.* **295,** 765.
Gregoriadis, G. (1977). *Nature (London)* **265,** 407.
Gregoriadis, G., and Allison, A. C. (1974). *FEBS Lett.* **45,** 71.
Gregoriadis, G., and Buckland, R. A. (1973). *Nature (London)* **244,** 170.
Gregoriadis, G., and Neerunjun, E. D. (1974). *Eur. J. biochem.* **47,** 179.
Gregoriadis, G., and Neerunjun, E. D. (1975a). *Biochem. Biophys. Res. Commun.* **65,** 537.
Gregoriadis, G., and Neerunjun, E. D. (1975b). *Res. Commun. Chem. Pathol. Pharmacol.* **10,** 351.
Gregoriadis, G., and Ryman, B. E. (1971). *Biochem. J.* **124,** 58.
Gregoriadis, G., and Ryman, B. E. (1972a). *Biochem. J.* **129,** 123.
Gregoriadis, G., and Ryman, B. E. (1972b). *Eur. J. Biochem.* **24,** 485.
Gregoriadis, G., Leathwood, P. D., and Ryman, B. E. (1974a). *FEBS Lett.* **14,** 95.
Gregoriadis, G., Putman, D., Louis, L., and Neerunjun, D. (1974b). *Biochem. J.* **140,** 323.
Gregoriadis, G., Swain, C. P., Wills, E. J., and Tavill, A. S. (1974c). *Lancet* **1,** 1313.
Gregoriadis, G., Dapergolas, G., and Neerunjun, E. D. (1976). *Biochem. Soc. Trans.* **4,** 256.
Gregoriadis, G., Neerunjun, E. D., and Hunt, R. (1977). *Life Sci.* **21,** 357.
Grotenhuis, I. M. (1966). *In* "Radioactive Pharmaceuticals" (G. A. Andrews *et al.*, eds.), CONF-651111, p. 205. U.S.A.E.C., Div. Tech. Inf., Springfield, Virginia.
Guclu, A., Ghose, T., Tai, J., and Mammen, M. (1976). *Eur. J. Cancer* **12,** 95.
Haest, C. W. M., de Gier, J., van Es, S. A., Verkleij, A. J., and van Deenen, L. L. M. (1972). *Biochim. Biophys. Acta* **288,** 43.
Halpern, B. N., Biozzi, G., Benacerrat, B., Stiffel, C., and Hillemand, B. (1956). *C. R. Seances Soc. Biol. Ses. fil.* **150,** 1307.
Harris, P. A., Watring, W. G., Lagasse, L. D., Byfield, J., Lee, Y.-T., and Block, J. (1975). *Proc. Am. Assoc. Cancer Res.* Abstr. No. 649.
Hayes, R. L., Nelson, B., Swartzendruber, D. C., Carlton, J. E., and Byrd, B. L. (1970). *Science* **167,** 289.
Haynes, D. H., and Kang, C. H. (1978). *In* "Liposomes and their Uses in Biology and Medicine" (D. Papahadjopoulos, ed.), p. 440. N.Y. Acad. Sci., New York.
Heath, T. D., Edwards, D. C., and Ryman, B. E. (1976). *Biochem. Soc. Trans.* **4,** 129.
Higasi, T., Nakayama, Y., Murata, A., Nakamura, K., Sugiyama, M., Kawaguchi, T., and Suzuki, S. (1972). *J. Nucl. Med.* **13,** 196.
Hilal, S. K., Michelsen, W. J., Driller, J., and Leonard, E. (1974). *Radiology* **113,** 529.
Hoffman, R. M., Margolis, L. B., and Bergelson, L. D. (1978). *In* "Liposomes and their Uses in Biology and Medicine" (D. Papahadjopoulos, ed.), p. 438. N.Y. Acad. Sci., New York.
Hsu, C.-T., Lin, J.-Y., and Tung, T.-C. (1974). *J. Formosan Med. Assoc.* **73,** 526.
Hurwitz, E., Levy, R., Maron, R., Wilchek, M., Arnon, R., and Sela, M. (1975). *Cancer Res.* **35,** 1175.
Iglewski, B. H., and Rittenberg, M. B. (1974). *Proc. Natl. Acad. Sci. U.S.A.* **71,** 2707.
Ihler, G. M., Glew, R. H., and Schnure, F. W. (1973). *Proc. Natl. Acad. Sci. U.S.A.* **70,** 2663.
Inbar, M., and Shinitzky, M. (1974). *Proc. Natl. Acad. Sci. U.S.A.* **71,** 2128.
Inoue, K. (1974). *Biochim. Biophys. Acta* **339,** 390.
Ito, Y., Okuyama, S., Sato, K., Takahashi, K., Sato, T., and Kanno, I. (1971). *Radiology* **100,** 357.
Jones, J. G., and Warner, C. G. (1972). *Brit. J. Industr. Med.* **29,** 169.
Juliano, R. L., and Stamp, D. (1975). *Biochem. Biophys. Res. Commun.* **63,** 651.
Juliano, R. L., and Stamp, D. (1976). *Nature (London)* **261,** 235.
Juliano, R. L., and Stamp, D. (1978). *Biochem. Pharmacol.* **27,** 21.

Kaplan, E., Mayron, L. W., and Graham, L. (1975). *Int. J. Nucl. Med. Biol.* **2,** 82.
Kaplan, N. O. (1976). *In* "Cancer Enzymology" (J. Schultz and F. Ahmad, eds.), p. 201. Academic Press, New York.
Karnovsky, M. J. (1967). *J. Cell Biol.* **35,** 213.
Kimelberg, H. K. (1976). *Biochim. Biophys. Acta* **448,** 531.
Kimelberg, H. K., Mayhew, E., and Papahadjopoulos, D. (1975). *Life Sci.* **17,** 715.
Kimelberg, H. K., Tracy, T. F., Jr., Biddlecome, J. M., and Bourke, R. S. (1976). *Cancer Res.* **36,** 2949.
Knudson, A. G., Jr., Di Ferrante, N., and Curtis, J. E. (1971). *Proc. Natl. Acad. Sci. U.S.A.* **68,** 1738.
Kobayashi, T., Tsukagoshi, S., and Sakurai, Y. (1975). *Gann* **66,** 719.
Kogan, A. Kh., and Kulitskaya, V. I. (1977). *Patol. Fiziol. Eksp. Ter.* **2,** 63.
Kramer, P. A. (1974). *J. Pharm. Sci.* **63,** 1646.
Kramer, P. A., and Burnstein, T. (1976). *Life Sci.* **19,** 515.
Kulpa, C. F., and Tinghitella, T. J. (1976). *Life Sci.* **19,** 1879.
Ladbrooke, B. D., Williams, R. M., and Chapman, D. (1968). *Biochim. Biophys. Acta* **150,** 333.
Landis, E. M. (1927). *Am. J. Physiol.* **82,** 217.
Landis, E. M., and Papenheimer, J. R. (1963). *Handb. Physiol., Sect. 2:* p. 961.
Lawaczek, R., Kainosho, M., and Chan, S. I. (1976). *Biochim. Biophys. Acta* **443,** 313.
Levy, H. B., Law, L. W., and Rabson, A. S. (1969). *Proc. Natl. Acad. Sci. U.S.A.* **62,** 357.
Levy, R., Hurwitz, E., Maron, R., Arnon, R., and Sela, M. (1975). *Cancer Res.* **35,** 1182.
Lin, J.-Y., Tserng, K.-Y., Chen, C.-C., Lin, L.-T., and Tung, T.-C. (1970). *Nature (London)* **227,** 292.
Lohmann-Matthes, M.-L. (1976). *In* "Immunobiology of the Macrophage" (D. S. Nelson, ed.), p. 463. Academic Press, New York.
McDevitt, D. G., and Nies, A. S. (1976). *Cardiovasc. Res.* **10,** 494.
McDougall, L. R., Dunnick, J. K., McNamee, M. S., and Kriss, J. P. (1974). *Proc. Natl. Acad. Sci. U.S.A.* **71,** 3487.
Magee, W. E., Goff, C. W., Schoknecht, J., Smith, M. D., and Cherian, K. (1974). *J. Cell Biol.* **63,** 492.
Magee, W. E., Talcott, M. L., Straub, S. X., and Vriend, C. Y. (1976). *Biochim. Biophys. Acta* **451,** 610.
Majno, G. (1965). *Handb. Physiol., Sect. 2: Circulation,* p. 2293.
Malinin, G. I., Gregory, W. D., Morelli, L., Sharma, V. K., and Houck, J. C. (1976). *Science* **194,** 844.
Marchesi, V. T., Tillack, T. W., Jackson, R. L., Segrest, J. P., and Scott, R. E. (1972). *Proc. Natl. Acad. Sci. U.S.A.* **69,** 1445.
Marks, T. A., and Venditti, J. M. (1976). *Cancer Res.* **36,** 496.
Marsden, N. V. B., and Ostling, S. G. (1959). *Nature (London)* **184,** 723.
Martin, F. J., and MacDonald, R. C. (1976). *J. Cell Biol.* **70,** 515.
Martius, C., Ganser, R., and Viviani, A. (1975). *FEBS Lett.* **59,** 13.
Mason, N., Thies, C., and Cicero, T. J. (1976). *J. Pharm. Sci.* **65,** 847.
Matas, A. J., Sutherland, D. E. R., Steffes, M. W., Mauer, S. M., Lowe, A., Simmons, R. L., and Najarian, J. S. (1976). *Science* **192,** 892.
Mayhew, E., Papahadjopoulos, D., Rustum, Y. M., and Dane, C. (1976). *Cancer Res.* **36,** 4406.
Mayhew, E., Papahadjopoulos, D., Rustum, Y., and Dave, C. (1978). *In* "Liposomes and their Uses in Biology and Medicine" (D. Papahadjopoulos, ed.), p. 436. N.Y. Acad. Sci., New York.

Meyers, P. H., Cronic, F., and Nice, C. M. (1963). *Am. J. Roentgenol., Radium Ther. Nucl. Med.* [N.S.] **90,** 1068.
Mosso, J. A., and Rand, R. W. (1973). *Ann. Surg.* **178,** 663.
Nakamura, T., Konno, K., Morone, T., Tsuya, N., and Hatano, M. (1971). *J. Appl. Phys.* **42,** 1320.
Neerunjun, D. E., and Gregoriadis, G. (1974). *Biochem. Soc. Trans.* **2,** 868.
Neerunjun, E. D., and Gregoriadis, G. (1976). *Biochem. Soc. Trans.* **4,** 133.
Nicholls, P., and Miller, N. (1974). *Biochim. Biophys. Acta* **356,** 184.
Nicolson, G. L., Robbins, J. C., and Hyman, R. (1976). *J. Supramol. Struct.* **4,** 15.
Noronha-Blob, L., Vengris, V. E., Pitha, P. M., and Pitha, J. (1977). *J. Med. Chem.* **20,** 356.
Pagano, R. E., and Huang, L. (1975). *J. Cell Biol.* **67,** 49.
Palade, G. F. (1953). *J. Appl. Phys.* **24,** 1424.
Papahadjopoulos, D., and Vail, W. J. (1978). *In* "Liposomes and their Uses in Biology and Medicine" (D. Papahadjopoulos, ed.), p. 259. N.Y. Acad. Sci., New York.
Papahadjopoulos, D., Nir, S., and Ohki, S. (1971). *Biochim. Biophys. Acta* **266,** 561.
Papahadjopoulos, D., Jacobson, K., Nir, S., and Isac, T. (1973). *Biochim. Biophys. Acta* **311,** 330.
Papahadjopoulos, D., Poste, G., and Mayhew, E. (1974a). *Biochim. Biophys. Acta* **363,** 404.
Papahadjopoulos, D., Mayhew, E., Poste, G., Smith, S., and Vail, W. J. (1974b). *Nature (London)* **252,** 163.
Papahadjopoulos, D., Poste, G., Vail, W. J., and Biedler, J. L. (1976). *Cancer Res.* **36,** 2988.
Papanastassiou, A. B., Bruni, R. J., White, E., and Levins, P. L. (1966). *J. Med. Chem.* **9,** 725.
Pappenheimer, A. M., Jr. (1977). *Annu. Rev. Biochem.* **46,** 69.
Parker, B. M., Andersen, D. C., and Smith, J. R. (1958). *Proc. Soc. Exp. Biol. Med.* **98,** 306.
Petriev, V. M., Bochkova, T. R., Khachirov, D. G., and Seryi, S. V. (1976). *Med. Radiol.* **21,** 39.
Poste, G., and Papahadjopoulos, D. (1976). *Proc. Natl. Acad. Sci. U.S.A.* **73,** 1603.
Potchen, E. J., Elliott, A. J., Segal, B. A., Studer, R., and Evens, R. G. (1971). *J. Surg. Oncol.* **3,** 593.
Prinzmetal, M., Simkin, B., Bergman, H. C., and Kruger, H. E. (1947). *Am. Heart J.* **33,** 420.
Rahman, Y. E., and Wright, B. J. (1975). *J. Cell Biol.* **65,** 112.
Rahman, Y. E., Cerny, E. A., Tollaksen, S. L., Wright, B. J., Nanc, S. L., and Thomson, J. F. (1974). *Proc. Soc. Exp. Biol. Med.* **146,** 1173.
Rahman, Y. E., Kilieleski, W. E., Buess, E. M., and Cerny, E. A. (1975). *Eur. J. Cancer* **11,** 883.
Rand, R. W., and Mosso, J. A. (1972). *Bull. Los Angeles Neurol. Soc.* **37,** 67.
Reese, T. S., and Karnovsky, M. J. (1967). *J. Cell Biol.* **34,** 207.
Regelson, W., and Munson, A. E. (1970). *Ann. N.Y. Acad. Sci.* **173,** 831.
Rhodes, B. A., and Wagner, H. N., Jr. (1969). *J. Nucl. Med.* **10,** 432.
Rhodes, B. A., Zolle, I., Buchanan, J. W., and Wagner, H. N., Jr. (1969). *Radiology* **92,** 1453.
Rifkind, R. A. (1966). *Am. J. Med.* **41,** 711.
Ring, G. C., Blum, A. S., Kurbatov, T., Mass, W. G., and Smith, W. (1961). *Am. J. Physiol.* **200,** 1191.
Robbins, J. C., Hyman, R., Stallings, V., and Nicolson, G. L. (1977). *J. Natl. Cancer Inst.* **58,** 1027.
Roerdink, F. H., Van Renswoude, A. J. B. M., Wielinga, B. Y., Kron, A. M., and Scherphof, G. L. (1976). *J. Mol. Med.* **1,** 257.

Rowland, G. F., O'Neill, G. J., and Davies, D. A. L. (1975). *Nature* (*London*) **255,** 487.
Rutman, R. J., Ritter, C. A., Avadhani, N. G., and Hansel, J. (1976). *Cancer Treat. Rep.* **60,** 617.
Ryman, B. E., Jewkes, R. F., Jeyasingh, K., Osborne, M. P., Patel, H. M., Richardson, V. J., Tattersall, M. H. N., and Tyrrell, D. A. (1978). *In* "Liposomes and their Uses in Biology and Medicine" (D. Papahadjopoulos, ed.), p. 281. N.Y. Acad. Sci., New York.
Saba, T. M. (1970). *Arch. Intern. Med.* **126,** 1031.
Salky, N. K., DiLuzio, N. R., Levin, A. G., and Goldsmith, H. S. (1967). *J. Lab. Clin. Med.* **70,** 393.
Scheffel, U., Rhodes, B. A., Natarajan, T. K., and Wagner, H. N., Jr. (1972). *J. Nucl. Med.* **13,** 498.
Scheu, J. D., Sperandio, G. J., Shaw, S. M., Landolt, R. R., and Peck, G. E. (1977). *J. Pharm. Sci.* **66,** 172.
Schmidt, V., Zapol, W., Prensky, W., Wonders, T., Wodinsky, I., and Kits, R. (1972). *Trans. Am. Soc. Artif. Intern. Organs* **18,** 45.
Schwope, A. D., Wise, D. L., and Howes, J. F. (1976). *In* "Narcotic Antagonists: The Search for Long-Acting Preparations" (R. Willette, ed.), p. 13. Natl. Inst. Drug Abuse, Rockville, Maryland.
Segal, A. W., Wills, E. J., Richmond, J. E., Slavin, G., Black, C. D. V., and Gregoriadis, G. (1974). *Br. J. Exp. Pathol.* **55,** 320.
Segal, A. W., Gregoriadis, G., and Black, C. D. V. (1975). *Clin. Sci. Mol. Med.* **49,** 99.
Segal, A. W., Gregoriadis, G., Lavender, J. P., Tarin, D., and Peters, T. J. (1976). *Clin. Sci. Mol. Med.* **51,** 421.
Senyei, A. E., Widder, K. J., and Czerlinski, G. (1978). *J. Appl. Phys.* **49,** 3578.
Sheagren, J. N., Block, J. B., and Wolff, S. M. (1967). *J. Clin. Invest.* **46,** 855.
Shearer, W. T. (1977). *Fed. Proc., Fed. Am. Soc. Exp. Biol.* **36,** 1254.
Shearer, W. T., and Parker, C. W. (1975). *J. Immunol.* **115,** 613.
Shearer, W. T., Philpott, G. W., and Parker, C. W. (1973). *Science* **182,** 1357.
Shearer, W. T., Philpott, G. W., and Parker, C. W. (1974). *J. Exp. Med.* **139,** 367.
Shearer, W. T., Philpott, G. W., and Parker, C. W. (1975). *Cell. Immunol.* **17,** 447.
Shier, W. T., Trotter, J. T., and Astudillo, D. T. (1976). *Int. J. Cancer* **18,** 672.
Sidman, K. R., Arnold, D. L., Steber, W. D., Nelsen, L., Granchelli, F. E., Strong, P., and Sheth, S. G. (1976). *In* "Narcotic Antagonists: The Search for Long-Acting Preparations" (R. Willette, ed.), p. 33. Natl. Inst. Drug Abuse, Rockville, Maryland.
Sirsi, M., and Bucher, K. (1953). *Experientia* **9,** 217.
Snyderman, R., and Mergenhagen, S. E. (1976). *In* "Immunobiology of the Macrophage" (D. S. Nelson, ed.), p. 323. Academic Press, New York.
Stahl, E., Dietz, R., and Gross, F. (1977). *Specialia* p. 333.
Stern, W. H., and Ernest, J. T. (1974). *Am. J. Ophthalmol.* **78,** 438.
Straub, S. X., Garry, R. F., and Magee, W. E. (1974). *Infect. Immun.* **10,** 783.
Studer, R., and Potchen, J. (1971). *Microvasc. Res.* **3,** 35.
Sullivan, M. F., and Kalwarf, D. R. (1976). *In* "Narcotic Antagonists: The Search for Long-Acting Preparations" (R. Willette, ed.), p. 27. Natl. Inst. Drug Abuse, Rockville, Maryland.
Szekerke, M., and Driscoll, J. S. (1977). *Eur. J. Cancer* **13,** 529.
Szekerke, M., Wade, R., and Whisson, M. E. (1972a). *Neoplasma* **19,** 199.
Szekerke, M., Wade, R., and Whisson, M. E. (1972b). *Neoplasma* **19,** 211.
Szymendera, J., Mioduszewska, O., Licinska, I., Czarnomska, A., and Lucka, B. (1977). *J. Nucl. Med.* **18,** 478.

Tanaka, T., Taneda, K., Kobayashi, H., Okumura, K., Muranishi, S., and Sezaki, H. (1975). *Chem. Pharm. Bull.* **23,** 3069.

Taplin, G. V., Johnson, D. E., Dore, E. K., and Kaplan, H. S. (1964). *J. Nucl. Med.* **5,** 259.

Tevethia, S. S., Zarling, J. M., and Flax, M. H. (1976). *In* "Immunobiology of the Macrophage" (D. S. Nelson, ed.), p. 509. Academic Press, New York.

Tillander, H. (1951). *Acta Radiol.* **35,** 62.

Tillander, H. (1956). *Acta Radiol.* **45,** 21.

Tillander, H. (1970). *IEEE Trans. Magn.* **mag-6,** 355.

Trouet, A., Deprez-de Campeneere, D., and de Duve, C. (1972). *Nature (London), New Biol.* **239,** 110.

Trouet A., Deprez-de Campeneere, D., de Smedt-Malengreaux, M., and Atassi, G. (1974). *Eur. J. Cancer* **10,** 405.

Tsou, K. C., Damle, S. B., Crichlow, R. W., Ravdin, R. G., and Blunt, H. W. (1967). *J. Pharm. Sci.* **56,** 484.

Tsujii, K., Sunamoto, J., and Fendler, J. H. (1976). *Life Sci.* **19,** 1743.

Turner, R. D., Rand, R. W., Bentson, J. R., and Mosso, J. A. (1975). *J. Urol.* **113,** 455.

Tyrrell, D. A., and Ryman, B. E. (1976). *Biochem. Soc. Trans.* **4,** 677.

Tyrrell, D. A., Richardson, V. J., and Ryman, B. E. (1977). *Biochim. Biophys. Acta* **497,** 469.

Utley, J., Carlson, E. L., Hoffman, J. I. E., Martinez, H. M., and Buckberg, G. D. (1974). *Circ. Res.* **34,** 391.

Wagner, H. N., Jr., Lio, M., and Hornick, R. B. (1963). *J. Clin. Invest.* **42,** 427.

Wagner, H. N., Jr., Jones, E., Tow, D. E., and Langan, J. K. (1965). *J. Nucl. Med.* **6,** 150.

Wagner, H. N., Jr., Stern, H. S., Rhodes, B. A., Reba, R. C., Hosain, R., and Zolle, I. (1969a). *Med. Radioisot. Scintigr. Proc. Symp., 1968* Vol. 2.

Wagner, H. N., Jr., Rhodes, B. A., Sasaki, Y., and Ryan, J. P. (1969b). *Inv. Radiol.* **48,** 374.

Warren, D. J., and Ledingham, J. G. G. (1974). *Cardiovasc. Res.* **8,** 570.

Warren, D. J., and Ledingham, J. G. G. (1975). *Clin. Sci. Mol. Med.* **48,** 51.

Weissmann, G., Bloomgarden, D., Kaplan, R., Cohen, C., Hoffstein, S., Collins, T., Gotlieb, A., and Nagle, D. (1975). *Proc. Natl. Acad. Sci. U.S.A.* **72,** 88.

Widder, K. J., Senyei, A. E., and Scarpelli, D. G. (1978a). *Proc. Soc. Exp. Biol. Med.* **158,** 141.

Widder, K. J., Senyei, A. E., Reich, S. D., and Ranney, D. F. (1978b). *Proc. Am. Assoc. Cancer Res.* **19,** 17.

Widder, K. J., Senyei, A. E., and Flouret, G. (1979). *J. Pharm. Sci.* **68,** 79.

Wisse, E. (1970). *J. Ultrastruct. Res.* **31,** 125.

Wisse, E., and Gregoriadis, G. (1975). *Res, J. Reticuloendothel. Soc.* **18,** 10a.

Woodruff, J. J. (1974). *Cell. Immunol.* **13,** 378.

Yesair, D. W., Bittman, L., and Schwartzbach, E. (1974). *Proc. Am. Assoc. Cancer Res.* p. 72 (Abstr. No. 285).

Zimmermann, U., Pilwat, G., and Riemann, F. (1975). *Biochim. Biophys. Acta* **375,** 209.

Zimmermann, U., Riemann, F., and Pilwat, G. (1976). *Biochim. Biophys. Acta* **436,** 460.

Zimmermann, U., Pilwat, G., and Esser, B. (1978). *J. Clin. Chem. Clin. Biochem.* **16,** 135.

Zolle, I., Rhodes, B. A., and Wagner, H. N., Jr. (1970). *Int. J. Appl. Radiat. Isot.* **21,** 155.

Zweifach, B. W., and Intaglietta, M. (1968). *Microvasc. Res.* **1,** 83.

cis-Diamminedichloroplatinum(II): A Metal Complex with Significant Anticancer Activity

DANIEL D. VON HOFF* AND MARCEL ROZENCWEIG†

National Cancer Institute
Bethesda, Maryland

I.	Introduction	273
II.	Discovery	274
III.	Chemical and Physiochemical Properties	274
	A. Pharmaceutical Data	275
IV.	Biological Properties	275
	A. Antimicrobial Activity	275
	B. Antiviral Activity	276
	C. Cytotoxic and Antineoplastic Activity	276
	D. Mutagenicity	276
	E. Immunosuppressive Properties	276
	F. Radiosensitizer Properties	276
V.	Mechanism of Action	277
VI.	Experimental Antitumor Activity	277
	A. Antitumor Activity Alone	277
	B. DDP Plus Other Agents	278
	C. DDP Analogs	279
VII.	Animal Toxicity	279
VIII.	Drug Metabolism and Distribution	281
	A. Studies in Animal Systems	281
	B. Studies in Man	282
IX.	Clinical Studies	282
	A. Phase I Studies	283
	B. Antineoplastic Activity by Tumor Type	284
	C. Toxicity in Man	290
X.	Summary and Conclusions	293
	References	294

I. Introduction

The Division of Cancer Treatment of the National Cancer Institute has sponsored clinical trials with *cis*-diamminedichloroplatinum(II) (DDP) since 1971. In the beginning, DDP was not considered clinically useful largely because of severe nausea and vomiting and dose-limiting renal

* Clinical associate, Pediatric Oncology Branch and Medicine Branch Division of Cancer Treatment.

† Special assistant, Office of Associate Director, Cancer Therapy Evaluation Program.

ISBN 0-12-032916-6

toxicity. However, recent developments have made the clinical use of platinum safer, and clinical trials with this agent have burgeoned.

The impressive antitumor activity of DDP against testicular, ovarian, and head and neck cancer makes the compound an extremely exciting prospect for future investigations. The purpose of this review will be to document the preclinical and clinical information now available. This information will lead to a number of suggestions for future clinical and preclinical investigations.

II. Discovery

In 1965, Rosenberg, Van Camp, and Krigas were investigating the effects of electrical fields on the growth processes of *Escherichia coli*. They noted that electrical current delivered between platinum electrodes did indeed inhibit growth of *E. coli*. However, they discovered that the growth inhibition was due to a variety of platinum-containing compounds released by the platinum electrodes rather than to the electrical field per se. These platinum-containing compounds were complexes of platinum, ammonium groups, and chlorine atoms (Rosenberg *et al.*, 1967a). Several of the platinum-containing complexes were tested in animal tumor systems and DDP was selected as having the best experimental antitumor activity (Rosenberg *et al.*, 1969; Rosenberg, 1973).

III. Chemical and Physiochemical Properties

cis-Diamminedichloroplatinum(II) has the empirical formula $PtCl_2H_6N_2$. Structurally, DDP is a complex formed by a central atom of platinum surrounded by chlorine atoms and ammonia groups in a cis relationship (Fig. 1). The chemical properties necessary for identifying the compound are listed in Table I (Rosenberg, 1973, 1975).

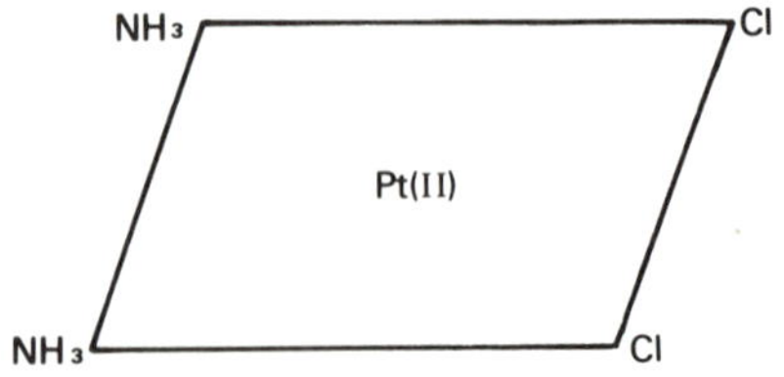

FIG. 1. *cis*-Diamminedichloroplatinum(II).

TABLE I

CHEMICAL PROPERTIES OF *cis*-DIAMMINEDICHLOROPLATINUM(II)

Description
Orange-yellow solid; melting point 207°C; molecular weight = 300.1.

Solubility
Water, 1 mg/ml; dimethylformamide (pure anhydrous), 24 mg/ml.

Ultraviolet absorption (0.8 mg/ml, 0.1 *N* HCl)
(Solution centrifuged before absorption measured)
max = 301 1 nm; *E* = 130 2 nm
min = 246 nm

Paper chromatography
Paper: Whatman No. 3 MM
Quantity spotted: 100r from DMF
Solvent systems: acetone/water, 9:1; acetone/water, 7:3
Detection: 1% $SnCl_2$ in 0.1 *N* HCl, freshly prepared

A. PHARMACEUTICAL DATA

Drug DDP will soon become a commercially available agent for use in specific circumstances. At the time of this writing the drug is available only to qualified oncologists through the Investigational Drug Branch of the National Cancer Institute. Two vial sizes are currently available: the 10-mg and the 25-mg vials. In the 10 mg size, DDP is supplied as a white lyophilized powder in a vial containing 10 mg of DDP, 90 mg of sodium chloride, 100 mg of mannitol (U.S.P.), and hydrochloric acid for pH adjustment. When the vial is reconstituted with 10 ml of sterile water for injection (U.S.P.) each milliliter of the resulting solution will contain 1 mg of DDP, 10 mg of mannitol (U.S.P.), and 9 mg of sodium chloride with a pH range of 3.5–4.5.

The intact vials are stable for at least 1 year when stored at refrigerated temperature (4°–8°C). The stability of the reconstituted solutions or solutions diluted further for clinical use is still somewhat controversial. At 22°C the reconstituted solution is stable for at least 8 hours.

IV. Biological Properties

A. ANTIMICROBIAL ACTIVITY

Rosenberg *et al.* (1965) discovered that platinum complexes present in low concentrations in nutrient medium could inhibit cell division of *E. coli* and cause the development of long filaments.

Further work by Howle and Gale (1970b), on a subcellular level revealed that *E. coli,* incubated in the presence of low concentrations of DDP, lost the ability to divide but retained the ability to grow along the long axis. Failure of cell division in the presence of an unimpeded growth rate further suggested that selective inhibition of DNA may occur with no appreciable action on RNA or protein synthesis.

Other investigators have also worked on the antimicrobial effects of DDP (Drobnik *et al.,* 1973; Rosenberg *et al.,* 1967a,b).

B. Antiviral Activity

cis-diamminedichloroplatinum(II) has been shown to inactivate papovavirus SV40 (Kutinova *et al.,* 1972).

C. Cytotoxic and Antineoplastic Activity

Drewinko and Gottlieb (1975) demonstrated that DDP kills human lymphoma cells in culture. It has a wide range of activity in a number of experimental tumor systems but these will be dealt with in detail in Section VI.

D. Mutagenicity

Beck and Brubaker (1975) demonstrated the mutagenic properties of DDP in *E. coli.*

E. Immunosuppressive Properties

A number of investigators have demonstrated DDP to be immunosuppressive in a variety of systems (Berenbaum, 1971) including suppression of graft-versus-host reactions (Khan and Hill, 1972b; Munster *et al.,* 1974), an effect on antibody plaque-forming spleen cells (Khan and Hill, 1971), an effect on the allograft reaction in mice (Brambilla *et al.,* 1974), an effect of skin grafts in mice (Khan *et al.,* 1972), and inhibition of lymphocyte blastogenesis in man (Khan and Hill, 1972a). This immunosuppressive effect of the drug is puzzling in light of the serious anaphylactic reactions seen when the drug is used clinically (von Hoff *et al.,* 1976).

F. Radiosensitizer Properties

A number of investigators have shown that DDP can act as a radiosensitizer (Merker *et al.,* 1977; Richmond and Powers, 1977; Douple *et al.,* 1977).

V. Mechanism of Action

The precise mechanism of action of DDP is not known. One well-established point is that DDP causes a primary lesion on cellular DNA (Rosenberg, 1977).

Howle and Gale (1970a) demonstrated that when a single intraperitoneal injection of DDP (10 mg/kg) was given to mice previously inoculated with Ehrlich ascites tumor cells, the patterns of subsequent synthesis of DNA, RNA, and protein measured *in vitro* were markedly different. Initially, there was a marked impairment of all three species but the inhibitory effect on the incorporation of thymidine into DNA persisted for 96 hours. These data were interpreted as indicating a selective inhibition by DDP of DNA *in vivo*.

Harder and Rosenberg (1970) utilized human amnion AV_3 cells and also measured the incorporation of labeled precursors of DNA, RNA, and protein synthesis in the presence and absence of DDP. They found that at lower concentrations *in vitro*, the complex selectively inhibited DNA synthesis (below $5 \mu M$), whereas at higher concentrations DDP extended its effective inhibition to RNA and protein synthesis as well.

From the foregoing information there has emerged a substantial volume of work on the mode of interaction of DDP with DNA. The chemical structure of DDP with the two labile chlorine atoms in the cis position is reminiscent of the mustard-type bifunctional alkylating agents. Roberts and Pascoe (1972) have shown that DDP does cross-link the complementary strands of DNA in HeLa cells, and other investigators have confirmed this interaction, including interstrand cross-linking, intrastrand cross-linking, and mono- and bifunctional attacks on the bases, particularly the purines (Mansey *et al.*, 1973; Munchausen and Rahn, 1975; Munchausen, 1974; Zwelling *et al.*, 1978).

Stone *et al.* (1974) have shown that there is a preferential attachment of DDP to G—C rich regions of the DNA. Interactions and reactions with the phosphate sugar chain are less likely reactions (Rosenberg, 1977).

VI. Experimental Antitumor Activity

A. Antitumor Activity Alone

cis-Diamminedichloroplatinum(II) has exhibited considerable experimental antitumor activity in a variety of tumor systems.

Rosenberg and colleagues (1969) reported the activity of DDP against L1210 mouse leukemia and sarcoma 180. Table II details the activity of DDP in the L1210 system in both the daily and intermittent schedules

TABLE II

cis-DIAMMINEDICHLOROPLATINUM(II) ACTIVITY AGAINST ASCITIC L1210 LEUKEMIA IN MICE AT VARIOUS DOSES AND DOSE SCHEDULES

Route[a]	Schedule[b]	Dose range (mg/kg/day)	Optimal dose (mg/kg/day)	Maximum ILS%[c]
IP	Day 1	2–16	16	55
IP	Q3H, day 1	0.5–4.0	2	78
IP	Days 1, 5, 9	1–8	8	78
IP	Q3H, days 1, 5, 9	0.125–1.0	1	111
IP	Days 1–5	0.5–4.0	4	78
IP	Days 1–9	0.5–4.0	2	78
PO	Days 1–9	2–16	8	28

[a] IP, intraperitoneal; PO, oral.

[b] Q3H, every 3 hours.

[c] Percent increase in life-span of treated L1210-bearing mice over that of untreated L1210-bearing mice.

(data from the Drug Research and Development Program, Division of Cancer Treatment, NCI). As can be appreciated from Table II, the compound shows a significant degree of activity over a variety of dosage schedules when given intraperitoneally. The drug has no activity in L1210 mouse leukemia when given orally. Judging from the L1210 system data, the drug is not schedule dependent.

Further investigations have shown activity in several experimental tumors, as noted in Table III, including several transplantable animal tumors, chemically induced primary tumors, and viral induced sarcoma (see references in Table III).

However, DDP failed to give responses in Walker 256 carcinosarcoma resistant to alkylating agents (Rosenberg, 1973).

B. DDP Plus Other Agents

DDP has been studied in combination with a number of other chemotherapeutic agents in the L1210 system. Sirica and colleagues (1971) reported synergism of cyclophosphamide and platinum combinations. Synergism with Iphosphamide was noted by Woodman and co-workers (1973), who also had reported synergy of ICRF-159 with DDP (Woodman *et al.*, 1971).

Some evidence of synergism of DDP with phosphoramide mustard, DIC (NSC 82196), cytosine arabinoside, hydroxyurea, 5-azacytidine, 6-thioguanine, vincristine, vinblastine, camptothecin, bleomycin, and emetine has been reported (Woodman *et al.*, 1973; Speer *et al.*, 1971; Merker *et al.*, 1977).

TABLE III

EXPERIMENTAL ANIMAL TUMOR SYSTEMS IN WHICH *cis*-DIAMMINEDICHLOROPLATINUM(II) IS ACTIVE

Type of tumor	Reference[a]
Transplantable animal tumors	
Lewis lung carcinoma	1
P388 leukemia	1
B16 melanoma	1
Ehrlich ascites tumor	1
Dunning ascitic leukemia	2
Walker 256 carcinosarcoma	2
Ependymoblastoma	3
Chemically induced primary tumors	
7,12-Dimethylbenzanthracene (DMBA)-induced rat mammary	4
N-(4-(5-Nitro-2-furyl)-2-thiazolyl) formamide (FANFT)-induced murine bladder cancer	5
Virally induced tumors	
Rous sarcoma	1

[a] Key to references: 1—Rosenberg (1973); 2—Kociba *et al.* (1970); 3—Geran *et al.* (1974); 4—Welsch (1971); 5—Soloway *et al.* (1974).

C. DDP ANALOGS

Merker and co-workers (1977) recently reviewed experimental antitumor activity of about 200 analogs of DDP. There were several compounds that have high antitumor activity against P388 leukemia but the therapeutic indices were not superior to the parent compound.

VII. Animal Toxicity

There are published reports of animal toxicity studies with DDP in dogs and monkeys. Table IV exhibits the essential quantitative toxicity information with the dog being the most sensitive large animal species (Schaeppi *et al.,* 1973).

The qualitative toxicity of DDP showed the kidney to be the principal target for the toxic actions of DDP. Dogs developed renal failure with azotemia, proteinuria, hypochloruria, and hypocalcemia. Dogs and monkeys experienced different histological changes; that is, there was acute tubular necrosis in dogs and interstitial nephritis in the monkeys (Schaeppi *et al.,* 1973).

A number of "protective" regimens have been devised to limit the heavy metal-like effect of DDP on the kidneys. Penicillamine was investi-

TABLE IV

cis-DIAMMINEDICHLOROPLATINUM(II) TOXICITY DATA IN BEAGLE DOG AND RHESUS MONKEY

	Dog				Monkey	
	Single dose		Daily, i.v. × 5		Daily, i.v. × 5	
Dose[a]	(mg/kg)	(mg/m^2)	(mg/kg)	(mg/m^2)	(mg/kg)	(mg/m^2)
HNTD	0.625	13.2	0.1875	3.87	0.156	1.94
TDL	1.25	22.5	0.375	7.75	0.313	8.0
TDH	2.5	47.3	0.75	14.9	1.25	15.9
LD	5.0	105.7	1.5	31.1	2.5	33.6

[a] *Highest nontoxic dose* (*HNTD*): The highest dose at which no hematological, chemical, clinical or pathological drug-induced alterations occurred; doubling this dose produces the aforementioned alterations.

Toxic dose low (*TDL*): The lowest dose to produce drug-induced pathological alterations in hematological, chemical, clinical, or morphological parameters; doubling this dose produces no lethality.

Toxic dose, high (*TDH*): The lowest dose to produce drug-induced pathological alterations in hematological, chemical, clinical, or morphological parameters; doubling this dose produces lethality.

Lethal dose (*LD*): The lowest dose to produce drug-induced death in any animals during the treatment or observation period.

gated by Higby and colleagues (1975), and Cvitkovic *et al.* (1977) employed with some success hydration and hydration plus mannitol to decrease the nephrotoxicity of DDP in dogs. Ward and co-workers (1977) demonstrated that furosemide diminished DDP toxicity in rats. Pera and Harder (1978) found furosemide pretreatment of rats gave higher kidney levels of DDP than did mannitol pretreatment or no pretreatment of the rats.

Very high doses of DDP produced prompt and severe emesis and diarrhea in both the dog and the monkey with the pathological correlate of these clinical signs consisting of a severe enterocolitis (Schaeppi *et al.*, 1973).

Additional toxicities of note include destruction of circulating lymphocytes and lymphoid atrophy, atrophy of the testes, prostate, and salivary glands as well as pancreatitis and myocarditis. Severe hypoplasia of the bone marrow was produced by high doses of the drug in both beagles and monkeys (Schaeppi *et al.*, 1973).

Despite occasional elevations of serum transaminases, no histopathology of the liver was induced in dogs or monkeys. No neurotoxicity has been noted in animals with the exception of a transient loss of hearing in monkeys receiving the drug (Schaeppi *et al.*, 1973). DDP has been shown to destroy hair cells of the organ of Corti of the rhesus monkey at a different site than that shown with another ototoxin, neomycin sulfate (Stadnicki *et al.*, 1975).

VIII. Drug Metabolism and Distribution

A. Studies in Animal Systems

In a study using radiolabeled platinum in tumored and nontumored mice, the highest concentrations of radioactivity were noted in the kidneys, liver, and spleen with the lowest uptake in the brain (Haeschelle and Van Camp, 1972; Lange *et al.*, 1972; 1973). Additional studies by Wolf and Manaka (1977) using ^{195m}Pt showed the skin of rats to be a major organ of DDP uptake. Although they found the concentration per gram of tissue was low for skin, muscle, and bone, these tissues took up a significant amount of the administered dose by virtue of their large organ/body mass ratios.

Litterst and colleagues (1976) examined the distribution and disposition of DDP following intravenous administration to beagle dogs. Plasma levels of DDP (as determined by atomic absorption spectrometry) demonstrated a biphasic clearance pattern with a rapid phase $T_{1/2}$ of less than 1 hour and a slow phase $T_{1/2}$ of nearly 5 days. Four hours after treatment, plasma levels fell by 90%, whereas 60–70% of the administered dose was recovered in the urine. They found DDP concentration to be highest in kidneys and liver, gonads, spleen, and adrenals. However of greatest interest was that platinum levels remained elevated in kidney, liver, ovary, and uterus for as long as 6 days post treatment. This information is of interest in the light of the clinical activity of DDP in ovarian cancer.

Circumstantial *in vitro* evidence of Litterst *et al.* (1977) suggests that DDP is highly protein bound, thus explaining its long second half-life.

Litterst and co-workers (1977) performed elegant comparative studies on pharmacokinetics in the rat, dogfish shark, and the beagle dog. After a single intravenous dose, the plasms concentration exhibited a biphasic decay with the short $T_{1/2}$ ranging from 20 minutes in the dog to 60 minutes in the shark, and the long $T_{1/2}$ from 2 days in the rat to 10 days in the shark. They noted the dog cleared the drug the fastest and the shark the slowest with 80% of the dose administered appearing in dog urine after 48 hours but only 10% of the dose appearing in shark urine after 6 days. In the rat the liver, kidneys and uterus contained large concentrations of platinum but not the testes. The shark displayed similar concentrations of DDP except that shark liver contained very little DDP.

B. Studies in Man

A number of pharmacokinetic studies in man have characterized the distribution and excretion of labeled DDP after a single intravenous dose. DeConti *et al.* (1973) showed plasma levels of radioactivity decayed in a biphasic manner with an initial plasma $T_{1/2}$ of 25–49 minutes and a second plasma $T_{1/2}$ of 58–73 hours. They found that more than 90% of the drug was protein bound during the excretion phase. Urinary excretion of the administered radioactivity was incomplete with only 27–45% of the radioactivity excreted in the first 5 days. It is unknown whether biliary excretion takes place in man. Piel and co-workers (1974) have shown that by the neutron activation analysis technique, platinum may still be detectable in tissue samples for as long as 4 months after administration.

Distribution data in man utilizing both nuclear medicine scans and analysis of autopsy material show high uptake of DDP in the kidneys (Hill *et al.*, 1975; Lange *et al.*, 1973), liver (Hill *et al.*, 1975; Lange *et al.*, 1973; Smith and Taylor, 1974), and intestine (Hill *et al.*, 1975; Smith and Taylor, 1974). Brain scans and tissue samples suggest poor penetration of the drug into the central nervous systems (Hill *et al.*, 1975; Lange *et al.*, 1973).

Hall and co-workers (1978) have investigated the pharmacokinetics of a continuous infusion of DDP (20 mg/m^2 daily for 5 days) after a loading dose of 5 mg/m^2. Plasma DDP concentrations ranged from 0.5–4.3 μg/ml during the infusion; DDP terminal plasma half-life ranged from 17.3 to 34.7 hours in patients with normal renal function. Mean cumulative urinary excretion of DDP was 34% of the administered dose in 8 days.

IX. Clinical Studies

Initial clinical studies with DDP began in 1971. Since the time of those studies, a tremendous number of clinical trials have emerged even though initially DDP was not a popular compound because of severe nausea, vomiting, and renal toxicity. Rozencweig and colleagues (1977) summarized the clinical information of DDP up until 1977. The following will be an all-inclusive update of that information.

In this section when discussing response rates the following terminology will apply. Partial remission (PR) denotes a greater than 50% measurable decrease in tumor area; lasting a minimum of 1 month or the occurrence of an M_2 marrow (5–25% blasts) in the case of leukemias. Complete remission (CR) denotes complete disappearance of measurable disease or an M_1 marrow (less than 5% blasts) lasting a minimum of 1 month.

A. Phase I Studies

Phase I involves toxicology studies designed to determine the maximum dose of drug tolerated by man.

In the early clinical trials, DDP was administered by a rapid intravenous infusion with a variety of dose schedules including biweekly, weekly, daily for 3 days, daily for 5 days, daily to tolerance, and continuous intravenous infusion for 5 days (see Table V). Two of the schedules most commonly used are 15–20 mg/m^2 daily for 5 days every 3–4 week schedules and 50–75 mg/m^2 once every 3 weeks.

In the early phase I trials, nausea and vomiting were severe, myelosuppression was minimal and transient, and renal functional impairment and ototoxicity were the significant dose-limiting toxicities (Higby *et al.*, 1973;

TABLE V

Phases I–II Studies with Various Dose Schedules of *cis*-Diamminedichloroplatinum(II)[a]

Dose schedule	Dose (mg/m^2)	No. treated patients	Reference[c]
Intermittent			1, 2, 3, 4, 5, 6
Biweekly ×6, then weekly	37[b]	5	7
Weekly	37–50	12	7, 8, 9
Every 2–3 weeks	30	22	10
Every 3 weeks	50–75	90	11, 12
Every 5 weeks	50	32	13
Daily			
Daily ×3, every 4 weeks	30	15	2, 3, 4, 10
Daily ×5, every 3–4 weeks	15–20	144	8, 9, 14, 15, 16
Various			
Daily to total dose of 46–259 mg/m^2	9–74[b]	26	17
Over 14 days, every 4 weeks	74–148[b]	86	18
Continuous infusion for 5 days	20	35	19

[a] Adapted from Rozencweig *et al.* (1977).

[b] Doses originally expressed in milligrams per kilogram body weight and converted to milligrams per square meter body surface area by a conversion factor of 37.

[c] Key to references: 1—DeConti *et al.* (1973); 2—Higby *et al.* (1973); 3—Rossof *et al.* (1972); 4—Talley *et al.* (1973); 5—Hayes *et al.* (1976); 6—Hayes *et al.* (1977); 7—Merrin (1976); 8—Higby *et al.* (1974); 9—Kamlaker *et al.* (1976); 10—Wiltshaw and Kroner (1976); 11—Bruckner *et al.* (1976); 12—Yagoda *et al.* (1976); 13—Kovach *et al.* (1973); 14—Nitschke *et al.* (1976); 15—Osieka *et al.* (1976); 16—Tekuzman *et al.* (1976); 17—Lippman *et al.* (1973); 18—Loeb *et al.* (1975); 19—Hall *et al.* (1978).

Lippman *et al.*, 1973; Rossof *et al.*, 1972; Talley *et al.*, 1973). These toxicities will be discussed in greater detail in Section IX,C.

It is unclear whether there are any advantages in terms of therapeutic index to any of the schedules noted in Table V. At this point in time there is no proven distinct advantage of one schedule over another.

Because of the severe nephrotoxicity associated with the early phase I clinical trials a number of methods have been introduced to alleviate the DDP-induced nephrotoxicity. These include continuous infusion of the drug (Hall *et al.*, 1978), intravenous hydration (Hill *et al.*, 1975; Piel and Perlia, 1975), and penicillamine (Higby *et al.*, 1975). The most exciting prophylactic measure was reported by Hayes *et al.* (1976, 1977) and by Merrin (1976). They noted an improved therapeutic index when DDP was given with intravenous fluid and a mannitol infusion with or without furosemide. With this method, higher doses of DDP could be administered (Hayes *et al.*, 1976, 1977). However, it is as yet unclear whether the higher-dose platinum is more effective than conventional doses of the drug.

B. Antineoplastic Activity by Tumor Type

1. *Testicular Cancer*

DDP has exhibited remarkable activity in nonseminomatous testicular tumors. Results of the use of DDP as a single agent, even in previously treated patients, have been quite impressive. Table VI shows that the response rate in individual series varies from 40–90% with a cumula-

TABLE VI

Single-Agent Activity of *cis*-Diamminedichloroplatinum(II) in Nonseminomatous Testicular Cancer

No. of evaluable patients	No. of remissions		Overall response rate (%)	Reference[a]
	Complete	Partial		
10	6	3	90	1
22	1	14	68	2
15	7	3	66	3
22	1	8	40	4
19	1	9	53	5–9
Total 88	16	37	60	

[a] Key to references: 1—Merrin (1976); 2—Osieka *et al.* (1976); 3—Higby *et al.* (1974); 4—Rossof *et al.* (1977); 5—Nitschke *et al.* (1976); 6—Hayes *et al.* (1977); 7—Chary *et al.* (1977); 8—Wiltshaw (1977); 9—Corder *et al.* (1977).

tive overall response rate of 60%. However, responses have generally been of short duration, none exceeding 1 year. There are insufficient data to determine the single-agent activity of DDP in the various histological subtypes of testicular cancer.

With an overall response rate of 60%, DDP is now recognized as one of the most active drugs in testicular cancer, and it therefore has been incorporated into combinations with other chemotherapeutic agents with remarkably good results. Table VII details the various combinations regimens investigated.

The basis for the active testicular cancer combinations is the vinblastine + bleomycin combination reported by Samuels and colleagues (1975a,b). Response rates with vinblastine + bleomycin have been reported as high as 76%. Einhorn *et al.* (1976) and Einhorn and Donahue (1977a) noted particularly good results when adding DDP to vinblastine + bleomycin: of 20 patients treated, 15 achieved a complete remission and 5 achieved a partial remission. In 7 of the patients the duration of remission exceeded 1 year and 2 partial responders had surgical removal of residual disease rendering them disease-free. The toxicity of the regimen was considerable, with 4 episodes of gram negative sepsis secondary to leukopenia and 1 septic death. These investigators recently updated their results (Einhorn and Donohue, 1977b) and in 47 evaluable patients

TABLE VII

cis-DIAMMINEDICHLOROPLATINUM(II) IN COMBINATION REGIMENS FOR TESTICULAR CANCER

Drug combination[a]	No. of evaluable patients	No. of remissions		Overall response rate (%)	Reference[b]
		Complete	Partial		
VLB–BLM	84	30	34	76	1, 2, 3
VLB–BLM–DDP	47	35	12	100	4
VLB–BLM–ACD	50	7	9	32	5
VLB–BLM–ACD–DDP	24	7	12	79	6
VLB–BLM–ACD–DDP–CTX	26	18	6	92	7
DDP–BLM	14	0	11	79	8
DDP–CTX	1	0	1	100	9
DDP–ADR	18	3	11	78	10, 11, 12

[a] ADR (adriamycin); BLM (bleomycin); CTX (cyclophosphamide); VLB (vinblastine); ACD (actinomycin-D).

[b] Key to reference: 1—Spiegel and Coltman (1974); 2—Samuels *et al.* (1975a); 3—Samuels *et al.* (1975b); 4—Einhorn and Donahue (1977a,b); 5—Wittes *et al.* (1976b); 6—Cvitkovic *et al.* (1975a); 7—Cvitkovic *et al.* (1976); 8—Cvitkovic *et al.* (1975b); 9—Piel and Perlia (1975); 10—Vogl *et al.* (1976); 11—Wallace *et al.* (1975); 12—Einhorn and Williams (1978).

they have reported a 72% complete remission rate and a 28% partial remission rate.

A recent Southwest Oncology Group study, reported by Samson and Stephens (1978), demonstrated a 56% complete and a 30% partial remission rate with the three-drug combination of vinblasting + bleomycin + DDP, thus demonstrating an excellent response rate in a cooperative group setting.

The Memorial Sloan Kettering Cancer Center has performed a series of clinical trials in testicular cancer using vinblastine + actinomycin D + bleomycin (the VAB regimen) with a 32% overall response rate (Wittes *et al.*, 1976b). They increased this response rate to 79% by adding DDP (the VAB II regimen; Cvitkovic *et al.*, 1975a). The VAB III regimen, which has recently been instituted, uses high-dose DDP (120 mg/m^2) and cyclophosphamide induction with a 92% overall response rate (Cvitkovic *et al.*, 1976). Bone marrow toxicity was acceptable with the VAB III regimen, and there have not been deaths secondary to leukopenia. Table VII also lists other DDP-containing regimens used in testicular cancer but the number of patients on each of these regimens is small.

2. *Ovarian Cancer*

Drug DDP has been used extensively and successfully for the treatment of advanced ovarian cancer. Table VIII details the single-agent activity of DDP in ovarian cancer with response rates varying from 13 to 26%. Wiltshaw and Kroner (1976) used both a low-dose intermittent 30-mg/m^2 and a 30-mg/m^2, daily for 3 days, dose of DDP. The low-dose schedule was less toxic, but they claimed similar antitumor effect. Remissions in patients with advanced disease have lasted from 3–15 months. Responses secondary to DDP are particularly impressive in that they occurred in patients who had become refractory to alkylating agents.

With the known single-agent activity of DDP, a number of combination regimens have emerged, as listed in Table VIII. However none have as yet been shown to be superior to DDP alone by a controlled prospectively randomized study. Nevertheless, preliminary results with these combinations look promising.

3. *Bladder Cancer*

A number of reports have documented the response rate of bladder cancer to DDP to be 33–60% (Yagoda *et al.*, 1976; Rossof *et al.*, 1977; Hayes *et al.*, 1977; Wallace and Higby, 1974; Soloway, 1978). This is an impressive response rate although in one trial all the responders had no prior chemotherapy (Yagoda *et al.*, 1976). Further work with DDP in combina-

TABLE VIII

cis-DIAMMINEDICHLOROPLATINUM(II) ALONE AND IN COMBINATION REGIMENS FOR OVARIAN CANCER

Drug(s)[a]	No. of evaluable patients	No. of remissions	Overall response rate (%)	Reference[b]
DDP	34	9	26	1
DDP	15	2	13	2
DDP	20	5	25	3, 4
DDP	20	5	25	5
DDP + ADR	42	21	50	6, 10
DDP + HMM	5	4	80	9
DDP + HMM + ADR	12	6	50	9
DDP + ADR + CTX + HMM	33	19	58	7, 8[c]
DDP + ADR + CTX	29	21	72	11
DDP + HMM + CTX + 5FU	—	—	—	[d]
DDP + CHL	—	—	—	[d]

[a] ADR (adriamycin); CTX (cyclophosphamide); HMM (hexamethylomelamine); 5FU (5-fluorouracil); CHL (chlorambucil).

[b] Key to references: 1—Wiltshaw and Kroner (1976); 2—Rossof *et al.* (1977); 3—Hayes *et al.* (1977); 4—Catane *et al.* (1977); 5—Bull *et al.* (1978); 6—Bruckner *et al.* (1977); 7—Vogl *et al.* (1978); 8—Kane *et al.* (1978); 9—Greenwald *et al.* (1978); 10—Briscoe *et al.* (1978); 11—Ehrlich *et al.* (1978).

[c] Includes both previously treated and previously untreated patients.

[d] Ongoing study.

tions for bladder cancer is proceeding (Troner and Hemstreet, 1978; Williams *et al.*, 1978).

4. *Head and Neck Cancer*

The activity of DDP alone and in combinations in head and neck cancer is detailed in Table IX. Activity of DDP in head and neck cancer was first noted by Krakoff and Lippman (1974) and confirmed by Hill *et al.* (1975) and Tekuzman *et al.* (1976).

Hayes *et al.* (1977) reported good responses with higher doses of DDP, with hydration, and with mannitol diuresis. Wittes and colleagues (1977) treated 26 patients with DDP alone with 2 complete responses and 6 partial responses. Responses lasted from 1–8+ months.

With this well-documented activity in a very refractory and difficult tumor to treat, DDP was put into the combination regimens outlined in Table IX. The results of these combination regimens look quite promising.

TABLE IX

cis-DIAMMINEDICHLOROPLATINUM(II) ALONE AND IN COMBINATION REGIMENS FOR HEAD AND NECK CANCER

Drug(s)[a]	No. of evaluable patients	No. of remissions	Overall response rate (%)	References[b]
DDP	64	22	34	1, 2, 3, 4, 8, 15
DDP + BLM	64	26	41	2, 5, 11, 13
DDP + ADR	11	5	45	6
DDP + BLM + MTX	57	37	65	7, 10, 12, 14[c]
DDP + BLM + VCR	16	6	38	9

[a] BLM (bleomycin); ADR (adriamycin); MTX (methatrexate); VCR (vincristine).

[b] Key to reference: 1—Hayes *et al.* (1977); 2—Wittes *et al.* (1975); 3—Krakoff and Lippman (1974); 4—Corder *et al.* (1977); 5—Randolf *et al.* (1977); 6—Bonomi *et al.* (1977); 7—Vogl and Kroner, (1977); 8—Wittes *et al.* (1977) 9—Amer *et al.* (1978); 10—Kaplan and Vogl (1978); 11—Hong *et al.* (1978); 12—Elias *et al.* (1978); 13—Bianco *et al.* (1978); 14—Caradonna *et al.* (1978); 15—Panettiere *et al.* (1978).

[c] High-dose methotrexate with leucovorin rescue.

5. *Prostate Cancer*

DDP has received some attention in the treatment of prostate cancer. Early results look interesting, but, considering the difficulties in measuring response in this tumor, they must be viewed cautiously. Further trials are needed with these interesting early results (Rossof *et al.*, 1977; Merrin, 1977d; Wallace and Higby, 1974). Perloff *et al.* (1977) have treated 17 patients with prostatic cancer with DDP + adriamycin and report a 53% response rate.

6. *Breast Cancer*

The activity of DDP in breast cancer has been explored by a number of investigators. Cumulative response rates utilizing a variety of dosages and schedules have been 3/56 (5%) (Wallace and Higby, 1974; Hayes *et al.*, 1977; Chary *et al.*, 1977; Catane *et al.*, 1977; Corder *et al.*, 1977; Hill *et al.*, 1975; Samal *et al.*, 1978; Bull *et al.*, 1978).

7. *Lung Cancer*

The single-agent activity of DDP in lung cancer is essentially not evaluable because too few patients with any one histological subtype of lung cancer have been treated with the drug. Published information gives the following response rates: 3/27 for adenocarcinomas of the lung; 0/5 for large cell; 0/4 for small cell; and 0/3 for anaplastic carcinomas of the lung (Rosoff *et al.*, 1976; Kvols *et al.*, 1978). Other phase II information lumped under "lung cancer" has been reported by Hayes *et al.* (1977), Corder *et al.* (1977), Hill *et al.* (1975), and Chary *et al.* (1977). A number of promising combination regimens have been reported in advanced non-small-cell lung cancer (Eagan *et al.*, 1977b, 1978; Gralla *et al.*, 1978; Higby *et al.*, 1977; Kvols *et al.*, 1978; Valdivieso *et al.*, 1978) and in small-cell lung cancer (Eagan *et al.*, 1977a; Sierocki *et al.*, 1978). Combinations of DDP with cyclophosphamide, adriamycin, or vinblastine and bleomycin have as yet yielded inconclusive results (Samson *et al.*, 1976; Piel and Perlia, 1975; Perlia and Stolbach, 1976; Vogl *et al.*, 1976; Wallace *et al.*, 1975; Mills *et al.*, 1977).

8. *Colon Cancer*

Patients with colon cancer have been treated with conventional-dose DDP (50 mg/m^2) (Kovach *et al.*, 1973) and with high-dose DDP (120 mg/m^2) (Samal *et al.*, 1978). The overall response rates for these regimens has been 0% (0/49 patients). Ellerby *et al.* (1974) have reported 3 responses in 8 patients with colon cancer treated with a combination of DDP + 5-fluorouracil.

9. *Childhood Tumors*

A number of investigators have reported activity of DDP in neuroblastoma patients (Kamalakar *et al.*, 1976, 1977; Talley *et al.*, 1973; Nitschke *et al.*, 1976; Tekuzman *et al.*, 1976) with 3 of 19 refractory patients showing objective responses. With this encouraging activity, a number of combination regimens for neuroblastoma including DDP are under study in cooperative groups.

Osteogenic sarcoma also seems to respond to DDP administration with 8 out of 24 patients achieving a remission in a number of trials (Ochs *et al.*, 1977; Catane *et al.*, 1977; Kamalakar *et al.*, 1977; Baum *et al.*, 1978). With this know activity the drug will be combined with other active agents for use in adjuvant cases of ostegenic sarcoma (Ettinger *et al.*, 1978).

10. *Miscellaneous Tumors*

Table X details the results with DDP used as a single agent in a variety of other types of tumor. There are too few evaluable patients to comment on drug activity. However, the activity of the agent looks interesting in melanoma, lymphoma, endometrial, thyroid, cervical cancer, hepatoma, and thymoma.

It is of great interest that the drug does not seem to have activity in ALL of childhood or in AML, although additional data would help firm up these conclusions. The drug has not yet been evaluated as a single agent

TABLE X

SUMMARY OF SINGLE-AGENT ACTIVITY OF *cis*-DIAMMINEDICHLOROPLATINUM(II) IN MISCELLANEOUS TYPES OF TUMORS

Tumor type	No. of evaluable patients	No. of responses	Reference[a]
Melanoma	29	5	1–3
Lymphoma (all types)	11	4	2, 4, 5
Hodgkins	7	2	3
Non-Hodgkins	28	7	3, 6, 7
Multiple myeloma	7	1	8, 4, 9, 1
Thyroid	1	1	10[b]
Endometrial	2	2	9
Hepatoma	3	1	8, 9
Gastric	2	0	3, 8
Pancreatic	1	0	8
Sarcoma (soft tissue)	23	0	5, 8, 4, 3, 2, 1
Renal	16	0	3, 10, 11
ALL (childhood)	37	2	7, 12
AML	35	2	4, 7
Adrenal	1	1	5
Thymoma	1	1	6
Wilms	2	1	5
Brain	1	0	9
Mesothelioma	1	0	3
Rhabdomyosarcoma	2	0	12
CML	2	0	7
CLL	3	0	7
Cervix	29	13	13, 14

[a] Key to references: 1—Chary *et al.* (1977); 2—Wiltshaw (1977); 3—Hayes *et al.* (1977); 4—Corder *et al.* (1977); 5—Tekuzman *et al.* (1976); 6—Talley *et al.* (1973); 7—Hill *et al.* (1977); 8—Catane *et al.* (1977); 9—Hill *et al.* (1975); 10—Wallace and Higby (1974); 11—Rossof *et al.* (1977); 12—Nitschke *et al.* (1976); 13—Thigpen and Shingleton (1978); 14—Cohen *et al.* (1978).

[b] Other trials have reported 3 more responders, but the total number of patients treated was not given.

in esophageal cancer, but DDP + bleomycin has been piloted in esophageal cancer with interesting results (Kelsen *et al.*, 1978).

C. TOXICITY IN MAN

The toxicities discovered in phase I, II, and III trials in man can be divided into renal, gastrointestinal, audiological, hematological, and miscellaneous categories.

1. *Nephrotoxicity*

Clearly the major dose-limiting toxicity of DDP, nephrotoxicity is dose-related and cumulative (Kovach *et al.*, 1973). It is manifested by elevations in BUN, creatinine, hyperuricemia, and decrease in creatinine clearance. It usually becomes irreversible with higher doses or with repeated courses of administration (Dentino *et al.*, 1977). The histopathology of the renal damage has been adequately documented in renal biopsies and post-mortem exam specimens. There is a focal acute tubular necrosis of the distal convoluted tubules and collecting ducts. The proximal convoluted tubules are also affected but to a lesser degree (Gonzales-Vitale *et al.*, 1977; Higby *et al.*, 1973; Rossof *et al.*, 1972; Lippman *et al.*, 1973; Yagoda *et al.*, 1976; Hardaker *et al.*, 1974).

The use of intravenous hydration along with mannitol infusions with or without furosemide has dramatically changed the nephrotoxicity problem associated with DDP. Hayes and colleagues (1976, 1977) noted that 3 mg/kg of DDP could be administered with infrequent and reversible elevations in serum creatinines. This is in contrast to patients receiving platinum without mannitol who have consistent and sometimes irreversible elevations in serum creatinines (Higby *et al.*, 1973). Gonzales-Vitale *et al.* (1977) have shown that the higher doses of DDP + mannitol and hydration attenuate the pathological changes in the kidney that are seen with conventional dose DDP. Merrin (1976) has also noted an absence of DDP-induced renal toxicity when DDP is given at doses of 1 mg/kg biweekly along with hydration, mannitol, and furosemide. At this point in time, although DDP + mannitol + hydration + furosemide is an attractive combination for the prevention of DDP-induced nephrotoxicity, it is still unclear whether the hydration itself, mannitol itself, or combination of these are necessary for a protective effect on the kidneys. It is clear that under certain circumstances, DDP can form complexes with mannitol (Eshaque *et al.*, 1977). In addition, furosemide has been reported to cause ototoxicity (Schwartz *et al.*, 1970) and could theoretically contribute to DDP-induced ototoxicity.

Clinical trials are currently underway to elucidate the importance of mannitol and hydration in the protection of the kidneys from the effects of DDP.

2. *Gastrointestinal*

Nausea and vomiting from DDP is a consistent side effect and can be very severe with a number of patients refusing further treatment because of these side effects (Higby *et al.*, 1974; Yagoda *et al.*, 1976; Lippman *et al.*, 1973). A number of methods have been attempted to reduce or alleviate the nausea and vomiting. Antiemetics have generally been ineffective. Nabilone, a derivative of Δ-9-tetrahydrocannabinol, has shown some effect in early trials (Nagy *et al.*, 1978). Continuous infusions have been said to decrease the nausea and vomiting (Hall *et al.*, 1978), but this information awaits further confirmation.

Minimal elevations in serum levels of glutamic oxalacetic transaminase were noted by Hill *et al.* (1975) and Hayes *et al.* (1977). Otherwise no hepatotoxicity of DDP has been noted.

3. *Ototoxicity*

Kovach and colleagues (1973) noted evidence of ototoxicity of DDP in about 30% of patients treated with an intravenous push dose of 50 mg/m^2 of DDP. Ototoxicity is manifested by tinnitus, subclinical hearing loss above the speech tones (4000–8000 Hz), or occasionally a decrease in the ability to hear conversational tones. Ototoxicity has been described without other DDP-induced toxicities (Piel *et al.*, 1974) and tinnitus has been described in the absence of audiogram abnormalities (Wiltshaw and Kroner, 1976). The reversibility of the ototoxicity is still controversial (Higby *et al.*, 1973; Hayes *et al.*, 1976, 1977; Lippman *et al.*, 1973).

As already mentioned, furosemide has been indicted as an ototoxic agent (Schwartz *et al.*, 1970) and its use with DDP could theorectically add to the ototoxicity of DDP.

4. *Myelosuppression*

Many researchers consider DDP as a nonmyelosuppressive drug. Doses of 50–60 mg/m^2 usually do not cause leukopenia according to Yagoda *et al.* (1976) and Kovach *et al.* (1973). However, other investigators have found that DDP does induce moderate myelosuppression including leukopenia, thrombocytopenia, and anemia particularly in patients with prior exposure to alkylating agents (Talley *et al.*, 1973; Lippman *et al.*, 1973).

5. *Miscellaneous Toxicities*

A number of investigators have reported anaphylactic-like reactions to DDP (Khan *et al.*, 1975; Von Hoff *et al.*, 1976; Hayes *et al.*, 1977). The reactions were comprised of tachycardia, wheezing, facial edema, and hypotension, all within a few minutes of drug administration. All reactions have been controlled by intravenous administration of antihistamines, steroids, and/or epinephrine. At the present time there are no skin tests that are predictive for this anaphlactic-like reaction. The clinical usefulness of the agent has necessitated premedicating some patients with steroids and antihistamine and "treating through" the reaction (Baum *et al.*, 1978; Wiesenfeld *et al.*, 1978). The usefulness of desensitization has not been explored.

Possible instances of neurotoxicity secondary to DDP have been reported by a number of investigators. These neurotoxicities include peripheral neuropathies (sensory and motor), seizures, loss of sensation of taste, intention tremor, postural hypotension (Bruckner *et al.*, 1977; Von Hoff *et al.*, 1978; Wiltshaw and Kroner, 1976; Kedar *et al.*, 1978).

Two instances of possible DDP-related cardiac effects have been reported including one episode of left bundle branch block (Wiltshaw and Carr, 1974) and an episode of congestive heart failure after DDP in a patient without prior evidence of heart disease (Talley *et al.*, 1973).

X. Summary and Conclusions

cis-Diamminedichloroplatinum(II) has been under study for 13 years and in clinical use for 7 years. It is an inorganic complex formed by a central atom of platinum surrounded by chlorine atoms and ammonia moieties. Its structure is unique in the field of cancerostatics. The drug possesses cytotoxic, antimicrobial, antiviral, immunosuppressive, mutagenic, and radiosensitizing properties in a variety of biological systems. It probably exerts its antitumor effects through an interaction with DNA, although the precise mechanism of action of this drug is uncertain at this time.

In toxicology studies, the dog and monkey were predictive for the nephrotoxicity, ototoxicity, nausea, and vomiting and myelosuppression seen with DDP. The animals did not predict the anaphylactic reactions and possible neurotoxicity seen in human trials.

The drug is active in a number of experimental tumor systems and exhibits synergism with a number of other cancerstatic agents. These synergistic interactions have not been fully exploited clinically.

It has remarkable activity in testicular, ovarian, bladder, and head and neck cancer. It is also active in a number of other tumor types, but more clinical trials are needed to confirm this activity.

Areas for future investigations with DDP include its use as a radiosensitizer, its intravesicular and intracavitary administration, adjuvant use of DDP in osteogenic sarcoma, bladder cancer, and head and neck cancer and further phase II and phase III trials. The area of analogs to DDP is burgeoning, but the question as to which compound(s) should undergo clinical trial is a difficult one.

Overall, DDP is a significant addition to the oncologists' armamentarium of useful chemotherapeutic agents.

References

Amer, M. H., Izbicki, R., and Al-Sarraf, M. (1978). *Proc. Am. Assoc. Cancer Res.* **19,** 312.

Baum, E., Greenberg, L., Gaynon, P., Krivit, W., and Hammond, D. (1978). *Proc. Am. Assoc. Cancer Res.* **19,** 385.

Beck, D. J., and Brubaker, R. R. (1975). *Mutat. Res.* **27,** 181.

Berenbaum, M. C. (1971). *Br. J. Cancer* **25,** 208.

Bianco, A. A., Taylor, S. G., IV, Reich, S. D., Merrill, J. M., and DeWys, W. D. (1978). *Proc. Am. Assoc. Cancer Res.* **19,** 380.

Bonomi, P. D., Mladineo, J., Wilbanks, G. D., and Slayton, R. (1977). *Proc. Am. Soc. Clin. Oncol.* **18,** 311.

Brambilla, G., Cavanna, M., and Maura, A. (1974). *Cancer Chemother. Rep.* **58,** 633.

Briscoe, K., Pasmantier, M., Brown, J., and Kennedy, B. J. (1978). *Proc. Am. Assoc. Cancer Res.* **19,** 378.

Bruckner, H. W., Cohen, C. J., Gusberg, S. B., Wallach, R. C., Kabakow, B., Greenspan, E. M., and Holland, J. F. (1976). *Proc. Am. Assoc. Cancer Res.* **17,** 287.

Bruckner, H. W., Cohen, C. C., Deppe, G., Kabakow, B., Wallach, R. C., Greenspan, E. M., Gusberg, S. B., and Holland, J. F. (1977). *J. Clin. Hematol. Oncol.* **7,** 619.

Bull, J. M., Anderson, T., Lippman, M. E., Cassidy, J. G., Gormley, P. E., and Young, R. C. (1978). *Proc. Am. Assoc. Cancer Res.* **19,** 87.

Caradonna, R., Paladine, W., Goldstein, J., Ruckdeschel, J., Hillinger, S., and Horton, J. (1978). *Proc. Am. Assoc. Cancer Res.* **19,** 401.

Catane, R., Douglass, H. O., Jr., and Mittelman, A. (1977). *Proc. Am. Assoc. Cancer Res.* **18,** 115.

Chary, K. K., Higby, D. J., Henderson, E. S., and Swinerton, K. D. (1977). *Cancer Treat. Rep.* **61,** 367.

Cohen, C. J., Castro-Marin, A., Deppe, G., Bruckner, H. W., and Holland, J. F. (1978). *Proc. Am. Assoc. Cancer Res.* **19,** 401.

Corder, M. P., Maguire, L. C., Witte, D. L., Panther, S. K., Lovett, J. M., and Dietz, B. J. (1977). *Proc. Am. Assoc. Cancer Res.* **18,** 344.

Cvitkovic, E., Wittes, R., Golbey, R., and Krakoff, I. H. (1975a). *Proc. Am. Assoc. Cancer Res.* **16,** 174.

Cvitkovic, E., Currie, V., Krakoff, I. H., and Golbey, R. (1975b). *Proc. Am. Assoc. Cancer Res.* **16,** 273.

Cvitkovic, E., Hayes, D., and Golbey, R. (1976). *Proc. Am. Assoc. Cancer Res.* **17,** 296.

Cvitkovic, E., Spaulding, J., Bethune, V., Martin, J., and Whitmore, W. F. (1977). *Cancer* **39,** 1357.

DeConti, R. C., Toftness, B. R., Lange, R. C., and Creasey, W. A. (1973). *Cancer Res.* **33,** 1310.

Dentino, M. E., Yum, M. N., Rohn, R. T., Einhorn, L. H., and Luft, F. C. (1977). *Proc. Am. Assoc. Cancer Res.* **18,** 116.

Douple, E. B., Richmond, R. C., and Logan, M. E. (1977). *J. Clin. Hematol. Oncol.* **7,** 585.

Drewinko, B., and Gottlieb, J. A. (1975). *Cancer Chemother. Rep.* **59,** 665.

Drobnik, J., Urbankova, M., and Krekulova, A. (1973). *Mutat. Res.* **17,** 13.

Eagan, R. T., Carr, D. T., Lee, R. E., Frytak, S., Rubin, J., and Coles, D. T. (1977a). *Cancer Treat. Rep.* **61,** 93.

Eagan, R. T., Ingle, J. N., Frytak, S., Rubin, J., Kvals, L. K., Carr, D. T., Coles, D. T., and O'Fallon, J. R. (1977b). *Cancer Treat. Rep.* **61,** 1339.

Eagan, R. T., Ingle, J. N., Frytak, S., and Rubin, J. (1978). *Proc. Am. Assoc. Cancer Res.* **19,** 78.

Ehrlich, C. E., Einhorn, L., and Morgan, J. L. (1978). *Proc. Am. Assoc. Cancer Res.* **19,** 379.

Einhorn, L. H., and Donohue, J. P. (1977a). *J. Urol.* **117,** 65.

Einhorn, L. H., and Donohue, J. P. (1977b). *Ann. Intern. Med.* **87,** 293.

Einhorn, L. H., and Williams, S. D. (1978). *Proc. Am. Assoc. Cancer Res.* **19,** 29.

Einhorn, L. H., Furnas, B. E., and Powell, N. (1976). *Proc. Am. Assoc. Cancer Res.* **17,** 240.

Elias, E. G., Chrétien, P. B., Monnard, E., and Wiernik, P. H. (1978). *Proc. Am. Assoc. Cancer Res.* **19,** 376.

Ellerby, R. A., Davis, H. L., Jr., Ansfield, F. J., and Ramirez, G. (1974). *Cancer* **34,** 1005.

Eshaque, M., McKay, M. J., and Theophanides, T. (1977). *J. Clin. Hematol. Oncol.* **7,** 338.

Ettinger, L. J., Douglas, H. O., Jr., Higby, D. J., Bjornsson, S., Mirdell, E. R., and Freeman, A. I. (1978). *Proc. Am. Assoc. Cancer Res.* **19,** 323.

Geran, R. I., Congleton, G. F., Dudeck, L. E., *et al.* (1974). *Cancer Chemother. Rep., Part 2* **4,** 53.

Gonzalez-Vitale, J. C., Hayes, D. M., Cvitkovic, E., and Sternberg, S. (1977). *Cancer* **39,** 1362.

Gralla, R. J., Critkovic, E., and Golbey, R. B. (1978). *Proc. Am. Assoc. Cancer Res.* **19,** 353.

Greenwald, E., Vogl, S. E., Kaplan, B. H., and Wollner, D. (1978). *Proc. Am. Assoc. Cancer Res.* **19,** 327.

Haeschelle, J. P., and Van Camp, L. (1972). *Adv. Antimicrob. Antineoplast. Chemother., Proc. Int. Congr. Chemother., 7th 1971* Vol. 2, p. 241.

Hall, S. W., Salem, P., Benjamin, R. S., Lu, K., Loo, T. L., Murphy, W. K., Wharton, J. T., and Bodey, G. O. (1978). *Proc. Am. Assoc. Cancer Res.* **19,** 417.

Hardaker, W. T., Jr., Stone, R. A., and McCoy, R. (1974). *Cancer* **34,** 1030.

Harder, H. C., and Rosenberg, B. (1970). *Int. J. Cancer* **6,** 207.

Hayes, D., Cvitkovic, E., Golbey, R., Scheiner, E., and Krakoff, I. H. (1976). *Proc. Am. Assoc. Cancer Res.* **17,** 169.

Hayes, D. M., Cvitkovic, E., Golbey, R. B., Scheiner, E., Helson, L., and Krakoff, I. H. (1977). *Cancer* **39,** 1372.

Higby, D. J., Wallace, H. J., Jr., and Holland, J. F. (1973). *Cancer Chemother. Rep.* **57,** 459.

Higby, D. J., Wallace, H. J., Jr., Albert, D., and Holland, J. F. (1974). *J. Urol.* **112,** 100.

Higby, D. J., Wallace, H. J., Jr., and Bekesi, J. G. (1975). *Proc. Am. Assoc. Cancer Res.* **16,** 131.

Higby, D. J., Wilbur, D., Wallace, H. J., Jr., Henderson, E. S., and Weiss, R. (1977). *Cancer Treat. Rep.* **61,** 869.

Hill, J. M., Loeb, E., MacLellan, A., Hill, N. O., Khan, A., and King, J. (1975). *Cancer Chemother. Rep.* **59,** 647.

Hill, J. M., Loeb, E., Pardue, A. S., Khan, A., Hill, N. O., King, J. J., and Hill, R. W. (1977). *J. Clin. Hematol. Oncol.* **7,** 681.

Hong, W. K., Bhutani, R., Shapshay, S., Craft, M. L., Ucmakli, A., Snow, M. N., Vaughn, C., and Strong, S. (1978). *Proc. Am. Assoc. Cancer Res.* **19,** 321.

Howle, J. A., and Gale, G. R. (1970a). *Biochem. Pharmacol.* **19,** 2757.

Howle, J. A., and Gale, G. E. (1970b). *J. Bacteriol.* **103,** 258.

Kamalakar, P., Wang, J. J., Higby, D., Freeman, A. I., and Wallace, H. J., Jr. (1976). *Proc. Am. Assoc. Cancer Res.* **17,** 283.

Kamalakar, P., Freeman, A. I., Higby, D. J., Wallace, H. J., and Sinks, L. F. (1977). *Cancer Treat. Rep.* **61,** 835.

Kane, R., Andrews, T., Bernath, A., Curry, S., Dixon, R., Gottlieb, R., Harvey, H., Kukrika, M., Lipton, A., Mortel, R., Ricci, J., and White, D. (1978). *Proc. Am. Assoc. Cancer Res.* **19,** 320.

Kaplan, B. H., and Vogel, S. E. (1978). *Proc. Am. Assoc. Cancer Res.* **19,** 323.

Kedar, A., Cohen, M. E., and Freeman, A. I. (1978). *Cancer Treat. Rep.* **62,** 819.

Kelsen, D. P., Cvitkovic, E., Bains, M., and Golbey, R. (1978). *Proc. Am. Assoc. Cancer Res.* **19,** 352.

Khan, A., and Hill, J. M. (1971). *Infect. Immun.* **4,** 320.

Khan, A., and Hill, J. M. (1972a). *Proc. Am. Assoc. Cancer Res.* **13,** 92.

Khan, A., and Hill, J. M. (1972b). *Transplantattion* **13,** 55.

Khan, A., Albayrak, A., and Hill, J. M. (1972). *Proc. Soc. Exp. Biol. Med.* **141,** 7.

Khan, A., Hill, J. M., Grater, W., Loeb, E., MacLellan, A., and Hill, N. O. (1975). *Cancer Res.* **35,** 2766.

Kociba, R. J., Sleight, S. D., and Rosenberg, B. (1970). *Cancer Chemother. Rep.* **54,** 325.

Kovach, J. S., Moertel, C. G., Schutt, A. J., Reitemeier, R. G., and Hahn, R. G. (1973). *Cancer Chemother. Rep.* **57,** 357.

Krakoff, I. H., and Lippman, A. J. (1974). *In* "Recent Results in Cancer Research" (T. A. Connors and J. J. Roberts, eds.), p. 183. Springer-Verlag.

Kutinova, L., Vonka, V., and Drobnick, J. (1972). *Neoplasma* **19,** 453.

Kvols, L. K., Eagan, R. T., Creagan, E. T., and Dalton, R. J. (1978). *Proc. Am. Assoc. Cancer Res.* **19,** 82.

Lange, R. C., Spencer, R. P., and Harder, H. C. (1972). *J. Nucl. Med.* **13,** 328.

Lange, R. C., Spencer, R. P., and Harder, H. C. (1973). *J. Nucl. Med.* **14,** 191.

Lippman, A. J., Helson, C., Helson, L., and Krakoff, I. H. (1973). *Cancer Chemother. Rep.* **57,** 191.

Litterst, C. L., Gram, T. E., Dedrick, R. L., Leroy, A. F., and Guarino, A. M. (1976). *Cancer. Res.* **36,** 2340.

Litterst, C. L., Torres, I. J., and Guarino, A. M. (1977). *J. Clin. Hematol. Oncol.* **7,** 169.

Loeb, E., Hill, J. M., MacLellan, A., Hill, N. O., Khan, A., King, J. J., Speer, R., and Ridgway, H. (1975). *Wadley Med. Bull.* **5,** 281.

Mansey, S., Rosenberg, B., and Thomson, A. J. (1973). *J. Am. Chem. Soc.* **95,** 1633.

Merker, P. C., Wodinsky, I., Mabel, J., Branfman, A., and Venditti, J. M. (1977). *J. Clin. Hematol. Oncol.* **7,** 301.

Merrin, C. (1976). *Proc. Am. Assoc. Cancer Res.* **17,** 243.

Merrin, C. (1977). *Proc. Am. Assoc. Cancer Res.* **18,** 100.

Mills, R. C., Maurer, L. H., Forcier, R. J., Grace, W. R., Burke, G. P., Karp, D. D., Smith, R. C., McIntyre, O. R., and Bean, C. (1977). *Cancer Treat. Rep.* **61,** 477.

Munchausen, L. L. (1974). *Proc. Natl. Acad. Sci. U.S.A.* **71,** 4519.

Munschausen, L. L., and Rahn, R. O. (1975). *Cancer Chemother. Rep.* **59,** 643.

Munster, A. M., Greenberg, P., Greenberg, S., Leary, A. G., and Gale, G. R. (1974). *Proc. Soc. Exp. Biol. Med.* **146,** 333.

Nagy, C. M., Furnas, B. E., Einhorn, L. H., and Bond, W. H. (1978). *Proc. Am. Assoc. Cancer Res.* **19,** 30.

Nitschke, R., Starling, K., Land, V., and Komp, D. (1976). *Proc. Am. Assoc. Cancer Res.* **17,** 310.

Ochs, J., Freeman, A., Douglass, H., and Sinks, L. (1977). *Proc. Am. Assoc. Cancer Res.* **18,** 167.

Osieka, R., Bruntsch, U., Gallmeier, W. M., *et al.* (1976). *Dtsch. Med. Wochenschr.* **101,** 191.

Panettiere, F. J., Lane, M., and Lehane, D. (1978). *Proc. Am. Assoc. Cancer Res.* **19,** 410.

Pera, M. F., and Harder, H. C. (1978). *Proc. Am. Assoc. Cancer Res.* **19,** 100.

Perlia, C. P., and Stolbach, L. (1976). *Proc. Am. Assoc. Cancer Res.* **17,** 27.

Perloff, M., Ohnuma, T., Holland, J. F., Kennedy, B. J., and Mills, R. C. (1977). *Proc. Am. Assoc. Cancer Res.* **18,** 333.

Piel, I. J., and Perlia, C. P. (1975). *Cancer Chemother. Rep.* **59,** 995.

Piel, I. J., Rayadu, G. V. S., and Perlia, C. P. (1974). *Proc. Am. Assoc. Cancer Res.* **15,** 111.

Randolph, V. L., Vallejo, A., Strong, E. W., and Wittes, R. E. (1977). *Proc. Am. Soc. Clin. Oncol.* **18,** 336.

Richmond, R. C., and Powers, E. L. (1977). *J. Clin. Hematol. Oncol.* **7,** 580.

Roberts, J. J., and Pascoe, J. M. (1972). *Nature (London)* **235,** 282.

Rosenberg, B. (1973). *Naturwissenschaften* **60,** 399.

Rosenberg, B. (1975). *Cancer Chemother. Rep.* **59,** 589.

Rosenberg, B. (1977). *J. Clin. Hematol. Oncol.* **7,** 817.

Rosenberg, B., Van Camp, L., and Krigas, T. (1965). *Nature (London)* **205,** 698.

Rosenberg, B., Renshaw, E., VanCamp, L., Hartwick, J., and Drobnik, J. (1967a). *J. Bacteriol.* **93,** 716.

Rosenberg, B., Van Camp, L., Grimley, E. B., and Thomson, A. J. (1967b). *J. Biol. Chem.* **242,** 1347.

Rosenberg, B., VanCamp, L., Trosko, J. E., and Mansour, V. H. (1969). *Nature (London)* **222,** 385.

Rossof, A. H., Slayton, R. E., and Perlia, C. P. (1972). *Cancer* **30,** 1451.

Rossof, A. H., Bearden, J. D., III, and Coltman, C. A., Jr. (1976). *Cancer Treat. Rep.* **60,** 1679.

Rossof, A. H., Talley, R. W., and Stephens, R. L. (1977). *Proc. Am. Assoc. Cancer Res.* **18,** 97.

Rozencweig, M., Von Hoff, D. D., Slavik, M., and Muggia, F. M. (1977). *Ann. Intern. Med.* **86,** 803.

Samal, B., Vaitkevicius, V., Singhakowinta, A., O'Bryan, R. M., Buroker, T., Samson, M., and Baker, L. (1978). *Proc. Am. Assoc. Cancer Res.* **19,** 347.

Samson, M. K., and Stephens, R. L. (1978). *Proc. Am. Assoc. Cancer Res.* **19,** 12.

Samson, M. K., Baker, L. H., Devos, J. M., Buroker, T. R., Isbicki, R. M., and Vaitkevicius, V. K. (1976). *Cancer Treat. Rep.* **60,** 91.

Samuels, M. L., Holoye, P. Y., and Johnson, D. E. (1975a). *Cancer* **36,** 318.

Samuels, M. L., Johnson, D. E., and Holoye, P. Y. (1975b). *Cancer Chemother. Rep.* **59,** 563.

Schaeppi, U., Heyman, I. A., Fleischman, R. W., Rosenkrantz, H., Ilievski, V., Phelan, R., Cooney, D. A., and Davis, R. D. (1973). *Toxicol. Appl. Pharmacol.* **25,** 230.

Schwartz, G. H., David, D. S., and Riggio, R. R. (1970). *N. Engl. J. Med.* **282,** 1413.

Sierocki, J. S., Golbey, R. B., and Wittes, R. E. (1978). *Proc. Am. Assoc. Cancer Res.* **19,** 352.

Sirica, A., Venditti, J. M., and Kline, I. (1971). *Proc. Am. Assoc. Cancer Res.* **12,** 4.

Smith, P. H. S., and Taylor, D. M. (1974). *J. Nucl. Med.* **15,** 349.

Soloway, M. S. (1978). *Proc. Am. Assoc. Cancer Res.* **19,** 366.

Soloway, M. S., Rose, D., and Weldon, T. (1974). *Proc. Am. Assoc. Cancer Res.* **15,** 7.

Speer, R. J., Lapis, S., Ridgway, H., Mayer, T. D., and Hill, J. M. (1971). *Wadley Med. Bull.* **1,** 103.

Spiegel, S. C., and Coltman, C. A., Jr. (1974). *Cancer Chemother. Rep.* **58,** 213.

Stadnicki, S. W., Fleischman, R. W., Schaeppi, U., and Merriam, P. (1975). *Cancer Chemother. Rep.* **59,** 467.

Stone, P. J., Kelman, A. D., and Sinex, F. M. (1974). *Nature (London)* **251,** 736.

Talley, R. W., O'Bryan, R. M., Gutterman, J. U., Brownlee, R. W., and McCredie, K. B. (1973). *Cancer Chemother. Rep.* **57,** 465.

Tekuzman, G., Kucuksu, N., and Ruacan, S. (1976). *Kanser* **6,** 17.

Thigpen, T., and Shingleton, H. (1978). *Proc. Am. Assoc. Cancer Res.* **19,** 332.

Troner, M., and Hemstreet, G. (1978). *Proc. Am. Assoc. Cancer Res.* **19,** 161.

Valdivieso, M., Burgess, M. A., and Bodey, G. P. (1978). *Proc. Am. Assoc. Cancer Res.* **19,** 409.

Vogl, S. E., and Kaplan, B. H. (1977). *Proc. Am. Soc. Clin. Oncol.* **18,** 316.

Vogl, S., Ohnuma, T., Perloff, M., and Holland, J. F. (1976). *Cancer* **38,** 21.

Vogl, S. E., Kaplan, H., Moukhtar, M., and Berenzweig, M. (1978). *Proc. Am. Assoc. Cancer Res.* **19,** 46.

Von Hoff, D. D., Slavik, M., and Muggia, F. M. (1976). *Lancet* **1,** 90.

Von Hoff, D. D., Reichert, C. M., Reddick, R., Ritch, P. S., Weisenthal, L., and Cuner, R. (1979). *Proc. Am. Assoc. Cancer Res.* (in press).

Wallace, H. J., Jr., and Higby, D. J. (1974). *In* "Recent Results in Cancer Research" (T. A. Connors and J. J. Roberts, eds.), p. 167. Springer-Verlag.

Wallace, H. J., Jr., Higby, D. J., Wilbur, D. W., and Cortes, E. P. (1975). *Proc. Am. Assoc. Cancer Res.* **16,** 244.

Ward, J. M., Grabin, M. E., LeRoy, A. F., and Young, D. M. (1977). *Cancer Treat. Rep.* **61,** 375.

Welsch, C. W. (1971). *Proc. Am. Assoc. Cancer Res.* **12,** 25.

Wiesenfeld, M., Reinders, E., Corder, M., and Yoo, T. J. (1978). *Proc. Am. Assoc. Cancer Res.* **19,** 343.

Williams, S. D., Rohn, R. J., Donohue, J. P., and Einhorn, L. H. (1978). *Proc. Am. Assoc. Cancer Res.* **19,** 316.

Wiltshaw, E. (1977). *J. Clin. Hematol. Oncol.* **7,** 616.

Wiltshaw, E., and Carr, B. (1974). *In* "Recent Results in Cancer Research" (T. A. Connors and J. J. Roberts, eds.), p. 178. Springer-Verlag.

Wiltshaw, E., and Kroner, T. (1976). *Cancer Treat. Rep.* **60,** 55.

Wittes, R. E., Brescia, F., Young, C. W., Magill, G. B., Golbey, R. B., and Krakoff, I. H. (1975). *Oncology* **32,** 202.

Wittes, R. E., Cvitkovic, E., and Strong, E. (1976a). *Wadley Med. Bull.* **6,** 85.

Wittes, R. E., Yagoda, A., Silvay, O., Magill, G. B., Whitmore, W., Krakoff, I. H., and Golbey, R. B. (1976b). *Cancer* **37,** 637.

Wittes, R. E., Cvitkovic, E., Shah, J., Gerold, F. P., and Strong, E. W. (1977). *Cancer Treat. Rep.* **61,** 359.

Wolf, W., and Manaka, R. C. (1977). *J. Clin. Hematol. Oncol.* **7,** 79.

Woodman, R. J., Venditti, J. M., Schepartz, S. A., and Kline, I. (1971). *Proc. Am. Assoc. Cancer Res.* **12,** 24.

Woodman, R. J., Sirica, A. E., Gang, M., Kline, I., and Venditti, J. M. (1973). *Chemotherapy* **18,** 169.

Yagoda, A., Watson, R. C., Gonzalez-Vitale, J. C., Grabstald, H., and Whitmore, W. F. (1976). *Cancer Treat. Rep.* **60,** 917.

Zwelling, L. A., Kohn, K. W., and Anderson, T. (1978). *Proc. Am. Assoc. Cancer Res.* **19,** 233.

Subject Index

A

Albumin microspheres
 distribution and targeting by, 235–237
 magnetically responsive, 239–259
 metabolism and toxicity of, 237–239
 preparation of, 233–235
Amino acid neurotransmitters, benzodiazepine effect on, 51–58, 83
γ-Aminobutyric acid, benzodiazepine effect on, 73
Amodiaquin, as antifilarial, 186
Ancylostoma caninum, diethylcarbamazine effects on, 163
Anesthetics, halogenated, pharmacology and toxicology of, 195–212
Anthelmintic resistance, 89–128
 biochemical aspects of, 110–113
 control of, 122–124
 definitions in, 91–95
 diagnosis of, 119–122
  by critical tests, 121–122
  by egg embryonation, 120
  by fecal egg counts, 119–120
  by larval culture, 120–121
 occurrence of, 95–103
  in cattle, 99–100
  in horses, 100–102
  in man, 102–103
  in sheep, 95–99
 physiology of, 103–113
  infectivity and pathogenicity, 104–105
  side- and cross-resistance, 105–109
 reversion in, 118–119
 selection for, 114–119
 standards for, 124
Antifilarial compounds, 129–193
 arsenical compounds, 181
 clinical uses of, 171–180
 broad-spectrum type, 184–186
 diethylcarbamazine, 130–132
 effects on
  adult worms, 156–158
  forms in insect vector, 158
  on infective larvae, 158–161
  microfilariae, 145–156
 organophosphorus compounds, 181–184
 resistance to, 161
 toxicity of, 164–171
Antimalarial drugs, 1–43
 drugs entering efficacy trails, 32–37
 phenanthrene methanols, 17–27
 quinazolines, 27–32
 quinoline methanols, 5–17
 terms relating to drug activity, 3–4
Antitumor agents, microsphere carriers for, 213–271
Arsenical compounds, as antifilarials, 181
Ascaris, diethylcarbamazine effects on, 163
Azacrine 5-oxide dihydrochloride, as antifilarial, 186

B

Behavior
 benzodiazepine effect on, 70–75
 mechanism, 80–82
Benzimidazole antihelmintics, efficiency of, 108
Benzodiazepines, 45–87
 binding sites for, 83
 biochemistry of, 50–61
 effects on
  amino acid neurotransmitters, 51–58
  behavior, 70–75
  corticosteroids, 58–61
  learning and memory, 75–76
  social relationships, 76–79
 historical background of, 46–50
 ionic movement of, 50, 82
 mechanisms of action of, 45–87
 neurohumors and, 46–50
  neuropharmacology of, 61–68, 83
  psychopharmacology of, 69–79, 83–84
Bladder cancer, DDP therapy of, 286–287
Brain
 benzodiazepine effect on, 61–68
  mechanism, 80–82

Breast cancer, DDT therapy of, 288
Bronchial asthma, diethylcarbamazine and, 145
Brugia malayi
  diethylcarbamazine treatment of, 172
    mass therapy, 174–180

C

C 9333-GO/CGP 4540, as antifilarial, 187
Cambendazole, resistance to, 114–116
Cattle, antihelmintic resistance in, 99–100
Centperazine, as antifilarial compound, 132
Children, tumors in, DDP therapy of, 289
Cerebellum, benzodiazepine effect on, 66–67
Colon cancer, DDP therapy of, 289
Corticosteroids, benzodiazepine effect on, 58–61
Cross-resistance, definition of, 95
Cuneate nucleus, benzodiazepine effect on, 64–66
Cysticercus sp., diethylcarbamazine effects on, 163

D

cis-Diamminedichloroplatinum (DDP), 273–298
  animal toxicity of, 279–281
  anticancer activity of, 284–290
  antitumor activity of, 277–279
  biological properties of, 275–276
  chemical and physicochemical properties of, 274–275
  clinical studies on, 282–290
  discovery of, 274
  mechanism of action of, 277
  metabolism and distribution of, 281–282
  toxicity in, 290–293
Diethylcarbamazine
  absorption and excretion of, 135–136
  anti-inflammatory effect of, 140–145
  chemical estimation of, 135
  chemical name for, 130
  clinical uses of, 171–180
  in cooking salt, 177–179
  deaths due to, 169–170
  effect on microfilariae, 152–156
  mass therapy using, 174–180
  metabolism of, 136–138
  pharmacology of, 138–145
  structure-activity relationships of, 130–132
  toxicity of, 164–171
Dithiazanine, as antifilarial, 186

E

Egg embryonation, anthelmintic resistance diagnosis by, 120
Encephalitis, in filariasis patients, 170–171
Enflurane
  metabolism of, 208
  pharmacology of, 207–208
  toxicity of, 208–209
Erythrocyte ghosts
  as antitumor agent carrier, 219–222
    distribution and targeting, 220–221
    metabolism, 221

F

Fasciola hepatica, diethylcarbamazine effects on, 163
Fecal egg counts, anthelmintic resistance diagnosis by, 119–120
Fenthion, as antifilarial, 183
Filariasis, new compounds for treatment of, 129–193
Fluroxene
  metabolism of, 204
  pharmacology of, 203–204
  toxicity of, 204–205

G

Glycine receptors, benzodiazepine effects on, 73
Guinea worm, diethylcarbamazine effects on, 162

H

Haemonchus contortus, Cambendazole selection of, 114–116
Halogenated anesthetics, pharmacology and toxicology of, 195–212
Halothane
  metabolism of, 200–201

pharmacology of, 198–200
toxicity of, 201–203
Haloxan, as antifilarial, 183
Head and neck cancer, DDP therapy of, 287
Hoechst antifilarial compounds, activity of, 132–135
Horses, antihelmintic resistance in, 100–102

I

Isoflurane
metabolism of, 210
pharmacology of, 209–210
toxicity of, 210–211

L

Larval culture, anthelmintic resistance diagnosis by, 120–121
Learning, benzodiazepine effects on, 75–76
Levamisole, as antifilarial, 184–185
Liposome
as antitumor agent carrier, 223–233
distribution and targeting, 226–230
metabolism, 230–231
preparation, 223–226
uses in chemotherapy, 231–233
Loa loa, diethylcarbamazine treatment of, 172
Lung cancer, DDP therapy of, 288–289
Lung worms, diethylcarbamazine effects on, 162

M

Magnetically responsive albumin microspheres
distribution and targeting by, 251–254
guidance of, 239–241
metabolism and toxicity of, 255–257
preparation of, 241–250
use in chemotherapy, 257–258
Malaria
drug therapy of, 1–43
plasmodial parasites causing, 3–5
Memory, benzodiazepine effects on, 75–76
Methoxyflurane
metabolism of, 206
pharmacology of, 205–206
toxicity of, 206–207
Metriphonate, as antifilarial, 181–182
Microspheres
as carriers for antitumor agents, 213–271
exposed carriers, 261–264
goals and problems in, 215–218

N

Necator americanus, drug resistance in, 102
Neurohumors, benzodiazepines and, 46–50
Nifurtimox, as antifilarial, 187
Nitrofurantoin, as antifilarial, 186

O

Onchocerca volvulus
diethylcarbamazine effects on, 154–155
clinical use, 173–174
mass therapy, 179–180
toxicity of, 165–169
drug resistance in, 103
Ovarian cancer, DDP therapy of, 286

P

Paragonimus westermani, diethylcarbamazine effects on, 163
Peripheral ganglia, benzodiazepine effect on, 61–62
Phosphodiesterase, benzodiazepine effects on, 73
Piperazine, effects on adult worms, 158
Plasmodial parasites
characteristics of, 3–5
life cycle of, 4
Prostaglandins diethylcarbamazine and, 144
Prostate cancer, DDP therapy of, 288

Q

Quinazolines, as antimalarial drugs, 27–32
Quinoline methanols, as antimalarial drugs, 5–17

R

Resistance, definition of, 91–95
Resistance factors, definition of, 95
Reversion, definition of, 95

S

Schistosomama mansoni, drug resistance in, 102–103
Serotonin, benzodiazepine effects on, 73
Setaria, diethylcarbamazine effects on, 161–162
Sheep, antihelmintic resistance in, 95–99
Side-resistance, definition of, 95
Social relationships, benzodiazepine effects on, 76–79
Spinal cord, benzodiazepine effect on, 62–64
Strongyloidiasis, diethylcarbamazine effects on, 162

T

Testicular cancer, DDP therapy of, 284–286
Thelazia sp., diethylcarbamazine effects on, 163
Tiguvon, as antifilarial, 183–184
Toxocara canix, diethylcarbamazine effects on, 162
Trichloroethylene
  metabolism of, 197
  pharmacology of, 196
  toxicology of, 197–198
Tropical eosinophilia, diethylcarbamazine therapy of, 180

W

WR 30, 090 antimalarial drug
  chemistry of, 5–7
  clinical studies on, 9–11
  pharmacology of, 8–9
  preclinical biology of, 7–8
  preclinical efficacy of, 6–7
WR 33, 063 antimalarial drug
  chemistry of, 17
  pharmacology of, 19–21
  preclinical efficacy of, 17–18
  preclinical toxicology of, 18–19
  structure of, 17
WR 122, 455 antimalarial drug
  chemistry of, 21
  clinical studies on, 24–25
  pharmacology of, 23–24
  preclinical efficacy of, 22
  preclinical toxicology of, 22–23
  structure of, 21
WR 142, 490 antimalarial drug
  chemistry of, 11
  clinical studies of, 15–17
  pharmacology of, 14–15
  preclinical efficacy of, 12–13
  preclinical toxicology of, 13–14
  structure of, 11
WR 158, 122 antimalarial drug
  chemistry of, 27–28
  clinical studies on, 31–32
  pharmacology of, 30–31
  preclinical efficacy of, 28–29
  preclinical toxicology of, 29
  structure of, 27
WR 171, 669 antimalarial drug
  chemistry of, 25
  clinical studies on, 26–27
  pharmacology of, 26
  preclinical efficacy of, 25
  preclinical toxicology of, 25–26
WR 180, 409 antimalarial drug
  chemistry of, 35
  clinical studies on, 37
  pharmacology of, 37–38
  preclinical efficacy of, 35
  preclinical toxicology of, 36
  structure of, 35
WR 184, 806 antimalarial drug
  chemistry of, 32
  clinical studies on, 34–35
  pharmacology of, 34
  preclinical efficacy of, 32–33
  preclinical toxicology of, 33
Wuchereria bancrofti
  diethylcarbamazine effects on, 152–153
    clinical use, 171–172